Health Effects of Dietary Fatty Acids

Edited By

Gary J. Nelson
Western Human Nutrition Research Center
U.S. Department of Agriculture, ARS
P.O. Box 29997
San Francisco, CA 94129

American Oil Chemists' Society
Champaign, Illinois

Preface

The chapters in this monograph are the distillations of the oral presentations made at the Short Course: Health Effects of Dietary Fatty Acids, held in Baltimore, MD, in April of 1990.

The ten years from 1975 to 1985 were the decade of the n-3 fatty acids in biomedical studies related to lipid metabolism, just as the previous ten years were the decade of the eicosanoids and the n-6 polyunsaturated fatty acids. This interest in n-3 polyunsaturated fatty acids was probably long over due, and provided much satisfaction to those investigators who had felt that n-3 fatty acids were an unduly neglected area of lipid research. Indeed, intense interest in the n-3 polyunsaturated fatty acids stimulated investigators to rethink the conventional wisdom about saturated, monounsaturated and n-6 polyunsaturated fatty acid. Even the controversy about the health effects of *trans* fatty acids was reemerging after several years of quiescence much to the surprise of several investigators who had assumed that this subject was resolved long ago. It occurred to me that limiting a short course to the health effects of dietary polyunsaturated fatty acids was inappropriate in 1990. There were reports that monounsaturated fatty acids were as effective as n-6 polyunsaturated fatty acids in lowering blood cholesterol levels. The controversy over the influence of stearic acid on blood cholesterol was rekindled by the report of Bonanome and Grundy suggesting that stearic acid did not raise blood cholesterol levels. Population based studies on fat consumption were being reexamined in view of recent mortality and morbidity statistics. Also there were several conflicting reports in the literature on the effect of n-3 fatty acid on blood cholesterol levels. Thus, a short course that attempted to bring the entire field of dietary fats and health into perspective seemed more appropriate than a more narrow approach limited to polyunsaturated fatty acids.

Once this was decided, it became necessary to provide a framework for prospective attendees in which to place the problem and some basic elements of fatty acid metabolism. Therefore, the opening session was devoted to these topics. The short course became almost self organizing, and the major subdivisions became various health conditions and not fatty acid classes. Cardiovascular disorders, cancer, immunology, etc. could be dealt with from the perspective of a person's total fat intake, not simply ones' consumption of n-3 or n-6 polyunsaturated fatty acids. Of course, any single presentation at the course might emphasize one class of fatty acids and its particular effect on a specific condition. Despite that, the reader of this monograph should find a comprehensive assessment of the state of our knowledge concerning the health effects of dietary fatty acids. The first section provides information on what the public is currently consuming, the general metabolism of dietary fats, and the function of essential fatty acids. The second and third sections cover the effect of dietary fatty acids on the cardiovascular system from hyperlipidemias through blood clotting and hypertension. In Section II, Dr. Hegsted, who has contributed much to this field over the years, gives a uniquely personal view of the role that dietary fatty acids play in the genesis of coronary heart disease using epidemiological data to make his case. Dr. Harris explains why there had been so much confusion over the effects of n-3 fatty acids blood cholesterol levels. (It depends on the lipoprotein phenotype of the individual). Dr. Nicolosi further explains this topic with particular emphasis on the metabolism of low density lipoproteins as influenced by dietary fat. This Section concludes with an assessment of the contributions of individual dietary fatty acids on blood cholesterol levels by Dr. Grundy, who himself has made major contributions to this subject.

The effects of dietary fatty acids on blood clotting and blood pressure are the topics covered in Section III. The dietary fatty acids most strongly influencing blood pressure appear to be saturated and n-6 polyunsaturated compounds. Dr. Knapp gives an overview of this topic and Dr. Iacono related his experience with clinical trials and field studies of dietary fat and blood pressure. Drs. Holub and Schoene lead one through the tangled web of platelet function and dietary fats to conclude this section. The next Section, IV, takes up the controversial subject of dietary fatty acids and cancer. This topic has generated much interest over the last decade or two, but, like many areas in the cancer field, it has, perhaps, yielded more heat than light. One will not find all the answers here, but you will get a feel for the issues and complexities of the subject.

The emerging area of dietary fatty acids and immune function is presented in Section V. This area, like the cancer field, is still controversial. The early promise that n-3 polyunsaturated fatty acids would provide efficacious treatment of several autoimmune diseases has not been fulfilled yet. Whether it ever will is dubious. Dr. Robinson and colleagues tell us the status of this potential treatment and provide an overview of this topic in Chapter 18. The last Section, VI, reviews the status of several other conditions that have been purported to either be ameliorated or induced by dietary fatty acids. Dr. Clandinin and associates discuss diabetes. Dr. Kremer describes the results of clinical trial with n-3 polyunsaturated fatty acids on the treatment of rheumatoid arthritis. Dr. Horrobin relates the therapeutic effects of gamma-linolenic acid on atopic eczema and diabetic neuropathy. This volume concludes with the review of the health effects of *trans* fatty acids by Dr. Emken.

This monograph was intended to be both a reference work for the active investigator and an overview for the professional who is not actively engaged in laboratory or clinical studies, but needs to know where this field is now and, perhaps, the major direction in which it is heading. Of course, only the reader can decide whether the editor and authors were successful in achieving that goal.

Acknowledgments

There are many people that have played an important part in getting this topic from the concept stage to this subsequent monograph. Ed Perkins asked me to organize a short course on Health Effects of Polyunsaturated Fatty Acids and it seemed an appropriate and timely topic. Previously, Bill Lands had organized a very successful meeting on n-3 fatty acids in 1987. As it takes time to organize a short course, the time between the two meetings was long enough to bring new and significant findings to the audience. I hope this conference and monograph will be as interesting and educational as its organizers envisioned it to be. Finally, I would like to thank the American Oil Chemists' Society, particularly Julie Cahill, who have been a tremendous help with the complicated logistic arrangements necessary to stage this course and the production of this monograph.

Gary J. Nelson
August 1990

AOCS Mission Statement

To be a forum for the exchange of ideas, information and experience among those with a professional interest in the science and technology of fats, oils and related substances in ways that promote personal excellence and provide for a high standard of quality.

Copyright @ 1991 by the American Oil Chemists' Society.
All rights reserved. No part of this book may be reproduced or transmitted in any form or by any means without written permission of the publisher.

Library of Congress Cataloging-in-Publication Data

Health effects of dietary fatty acids / edited by Gary J. Nelson.
    p. cm.
    Based on the oral presentation made at the short course, held in Baltimore, Md., Apr. 1990.
    Includes bibliographical references and index.
    ISBN 0-935315-44-6
    1. Fatty acids in human nutrition—Congresses. 2. Fatty acids—Health aspects—Congresses. I. Nelson, Gary J. II. American Oil Chemists' Society.
    [DNLM: 1. Dietary Fats—adverse effects—congresses. 2. Disease—etiology—congresses. 3. Fatty Acids—adverse effects—congresses. QU 85 H434 1990]
QP752.F35H4 1991
616.3'9—dc20
DNLM/DLC   91-4567
for Library of Congress   CIP

Contents

Preface i

Section I: Composition, Function and Metabolism of Dietary Fatty Acids

Chapter 1 **Fatty Acid Composition of Present Day Diets**
—*Nancy D. Ernst* 1

Chapter 2 **Metabolism of Dietary Fatty Acids**
—*Howard Sprecher* 12

Chapter 3 **The Function of Essential Fatty Acids**
—*William E.M. Lands, Anna Morris, and Bozena Libelt* 21

Chapter 4 **Are N-3 Polyunsaturated Fatty Acids Essential for Growth and Development?**
—*Susan E. Carlson* 42

Section II: Effect of Dietary Fatty Acids on the Cardiovascular System: Hyperlipidemia and Lipoproteins

Chapter 5 **Dietary Fatty Acids, Serum Cholesterol and Coronary Heart Disease**
—*D.M. Hegsted* 50

Chapter 6 **Effects of Dietary Fatty Acids on Cholesterol, Triglyceride and Lipoprotein Distribution**
—*William S. Harris* 69

Chapter 7 **Effect of Dietary Fat Saturation on Low Density Lipoprotein Metabolism**
—*Robert J. Nicolosi, Arthur F. Stucchi, and Joseph Loscalzo* 77

Chapter 8 **Which Saturated Fatty Acids Raise Plasma Cholesterol Levels?**
—*Scott M. Grundy* 83

Section III: Effect of Dietary Fatty Acids on the Cardiovascular System: Blood Pressure and Blood Clotting

Chapter 9 **Effects of Dietary Fatty Acids on Blood Pressure: Epidemiology and Biochemistry**
—*Howard R. Knapp* 94

Chapter 10	**The Effect of ω 6 Dietary Fatty Acids on Blood Pressure** —*James M. Iacono*..107
Chapter 11	**Effect of Dietary Omega-3 Fatty Acids on Blood Platelet Reactivity** —*Bruce J. Holub*...122
Chapter 12	**Dietary Fatty Acids and Platelet Function: Mechanisms** —*Norberta W. Schoene*..129

Section IV: Relationships Between Dietary Fatty Acid and Cancer

Chapter 13	**Correlations Between Fatty Acid Intake and Cancer Incidence** —*Maureen M. Henderson*...136
Chapter 14	**Fatty Acid Metabolism and Biochemical Mechanisms in Cancer** —*Rashida A. Karmali*...150
Chapter 15	**Omega-3 Fatty Acids as Anticancer Agents** —*Bandaru S. Reddy*...157

Section V: Effects of Dietary Fatty Acids on the Immune System

Chapter 16	**Effect of Dietary Fats and Eicosanoids on Immune System** —*Simin Nikbin Meydani*..167
Chapter 17	**Effect of Dietary Fatty Acids on Cell Mediated Immune System** —*Darshan S. Kelley*..184
Chapter 18	**Suppression of Autoimmune Disease by Purified N-3 Fatty Acids** —*Dwight R. Robinson, Li-Lian Xu, Walter Olesiak, Sumio Tateno, Christopher T. Knoell, and Robert B. Colvin*........203

Section VI: Other Effects of Dietary Fatty Acids on Health

Chapter 19	**Relationship Between Diet Fat, Plasma Membrane Composition and Insulin Stimulated Functions in Adipocytes** —*M.T. Clandinin, C.J. Field, M. Toyomizu, A.B.R. Thomson, and M.L. Garg*..........................209
Chapter 20	**Studies of Dietary Supplementation with Omega-3 Fatty Acids in Patients with Rheumatoid Arthritis** —*Joel M. Kremer*...223
Chapter 21	**Therapeutic Effects of Gamma-linolenic Acid (GLA) as Evening Primrose Oil in Atopic Eczema and Diabetic Neuropathy** —*David F. Horrobin*..234

Chapter 22 **Do *Trans* Acids Have Adverse Health Consequences?**
—*E.A. Emken*..245

List of Contributors...265

Index...269

Chapter One
Fatty Acid Composition of Present Day Diets

Nancy D. Ernst, M.S., R.D.
National Heart, Lung, and Blood Institute
National Institutes of Health
7550 Wisconsin Avenue, Room 204
Bethesda, MD 20892

Trends in Individual Consumption of Fats

The average percentage of calories from fat in current diets may be lower than was evidenced 10 years ago. A somewhat decreasing fat intake over the past several years is shown in various survey data, with the exception of the National Health and Nutrition Examination surveys (NHANES), (1-3) (Table 1-1). The NHANES I, 1971-74, and NHANES II, 1976-80, show fat intake as 37-38% calories, for men and women. The USDA's National Food Consumption Survey (NFCS), 1977-78 show fat intake as 41-42% calories. In 1985, the U.S. Department of Agriculture

TABLE 1-1

KCalories and Total Fat Intake, as Percentage of Kilocalories
National Health and Nutrition Examination Survey (NHANES)
Nationwide Food Consumption Survey (NFCS)
and Continuing Survey of Food Intakes by Individuals

	NHANES I 1971-74		NFCS 1977-78		NHANES II 1976-80		CSFII 1985-86	
	Fat	KCal	Fat	KCal	Fat	KCal	Fat	KCal
Men								
30-39	37	2,668	42	2,382	37	2,554	36	2,484
40-49	37	2,428	42	2,341	38	2,421	37	2,384
Women								
30-39	37	1,610	41	1,571	37	1,596	37	1,648
40-49	37	1,552	42	1,562	38	1,531	37	1,541

(USDA) survey of individuals show that for ages 19 to 50, the percentage of calories from fat was 37% and 36% for women and men, respectively. These same data indicate that saturated fatty acids, as percentage of calories, average about 13.2% for men and women. The monounsaturated fatty acids account for 13.5 to 13.8% of calories, and polyunsaturated fatty acids account for 6.8 to 7.3% of calories in the diets of adults, ages 19 to 50 (5-7). Both of the NHANES surveys portray energy intake for men, ages 30-49 as about 2500-2600 calories and for women as about 1600 calories. In comparison, the USDA survey data reflect similar energy for women but somewhat lower caloric intake for men. For men ages 30-49, the intake was about 2400 calories.

These data may be compared with several studies conducted over the past several decades that were supported by the National Heart, Lung, and Blood Institute (NHLBI). Slight differences in intake are apparent for several nutrients, including total calories, percent of calories from fat, and percent of calories from saturated fatty acids (SFA).

Fatty acid intake is not available from the survey conducted in the 1970s by USDA (4) nor NHANES (1-3). However, the NHLBI-sponsored studies (8-11) show a slight and gradual decrease in SFA during the past decades (Table 1-2). Substantial differences are noted in the percent of calories from PFA and the P/S ratio. The PFA accounted for approxi-

TABLE 1-2

Mean Kilocalories and Fat Intake, for Men
NHLBI-Supported Studies
1963-1975

Study	Age Years	K.Calories	Fat % of KCalories	SFA	PFA	P/S Ratio
Diet-Heart (1963-64)	45-54	2565	40.4	15.6	3.9	0.3
Framingham (1960-64)	45-54	2666	39.7	15.2	5.6	0.4
	55-64	2563	38.4	14.9	5.2	0.4
LRC[a] (1972-75)	45-49	2612	40.2	14.8	6.9	0.5
	50-54	2492	39.6	14.6	6.8	
MRFIT[b] (1973-75)	35-57	2488	40.4	14.0	6.4	0.5

[a]Lipid Research Clinics
[b]Multiple Risk Factor Intervention Trial

mately 7% of calories in the 1985-86 USDA survey data, as well as in the studies sponsored by the NHLBI in the 1970s. This compares with 3.9% reported by the National Diet Heart Study which was conducted in the early 1960s.

Information on the stearic fatty acid content calculated from women in the USDA 1985 survey data mentioned previously indicate that of the 67g of total fat intake in the diets of women, ages 19-50, about 5.6g was stearic fatty acid (12).

Trends in Fats Available in the Food Supply

In reviewing estimates of fats in the food supply (13), it is recognized that estimates do not account for losses after food is measured, such as during processing, marketing or cooking. This is particularly relevant to fats, since previous calculations predict that about one-fourth of the fat in the food supply is wasted (14). The waste portion of fats and oil has increased during the past decade with the growth in away-from-home eating places, especially fast food places. The quantity of used frying fat disposed of by restaurants and processed by renderers for use in animal feed, pet food, industrial operations, and for export has been estimated to be about 10% of the 1988 disappearance of food fats and oils (13). Another influencing factor on fat available in the food supply is the current practice to trim exterior fat from beef cuts before retail sale (15). To what extent this substantial increase in the amount of fat trimmed affects the amount of beef fat consumed is unknown. In previous times, perhaps consumers removed the fat now being trimmed by meat packers and food distributors. Thus, we should regard food supply data as indicators of trends in fats and oils sold for human food. Such data are considered to be an over estimation of the fats consumed (13).

As indicated by data reviewed in the 1989 nutrition monitoring report (16), the major change in fat available in the supply is in the type of fat. This is manifest primarily as an increase in monounsaturated fat (24%) and polyunsaturated fat (94%). This is accounted for by fat from vegetable sources. Since the late 1940s, the percent of calories available from total fat has increased from 38 to 43% with the saturated fatty acids in the food supply decreasing only slightly from 17 to 16% of calories (16).

Data from the U.S. Food Supply Series (17) provide information on the omega-3 fatty acids. These data indicate that in the period 1947-49 through 1985 the amount of the two major omega-3 fatty acids found in fish was the same in 1985 as in 1935-39, about 50 mg per capita. This

Per Capita Consumption of Meat, Poultry, Fish U.S., 1967-1989

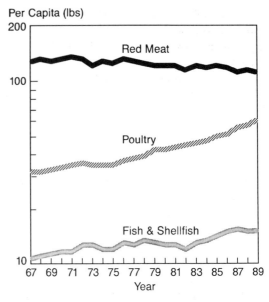

Fig. 1-1. Per Capita Consumption of Meat, Poultry, Fish U.S., 1967-1989.

probably reflects a decreased use of canned salmon and sardines, as well as cured fish. The amount of linolenic acid, from plant sources, increased from 1.6g per capita to 2.8g per capita per day. These changes reflect the increased consumption of soybean oil that occurred over this period of time. To a lesser degree, increased use of beef and poultry contributed to the upward trend.

Trends in Available Foods Contributing to Fat Intake

Data for food availability from 1967 to present shows noteworthy changes in foods that are important sources of fat and fatty acid intake. In terms of percentage changes, increases occurred (in descending order) for lowfat milks, vegetable fats and oils, cheese, poultry, fish, and nuts. Decreases occurred for whole milk, animal fat, eggs, cocoa, and meat—mainly beef (16).

The trend toward more poultry and fish consumption with no increase in meat consumption is shown in Figure 1-1. Per capita, in 1989, Americans averaged 18 pounds less red meat, 28 pounds more poultry and 2 pounds more fish and shellfish than in 1967. Estimates for 1989 and forecasts for 1990 put red meat and beef, per capita, at the lowest

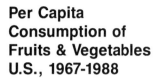

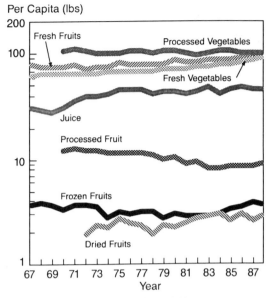

Fig. 1-2. Per Capita Consumption of Dairy Products U.S., 1967-1988.

levels since the early 1960s. In 1989 the beef consumption was 65 pounds per capita or 2.85 ounce per day compared with 60 pounds poultry or 2.63 ounces per day. Thus poultry consumption was 8% less than beef in 1989 (13).

In 1988, the per capita consumption of fish was one-quarter that of poultry—that is .66 oz per day or 15 pounds per year. This reflects a slight decline over 1987 and the first decrease since 1981. This is consistent with increased prices, lower imports, record high exports and food safety concerns. The Consumer price index for fish and shellfish in this one year period 1987-88 rose 6%, compared with 7.5% for poultry and 4.7% for all food items (13).

The supply data, Figure 1-2, show for dairy products, a substantial and steady substitution of lowfat milk for whole milk has occurred between 1967 and 1988 (13). Whole milk decreased to 47% of beverage milk down from 84% in 1967. Thus lowfat and skim milk comprised 53% of all beverage milk in 1988. However more cream products are being consumed, the supply data indicate 7.2 pounds per person in 1988, compared with 5 pounds in 1979. There is some evidence that increased consumption is concentrated in the ingredient and away from home

Per Capita Consumption of Dairy Products U.S., 1967-1988

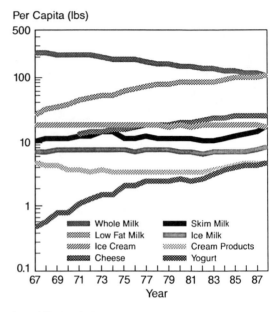

Fig. 1-3. Per Capita Consumption of Fruits & Vegetables U.S., 1967-1988.

markets. Pizza sales and convenience items are probably the major forces influencing this trend (13).

It is also useful to consider the supply data (13) for availability of foods that influence the fatty acid content of the diet by displacement of fats. Such foods include fruits, vegetables, and cereals. Per capita consumption of fresh fruits and vegetables was higher in 1988, compared with the previous two decades, see Figure 1-3. Fruit consumption in 1988 was 94 pounds per person, compared with 73 pounds in 1970-72. As one example, raisins and currents were up one pound in this time period due to consumption of cereals, bakery items, and snacks. Nine fresh vegetables reached a record high consumption in 1988, 27% above that of 1967. Those vegetables increasing by the largest amount were lettuce, onions, carrots, tomatoes, and broccoli. Finally cereals have increased dramatically in recent years. Part of the increase is attributed to a demographic influence of an aging U.S. population. Households which are headed by those 45 years are older spent 36% more for cereals and bakery products than younger households (13).

Trends in the Contribution of Fats from Individual Foods in the Food Supply

The food supply data show that from the late 1940s to the present there was little change in the contribution of total fat from meat, poultry and fish (14). There has been a shift in choices within the group. Meat has decreased by 3% while poultry and fish have increased by 3%. The contribution of dairy products to total fat has decreased by 6.6%. Within the fats and oils group, animal fats have decreased by 3% and vegetable oils increased 11.9%. A focus on saturated fat, shows that since the late 1940s the contribution of meat, poultry and fish increased by 4.7 percentage points. The percentage increase of monounsaturated fatty acids, and polyunsaturated fatty acids contributed by salad, cooking, and other edible oils were 11 and 20 percentage points (14).

Trends in Individual Consumption of Foods Contributing to Fat Intake

Food consumption data for individuals has been used to consider those foods which contribute to the intake of fat and fatty acids. The two methods used are "food group" or "ingredient foods" (18-19). Using a "food group" approach which classifies foods by their major ingredients, about 50 to 55% of the fat and 55 to 60% of the SFA was estimated to come from meat, poultry, fish, egg and dairy products, and from mixed dishes containing these animal products as major ingredients (18), (Figure 1-4). These estimates include fats of other origins, such as frying fats and salad dressings, used in preparation of these foods. The estimates exclude the fat and SFA from the animal products in a mixed dish included in another food group, for example the meat and cheese included in spaghetti or pizza. An "ingredient approach," that separates foods into their ingredients has also been used to estimate sources of fat, although the analyses is limited to women's diets. These preliminary data, show that about 50% of the fat and about 59% of SFA came from meat, poultry, fish, egg and dairy products (Figure 1-5). The ingredient approach also showed that fats and oils added at the table or in food processing and preparation accounted for at least 33% of the fat in women's diet (19).

The palm, palm kernel and coconut oils, ("tropical oils"), contain as high, or higher proportions of SFAs than animal fats (15). In 1985, these tropical oils provided about 3% of the total amount of fat in the food supply (18). Current intakes, of the three tropical oils combined, by the

Total Fat

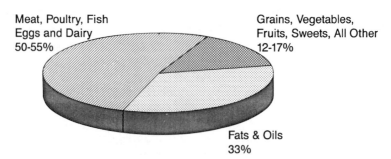

Fig. 1-4. Food Sources Percentage Contribution of Total Fat in Diet.

Saturated Fatty Acids

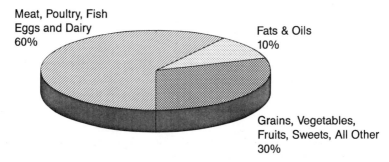

Fig. 1-5. Food Sources Percentage Contribution of Saturated Fatty Acids.

U.S. population are estimated to be about 2 to 4 gram per person per day. These estimates represent less than 4% of total fat intake, less than 2% of daily energy intake, and 8% or less of the SFA intake (18).

Factors Associated with Fat Intake

There is little data to clearly establish a profile of the variation in fat intake. It was reported by Harris and Welsh (19) that higher income women had a lower percentage of total fat intake from meat, poultry and fish than for lower income women. The proportion of fat from milk and milk products differed little by income. The higher income had a greater intake of lowfat milk, but ate more cheese and cream desserts. The greatest difference was in the fats and oils group with higher income women having a higher intake of salad dressings, and butter or margarine.

It is acknowledged that traditional and nontraditional demand determinants have influenced trends in consumption of foods that influence the fatty acid composition of our diets (13). These include changes in real income, that is income adjusted for inflation, and shifts in the demographic composition of households. Contributing factors to changes in food patterns are changes in lifestyles, technological developments, advertisements, and concern for nutrition and health. Recommendations by public health officials on diet and health (20-25) have also influenced food availability and consumption patterns.

In summary, we have reviewed food supply trends in fat from food sources and noted marked variation from commodity to commodity during the 20-year period from 1967 to 1989. There was a rise in the consumption of some reduced or low-fat products, such as low-fat milk and fish, but there was increased use of high-fat foods, such as cheese and fats used in cooking of both vegetable and animal origin. There is a movement among food producers, processors, and manufacturers toward lowering the fat content. This mostly consists of the physical removal of fat in the food production process, such as closely trimmed retail cuts of beef.

A primary interest of consumers is convenience, thus the intake of processed foods continues to increase since processed foods generally require less preparation time. Such food market trends are reflected in the intake of fats in processed foods such as mixtures, baked goods, carry-out items, and partially prepared foods that require little additional preparation at home. In contrast there is a decrease in the intake of visible, separable fats.

A look at food supply data provides information on an additional trend with potential nutrition implications, that is the increase in crop-derived foods compared with foods from animal products. Between 1967 and 1988, crop-derived foods increased 16%, while animal-based foods increased only 5% on a per-capita basis. Yet, in 1988, the per capita consumption of meat, poultry and fish reached a record high of 187 pounds per person per year, a 15-pound increase from the 1967 level

(13). It will be interesting to continue to monitor food trends which obviously have potential to markedly influence the fatty acid composition of our future dietary patterns.

References

1. Dietary Intake Findings—United States, 1971-74. Vital and Health Statistics, Series 11, No. 202. Department of Health, Education, and Welfare. Hyattsville, MD Publication No. (URA)77-1647 (1977).
2. Abraham, S., Carroll, M.D., Johnson, C.L., Dresser, C.M., Vital and Health Statistics Series 11, No. 209, DHEW Publication No. (PHS)79-1657. U.S. Department of Health, Education, and Welfare, Public Health Service, National Center for Health Statistics (1979).
3. Carroll, M.D., Abraham, S., Dresser, C.M., Vital and Health Statistics Series 11, No. 231, DHHS Publication No. (PHS) 83-1681. U.S. Department of Health and Human Services, Public Health Service, National Center for Health Statistics (1983).
4. U.S. Department of Agriculture. Nationwide Food Consumption Survey. 1977-78. Report No. I-2. Consumer Nutrition Division, Human Nutrition Information Service, Hyattsville, MD, pp. 439 (1984).
5. Human Nutrition Information Service. Nationwide Food Consumption Survey. Hyattsville, MD: U.S. Department of Agriculture, CSFII Report No. 85-1 (1985).
6. Human Nutrition Information Service. Nationwide Food Consumption Survey. Hyattsville, MD: U.S. Department of Agriculture, CSFII Report No. 85-4 (1985).
7. Human Nutrition Information Service. Nationwide Food Consumption Survey. Hyattsville, MD: U.S. Department of Agriculture, CSFII Report No. 85-3 (1985).
8. The Lipid Research Clinics Population Studies Data Book. Volume II. The Prevalence Study—Nutrient Intake. U.S. Department of Health and Human Services, U.S. Government Printing Office, Washington, DC, (1982).
9. The National Diet Heart Study Final Report. National Diet Heart Study Research Group, Circulation 37(Suppl 1):1-428 (1968).
10. In An Epidemiological Investigation of Cardiovascular Disease. (W.B. Kannel and T. Gordon, eds). Section 24, Bethesda, MD: National Institutes of Health (1970)
11. The Multiple Risk Factor Intervention Trial (MRFIT): A national study of primary prevention of coronary heart disease. JAMA 235:82-7 (1976).
12. Human Nutrition Information Service, U.S. Department of Agriculture (Personal Communication to the author). Hyattsville, MD: U.S. Department of Agriculture, CSFII Report No. 85-4 (1985).
13. Putnam, J.J., 1966-88, U.S. Department of Agriculture. Economic Research

Service, Statistical Bulletin No. 773, in press.
14. Rizek, R.L., *et al.* In Dietary Fats and Health, edited by E.G. Perkins and W.J. Visek, American Oil Chemists' Society, Champaign, IL (1983).
15. National Research Council, Committee on Technological Options to Improve the Nutritional Attributes of Animal Products, Board on Agriculture. Washington, DC: National Academy Press (1988).
16. Life Sciences Research Office, Federation of American Sciences for Experimental Biology: DHHS Publication No. (PHS) 89-1255. Public Health Service. Washington. U.S. Government Printing Office (1989).
17. Raper, N., Personal communication to author.
18. Park, Y.K., and Yetley, E.A. (1990) Am J Clin Nutr 51:738-48.
19. Harris, S., and Welsh, S. (1989) Nutrition Today 24(6):20-28.
20. U.S. Department of Agriculture/U.S. Department of Health and Human Services. Nutrition and Your Health: Dietary Guidelines for Americans, 2nd ed. Home and Garden Bulletin No. 232. Washington, DC: U.S. Government Printing Office (1985).
21. National Cholesterol Education Program. (1988) Arch Intern med 148:36-69.
22. U.S. Department of Health and Human Services. Public Health Service. Surgeon General's Report on Nutrition and Health. Washington, DC: U.S. Department of Health and Human Services, Public Health Service, Pub. No. (PHS) 88-50210. (1988).
23. National Research Council. Diet and Health: Implications for Reducing Chronic Disease Risk. Washington, DC: National Academy Press (1989).
24. National Research Council. Subcommittee on the Tenth Edition of the RDAs. Recommended Dietary Allowances. 10th Edition. Food and Nutrition Board, Commission on Life Sciences, National Academy Press (1989).
25. Report of the National Cholesterol Education Program Expert Panel on Population Strategies for Blood Cholesterol Reduction (Population Panel), in press.

Chapter Two

Metabolism of Dietary Fatty Acids

Howard Sprecher

Department of Physiological Chemistry
The Ohio State University, Columbus, Ohio 43210

The types of unsaturated fatty acids found in membrane lipids are in part regulated by the type of dietary fat that is fed as well as how fatty acids are modified prior to their acylation into lipids via a number of different pathways. The primary objective of this review is to discuss some of the factors regulating polyunsaturated fatty acid biosynthesis and in addition to focus on some of the differences in (n-3) and (n-6) polyunsaturated fatty acid metabolism. It is now accepted that there are four families of unsaturated fatty acids. These pathways are depicted in Figure 2-1. According to these pathways both linoleate and linolenate are metabolized to 22-carbon polyunsaturated acids via an alternating series of position specific desaturases and chain elongating enzymes. In addition, the process of partial degradation or retroconversion also may play a role in modifying certain polyunsaturated fatty acids. The

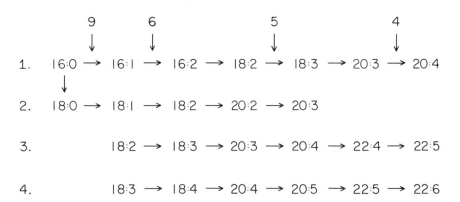

Fig. 2-1. Pathways for the biosynthesis of the four families of polyunsaturated fatty acids.

next three sections will briefly review the role played by these three types of reactions in modifying dietary acids.

Desaturation

It is generally assumed that only three position specific desaturases are used in PUFA biosynthesis. These enzymes introduce double bonds at the 6-, 5- and 4-positions. The presence of different enzymes is usually assumed to be fact only when a protein is isolated and shown to catalyze a specific reaction. This type of information is generally lacking for the 6-, 5-, and 4-desaturases. Indeed, much of our basic knowledge about these three desaturases may be inferred information that is based on elegant studies of the 9-desaturase. This enzyme converts stearate and palmitate respectively to oleate and palmitoleate and is not used in (n-6) or (n-3) polyunsaturated fatty acid biosynthesis. It has long been recognized that the activity of the 9-desaturase is depressed by fasting while its activity is increased by dietary carbohydrate and insulin (1,2). These findings were based primarily on rate studies with microsomal preparations and suggest that this enzyme is a lipogenic enzyme whose primary function is to participate in the conversion of carbohydrate to fat. In 1974 the 9-desaturase was isolated from rat liver microsomes and shown to have a molecular weight of 53,000 (3). The absolute requirement for cytochrome b_5 and cytochrome b_5 reductase in a reconstituted system was also established at that time. Subsequent studies established that the enhanced activity of the enzyme in response to dietary carbohydrate correlated with an increase in the mRNA which codes for the desaturase (4). This mRNA has now been used to sequence the cDNA that codes for this enzyme (5).

The 6-desaturase was partially purified in 1981 and its requirement for cytochrome b_5 and cytochrome b_5 reductase was established at that time (6). The 5-desaturase is usually assayed by incubating a suitable acyl-CoA with microsomes. However, Pugh and Kates (7) showed that choline phosphoglycerides containing 8,11,14-20:3 at the sn-2 position were desaturated to a choline phosphoglyceride containing esterified arachidonate. We showed that a number of fatty acids with their first double bond at position-11 were desaturated at position-5 rather than at position-8 (8). The 5-desaturase has never been solubilized so it is not known if a single protein can catalyze the above three types of reactions.

It is also in theory possible that linoleate and linolenate could be metabolized according to the following pathways: 9,12-18:2 → 11,14-20:2 → 8,11,14-20:3 → 5,8,11,14-20:4 and 9,12,15-18:3 → 11,14,17-20:3 →

8,11,14,17-20:4 → 5,8,11,14,17-20:5. This pathway implies that the 18-carbon unsaturated acids are initially chain elongated prior to desaturation at position-8. We showed that 11,14-20:2 and 11,14,17-20:3 were desaturated at position-5 to yield respectively 5,11,14-20:3 and 5,11,14,17-20:4 (8). These are dead end metabolites and thus show that 20:4(n-6) and 20:5(n-3) are made only as depicted in Figure 2-1.

There is no question that dietary linoleate and linolenate are converted respectively to 22:5(n-6) and 22:6(n-3). However, very little information is available about the putative 4-desaturase which uses 22:4(n-6) and 22:5(n-3) as substrates. We reported that microsomes from rats fed an essential fatty acid deficient diet converted small amounts of 22:4(n-6) to 22:5(n-6) (9). However, Ayala *et al.* (10) found that testes and liver microsomes from rats fed a chow diet did not desaturate 22:4(n-6). The regulation of the activity of this important enzyme is poorly understood relative to its potential importance. Brain and retina lipids in particular both contain high levels of 22:6(n-3) and it has never been established whether the 22:6(n-3) in these lipids is made in liver and transported to these tissues or whether the majority of 22:6(n-3) is made immediately prior to acylation in brain and retina.

Chain Elongation

Figure 2-2 shows the general pathway of microsomal fatty acid chain elongation. According to this pathway, an acyl-CoA condenses with malonyl-CoA to yield a β-keto compound. The β-keto compound is then reduced with either NADH or NADPH to yield a β-hydroxy intermediate which is dehydrated and following nucleotide dependent reduction yields the fully chain elongated product. The true substrates for all reactions are the acyl-CoA derivatives (11). Inhibitor studies (12), dietary or hormonal modification prior to the sacrifice of the animals (12,13), as well as differential less of enzyme activity when microsomes are treated with proteolytic enzymes (13), support the hypothesis that microsomes contain two or perhaps three condensing enzymes. The respective β-keto acyl-CoA derivatives are then channeled into a common set of enzymes to complete the chain elongation process. The validity of this later hypothesis is based on competitive substrate studies (15), and the observation that the overall rate of condensation equals that of chain elongation, and the finding that rates subsequent to condensation are much more rapid than is the initial malonyl-CoA dependent reaction (12). It should be noted that the conversion of linoleate to 22:5(n-6) requires two chain elongation steps - i.e. 18:3(n-6) → 20:3(n-6)

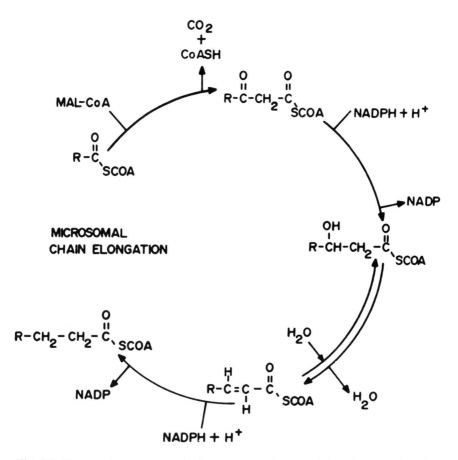

Fig. 2-2. The reaction pathway for the microsomal malonyl-CoA dependent chain elongation of fatty acids.

and 20:4(n-6) → 22:4(n-6). In a similar way 18:4(n-3) and 20:5(n-3) are substrates for chain elongation in the synthesis of 22:6(n-3). It is not known if a single condensing enzyme uses both 18- and 20-carbon unsaturated acids as primers.

Retroconversion

It has long been recognized that 20-carbon (n-3) and (n-6) acids are acylated into membrane lipids when 22-carbon (n-6) and (n-3) acids

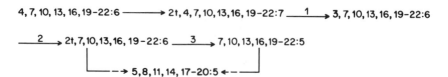

Fig. 2-3. Pathway for the partial β-oxidation of 4,7,10,13,16,19-docosahexaenoic acid showing where 2,4-dienoyl-CoA reductase (1), Δ^3-cisΔ^2-trans-enoyl-CoA isomerase (2) and intra-mitochondrial nucleotide dependent reduction (3) are used in this process.

are included in the diet (16). In fact, it is possible to detect prostacylin I_3 in the urine of humans when 22:6(n-3) is fed (17). This partial degradation or retroconversion is really partial β-oxidation that takes place in mitochondria or peroxisomes. This pathway, as elucidated by Kunau and Schulz (18), is illustrated in Figure 2-3 for the catabolism of 22:6(n-3). Initially 22:6(n-3) is a substrate for a flavin linked enzyme to introduce a *trans* double bond at position-2. The conjugated diene is then reduced via a nucleotide dependent reductase—i.e. 2,4-dienoyl-CoA reductase—to give an acid with its first double bond at position-3. The enzyme $\Delta 3$-*cis*-$\Delta 2$-*trans* enoyl-CoA isomerase then catalyzes the transfer of the double bond to the 2-*trans* position. Intramitochondrial nucleotide dependent reduction then gives 22:5(n-3). Alternatively, some of the 2-*trans*, 7,10,13,16,19-22:6 is catabolized via β-oxidation to yield 20:5(n-3). For reasons which are not understood some of the 20:5(n-3) is acylated rather than being completely catabolized. It should be noted that the enzymes 2,4-dienoyl-CoA reductase and $\Delta 3$ *cis*-$\Delta 2$ *trans* enoyl-CoA isomerase are only used in the catabolism of unsaturated fatty acids. The latter enzyme is used every time a double bond is encountered while the former enzyme is used only when double bonds are at even numbered carbon atoms.

Regulation of 22-Carbon Unsaturated Fatty Acid Biosynthesis

Table 2-1 compares the unsaturated fatty acid composition of liver ethanolamine phosphoglycerides when weanling rats were fed either a chow diet, a diet containing 3% ethyl linoleate or ethyl linolenate as the sole source of fat or 1.5% of each of the ethyl esters (19). In the chow fed animal this lipid and other phospholipids contain large amounts of 20:4(n-6) but only small amounts of 22:4(n-6) and 22:5(n-6). Converse-

TABLE 2-1
Unsaturated fatty acid composition of liver ethanolamine phosphoglycerides after feeding rats a chow diet or various ethyl esters

Component	Chow	18:2(n-6)	18:3(n-3)	18:2(n-6) 18:3(n-3)
18:2(n-6)	7.7	5.1	1.3	3.6
18:3(n-3)	—	—	0.7	—
20:4(n-6)	30.3	35.8	4.5	18.6
20:5(n-3)	1.1	—	19.3	5.4
22:4(n-6)	0.2	0.9	—	0.1
22:5(n-6)	—	5.8	0.1	0.3
22:5(n-3)	1.5	—	3.5	2.4
22:6(n-3)	10.3	2.4	17.6	19.4

TABLE 2-2
Percent distribution of radioactive fatty acids in total phospholipids when hepatocytes from chow fed and essential fatty acid deficient rats were incubated with either [3-^{14}C]labeled 7,10,13,16-docosatetraenoic or 7,10,13,16,19-docosapentaenoic acids

Component	Chow Fed	Fat Free
	[3-^{14}C]22:4(n-6)	
22:4(n-6)	21	20
20:4(n-6)	79	70
22:5(n-6)	—	10
	[3-^{14}C]22:5(n-3)	
22:5(n-3)	57	39
20:5(n-3)	43	33
22:6(n-3)	—	27

ly, membrane lipids generally contain 22:5(n-3) and large amounts of 22:6(n-3). When linoleate is fed the membrane lipids contain only relatively small amounts of 22:4(n-6) and 22:5(n-6) even though it would seem that an adequate amount of 20:4(n-6) was potentially available for their biosynthesis. As expected, when linolenate was fed alone the membrane lipids contain large amounts of 22:6(n-3). However, when equal amounts of the two esters were fed there is a clear preference for converting 18:3(n-3) to 22:6(n-3) and acylating it into membrane lipids versus the analogous reaction sequence for linoleate. Clearly different mechanisms *in vivo* are involved in dictating what regulates the conversion of 20:5(n-3) to 22:6(n-3) followed by their acylation, versus the metabolism of 20:4(n-6) to the analogous 22-carbon (n-6) acids followed by their esterification. These differences are not explained by enzymatic studies. We found that 20:4(n-6) and 20:5(n-3) were chain elongated at about the same rates - i.e. 1.1 and 1.3 nmols/min/mg of rat liver microsomal protein. Lands et al. (20) reported that 20:4 (n-6) and 20:5(n-6) were acylated at about the same rates when 1-acyl-2-*sn*-glycero-3-phosphocholine was the acceptor. *In vivo* the synthesis and acylation of specific 22-carbon acids into membrane lipids is thus not solely dependent on specificities for anabolic processes. Table 2-2 defines how [3-^{14}C] labeled 22:4(n-6) and 22:5(n-3) are metabolized when they are incubated with hepatocytes from rats raised on a chow diet or a diet devoid of fat. Both 22-carbon acids were substrates for retroconversion. However, more 22:4(n-6) was retroconverted to 20:4(n-6) followed by its esterification when compared to the analogous metabolism of 22:5(n-3). There is thus a tendency to retroconvert 22:4(n-6) while 22:5(n-3) is preferentially acylated. In hepatocytes from chow fed rats it was not possible to detect any product of the 4-desaturase in phospholipids. In rats fed a fat free diet both substrates were also desaturated. In these studies more 22:5(n-3) than 22:4(n-6) was desaturated. These cell studies thus show that 22:4(n-6) and 22:5(n-3) are metabolized with differenct specificities. In addition, they show that the process of retroconversion may play a real role in defining what specific 22-carbon acids are available for acylation.

Frequently, 22:5(n-6) and 22:6(n-3) are considered to be the end product of linoleate and linolenate metabolism. However, retina (21) and brain lipids (22) in particular accumulate significant amounts of (n-6) and (n-3) unsaturated acids which contain as many as 36 carbon atoms and six double bonds. Clearly unique specificities must exist for the synthesis and acylation of this unique class of compounds.

Conversion of Linoleate and Linolenate to 20-Carbon Acids

When rats are maintained on a chow diet their membrane lipids do not contain high levels of 18:3(n-6) or 20:3(n-6) even though these two acids are obligatory intermediates in the synthesis of arachidonate. The lack of these acids in membrane lipids cannot be explained by rates of reactions for desaturation, chain elongation or acylation. Our recent studies suggest that some linoleate may be channeled directly to arachidonate without intracellular mixing of 18:3(n-6) and 20:3(n-6) (23). If this is true, then a somewhat different mechanism exists for regulating linolenate metabolism. As shown in Table 2-1, very little 18:3(n-3) accumulates in membrane lipids even when it is fed as a sole source of fat. This may be due, in part, to its very rapid and selective mitochondrial β-oxidation (24). Chow fed rats only accumulate 22:5(n-3) and 22:6(n-3) while some 20:5(n-3) does accumulate when 18:3(n-3) is fed as the sole source of fat. However, neither 18:4(n-3) nor 20:4(n-3) accumulate in membrane lipids when linolenate is the sole source of fat. These studies suggest that when low levels of linolenate are fed, as is found in rat chow, that it is channeled all the way to 22:5(n-3) and 22:6(n-3) and then acylated. Conversely, arachidonic acid synthesis, as measured by lipid compositional studies, is in general the major end point of linoleate metabolism.

Acknowledgment

These studies were supported in part by NIH Grants DK20387 and DK18844.

References

1. Gellhorn, A. and Benjamin, W. (1964) Biochim. Biophys. Acta 84, 167-175.
2. Oshino. N. and Sato, R. (1972) Arch. Biochem. Biophys. 149, 369-377.
3. Strittmatter, P., Spatz, L., Corcoran, O., Rogers, M.J., Setlow, B. and Redline, R. (1974) Proc. Natl. Acad. Sci. USA 71, 4565-4569.
4. Thiede, M.A. and Strittmatter, P. (1985) J. Biol. Chem. 260, 14459-14463.
5. Thiede, M.A., Ozols, J. and Strittmatter, P. (1986) J. Biol. Chem. 261, 13230-13235.
6. Okayasu, T., Nagao, M., Ishibashi, T., and Imai, Y. (1981) Arch. Biochem. Biophys. 206, 21-28.
7. Pugh, E.L. and Kates, M. (1977) J. Biol. Chem. 252, 68-72.
8. Sprecher, H. and Lee, C-J. (1975) Biochim. Biophys. Acta 388, 113-125.
9. Bernert, J.T. and Sprecher, H. (1975) Biochim. Biophys. Acta 398, 354-363.
10. Ayala, S., Gaspar, G., Brenner, R.R., Peluffo, R.O. and Kunau, W. (1973) J. Lipid Res. 14, 296-305.
11. Bernert, J.T. and Sprecher, H. (1979) Biochim. Biophys. Acta 573, 436-442.
12. Bernert, J.T. and Sprecher, H. (1977) J. Biol. Chem. 252, 6736-6744.
13. Suneja, S.K., Osei, P., Cook, L., Nagai, M.N. and Cinti, D.L. (1990) Biochim. Biophys. Acta 1042, 81-85.
14. Prasad, M.R., Nagai, M.N., Ghesquier, D., Cook, L. and Cinti, D.L. (1986) J.

Biol. Chem. 261, 8213-8217.
15. Nagai, M.N., Cook, L., Prasad, M.R. and Cinti, D.L.(1986) Biochem. Biophys. Res. Commun. 140, 74-80.
16. Sprecher, H. and James, A.T. in Geometrical and Positional Fatty Acid Isomers, edited by E.A. Emken and H.J. Dutton, American Oil Chemists Soc., Champaign, Illinois, 1979, pp. 303-338.
17. Fischer, S., Vischer, A., Preac-Mursic, V. and Weber, P.C. (1987). Prostaglandins 34, 367-375.
18. Schulz, H. and Kunau, W.H. (1987) Trends Biochim. Sci. 12, 403-406.
19. Weiner, T.W. and Sprecher, H. (1984) Biochem. Biophys. Acta 792, 293-303.
20. Lands, W.E.M., Inoue, M., Sugiura, Y. and Okuyama, H. (1982) J. Biol. Chem. 257, 14968-14972.
21. Aveldano, M.I. and Sprecher, H. (1987) J. Biol. Chem. 262, 1180-1186.
22. Robinson, B.S., Johnson, D.W. and Poulos, A. (1990) Biochem. J. 265, 763-767.
23. Voss, A.C. and Sprecher, H. (1988) Lipids 23, 660-665.
24. Clouet, P., Niot, I. and Bezard, J. (1989) Biochem. J. 263, 867-873.

Chapter Three

The Function of Essential Fatty Acids

William E.M. Lands, Anna Morris, and Bozena Libelt

Department of Biological Chemistry
University of Illinois at Chicago
1853 West Polk St., A312-CMW
Chicago, IL 60612

M any published reports provide detailed lists of the abundances of the different fatty acids that are maintained in rat tissues. The reports provide evidence that different enzymes act together to maintain steady state compositions of fatty acids in cellular lipid (1). The esterifying enzymes tend to place saturated fatty acids (SFA) at the sn-1 position of glycerolipids (Figure 3-1). Therefore, the saturated fatty acids (SFA) at the sn-1 position constitute nearly one-half of the fatty acids in diacyl-phosphoglycerides (ca. 40 to 45%) and about one-third of the fatty acids in triacylglycerols (ca 25 to 35%). In contrast, the 16- and 18-carbon unsaturated fatty acids (UFA) are esterified at the sn-2 position during *de novo* synthesis and the 20- and 22-carbon highly unsaturated fatty

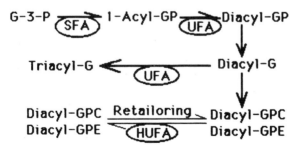

Fig. 3-1. General Selectivities in Lipid Synthesis Saturated fatty acids. Saturated fatty acids (SFA), C-16 and C-18 unsaturated fatty acids (UFA) and C-20 and C-22 highly unsaturated fatty acids (HUFA) are incorporated during glycerolipid biosynthesis.

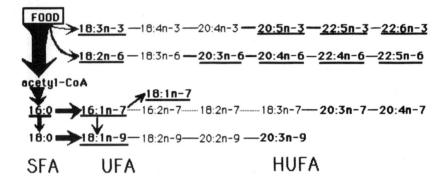

Fig. 3-2. Exogenous and Endogenous Fatty Acids.
A large influx of carbohydrate and protein provides most of the acetyl CoA for the synthesis of endogenous acids.

acids (HUFA) at the sn-2 position during the retailoring process (Figure 3-1). Slightly different activities of the *de novo* and retailoring enzymes in different tissues appear to produce different proportions of UFA and HUFA in different tissues. As a result, the fatty acid composition in each tissue can reflect both the selectivity of the enzymes and the relative abundances of the different acids available to the enzymes (2). These general enzyme slectivities appear to be similar for either rat or human tissue. Although alterations in dietary fat can influence the maintenance levels, a strong influence of the general esterification selectivity with the endogenous fatty acids seems likely to cause the strikingly similar overall compositional patterns for fatty acids in lipids of human tissues world-wide (3) and for the similarity of the fatty acid patterns in the lipids of rats and humans.

In the absence of any dietary fat, tissue lipids have small amounts of n-3 and n-6 fatty acids (apparently acquired from maternal supplies), and most of the fatty acids in tissue lipids (about 90%) are the endogenous acids (4,5) synthesized from acetate: 14:0, 16:0, 18:0, 16:1n-7, 18:1n-7 and 18:1n-9 (Figure 3-2). In addition to these acids, rat tissues can also accumulate and maintain significant amounts of 20- and 22-carbon highly unsaturated fatty acids (HUFA), 20:3n-9, 20:3n-7 (6) and 20:4n-7 (7,8). The pattern that is maintained among these fatty acids (Figure 3-2) is created by the relative rates of synthesis of the various acids from their carbohydrate and amino acid precursors (which customarily comprise the major source of dietary calories and cellular acetylcoenzyme A). Continued hydrolysis and replacement of tissue lipid esters maintains the proportions of saturated (14:0, 16:0, 18:0), unsaturated (16:1n-7, 18:1n-7 and 18:1n-9) and highly unsaturated fatty acids (20:3, 20:4) in accord with the general selectivities of esterification and oxidation during fatty acid and glycerolipid metabolism (1).

When the diet includes polyunsaturated fatty acids of either the n-3 or n-6 type (which cannot be synthesized *de novo* in animal tissues), there is a marked displacement of the "endogenous" type of HUFA (20:3n-9, 20:4n-7) by new HUFA of the n-3 type (20:5n-3, 22:5n-3, 22:6n-3) or the n-6 type (20:3n-6, 20:4n-6, 22:4n-6, 22:5n-6) derived from dietary 18:3n-3 and 18:2n-6, respectively. For example, with a rat chow diet (9), a pattern of tissue acids is maintained which includes relative amounts of 14:0, 16:0, 18:0, 16:1n-7, 18:1n-7 and 18:1n-9, that are rather similar to those seen with a fat-free diet, but with 18:2n-6 apparently displacing 18:1n-7 and 18:1n-9 and with 20:4n-6 displacing 20:3n-9, 20:3n-7 and 20:4n-7. The early recognition (10) that the dietary n-3 acid (18:3n-3) can inhibit the elongation and desaturation of 18:2n-6 to 20:4n-6 was extended to a thorough demonstration of competitive metabolic interactions between polysaturated fatty acids of the n-3, n-6 and n-9 types (4,5).

Because the 20-carbon highly unsaturated fatty acids (HUFA) play important roles as precursors and antagonists of eicosanoid biosynthesis (11,12), altering the abundance of dietary precursors of these HUFA seems certain to influence a tissue's capacity to form eicosanoids. An altered capacity seems likely to affect the frequency and severity of eicosanoid-related disorders (13). Such a possible influence makes it important to understand in more detail how tissues maintain their typical levels of n-3 and n-6 HUFA and to understand how much those levels may be influenced by different amounts of dietary polyunsaturated fatty acids. If we can understand the basic processes and selectivities by which rat tissues maintain their characteristic patterns of fatty acids, we can then test the extent to which that understanding could be applied to interpreting the patterns of fatty acids in lipids of humans.

This report describes the results of dietary studies with rats that establish quantitative relationships among dietary and endogenous tissue fatty acids for these experimental animals. The results are expressed in the form of algebraic equations that may be useful for estimating the different compositions of fatty acids in tissues which result from altered dietary intakes. Further experience with the equations may eventually permit using analyses of compositions of fatty acids in tissues to estimate the average dietary intakes of n-3 and n-6 acids.

General Maintenance of Animals

Pregnant Sprague-Dawley rats (from Sasco, Inc., Oregon, Wisconsin) were maintained at 70-72°C, 40% humidity and 12 hr light-dark cycle in the Biological Resources Laboratory of the University of Illinois at Chicago. They were fed one of the defined diets described in Table 3-1 from the time of their arrival in the facility until after the weaning period when the pups were placed in separate cages and maintained on the same diet as their parent until they reached approx. 500g (males) or approx 300g (females).

TABLE 3-1
Fatty Acid Composition of the Diets

	Weight %						
Component	0	A	B	C	D	Fl	Co
18:1	0.00	80.17	77.40	70.95	48.56	21.20	28.38
18:2	0.00	3.67	4.88	6.01	13.12	18.68	58.46
18:3n-3	0.00	0.00	2.37	8.08	25.03	51.18	1.13
Other acids	0.00	16.15	15.36	14.96	13.29	8.94	12.02
Diet(n-3/n-6)	0.00	0.00	0.49	1.34	1.91	2.74	0.02
en%18:2n-6	0.00	0.33	0.44	0.55	1.19	4.11	12.86
en%18:3n-3	0.00	0.00	0.22	0.73	2.28	11.26	1.25
en%PUFA	0.00	0.33	0.66	1.28	3.47	15.37	13.11

Fatty Acid Composition of Triglycerides

The average overall fatty acid compositions maintained in the triglycerides of three different tissues (plasma, liver, adipose) were similar to each other irrespective of the sex of the animals or the different diet fed; about 25% saturated fatty acids (SFA), 70% 16- and 18-carbon unsaturated fatty acids (UFA), and 2 to 5% HUFA. A decrease in the synthesis of endogenous fatty acids from dietary carbohydrate and protein was evident in the decreased amounts of the n-7 fatty acids that were maintained in tissue triglycerides as the amount of dietary fat increased. With

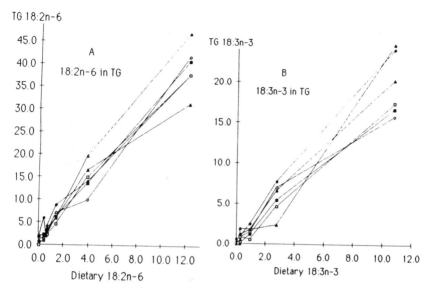

Fig. 3-3. Maintenance Levels of Polyunsaturated Fatty Acids in Triglycerides of Rat Tissues A.-Linoleate maintained in triglycerides of adipose (O), liver (□), plasma (△) of male (open symbols) and female (solid symbols) rats is shown in relation to the energy percent of 18:2n-6 provided in the diet. B.-Linolenate maintained in triglycerides in relation to the energy percent of 18:3n-3 provided in the diet (symbols as in Fig. 3-3).

the fat-deficient diet, the n-7 acids were about 38% of triglyceride UFA, whereas they were about 25% of UFA with 10 en% fat and only about 5% of UFA with 20 en% fat. The proportion of triglyceride UFA in the form of n-7 acids was similar for all three tissues, and it was slightly higher in the triglycerides of male rats. Only at the highest level of dietary polyunsaturated fat were appreciable amounts of HUFA accumulated in the plasma and liver triglycerides. The approximate value for 20:5n-3 maintained by 10 en% dietary 18:3n-3 was about 3%, and that for 20:4n-6 maintained by 12 en% dietary 18:2n-6 was about 5%. In contrast, adipose tissue of males and females consistently maintained very low amounts of HUFA in triglycerides with all diets, reaching maximal values of about 1 with diets Fl and Co.

With higher amounts of 18:2n-6 and 18:3n-3 in the diet, the rat tissues maintained progressively higher levels of these acids in triglycerides (Figure 3-3). The linear trend was similar for plasma, liver, and adipose, (with no significant difference between males and females) and fit the following equations.

$$\text{Triglyceride wt\% 18:2n-6} = 3.2 \times \text{dietary en\% 18:2n-6} \quad [1a]$$

$$\text{Triglyceride wt\% 18:3n-3} = 1.8 \times \text{dietary en\% 18:3n-3} \quad [1b]$$

These consistent linear trends for the maintenance levels of 18:2n-6 and 18:3n-6 in triglycerides appeared to be independent of the amounts of other fatty acids in the diets or the proportion of total calories as fat.

Fatty Acid Composition of Phospholipids

The general pattern of fatty acids was similar for the phospholipids of plasma (Figure 3-4), liver, and erythrocytes, and the values for males and females were also similar; averaging approximately 42% SFA, 32% UFA and 25% HUFA. The HUFA were less abundant in the phospholipids of plasma (20%) than in red cells (28%) or liver (31%). Greater amounts of UFA in plasma phospholipids accompanied the lower HUFA, maintaining the customary balance of nearly equal amounts of total saturated and unsaturated fatty acids that occur with the two esterified hydroxyls of phosphoglycerides.

Rather than fitting a linear relationship with dietary precursors as seen for 18:2n-6 and 18:3n-3 in tissue triglycerides, the amounts of n-3 and n-6 HUFA that were maintained in phospholipids fit a competitive hyperbolic realtionship to the dietary supply of precursors.

$$Response = \frac{V_{max}}{1 + \dfrac{K_s}{en\%S}\left(1 + \dfrac{en\%I}{K_i}\right)} \quad [2]$$

Trial and error fitting of the data to Equation 2 indicated that very small amounts of dietary fatty acid (ca 0.1 en%) permitted the hyperbolic equation to fit the observed results. Further trial and error fitting of these data led us to add a term, C_o, to describe the influence of other dietary fatty acids upon the resultant tissue HUFA contents. Also, another term, K_s, was added to modify the shape of the hyperbola to better fit the observed shape. With these modifications, we used the three forms of Equation 3 to examine the degree to which dietary n-3 and n-6 nutrients could predict the observed fatty acid compositions. In these equations C_3, C_6 and C_o function analogous to Km or Ki values for n-3, n-6, and other types of dietary fatty acids, whereas the dimensionless constant, K, in equation 3c is a selected value of the ratio of [C_9/en%9] that fits the equation to 20:3n-9 in the tissue. The fitted value of K was 0.2 for plasma and 0.3 for erythrocytes of males and females; whereas for liver phospholipids, it was 0.4 for males and 0.5 for females.

$$n\text{-}3 \ as \ \%HUFA = \frac{100}{1+\dfrac{C_3}{en\%_3} \quad 1+\dfrac{en\%_6}{C_6} + \dfrac{en\%_0}{C_0} + \dfrac{en\%_3}{K_s}} \quad [3a]$$

$$n\text{-}6 \ as \ \%HUFA = \frac{100}{1+\dfrac{C_6}{en\%_6} \quad 1+\dfrac{en\%_3}{C_3} + \dfrac{en\%_0}{C_0} + \dfrac{en\%_6}{K_s}} \quad [3b]$$

$$n\text{-}9 \ as \ \%HUFA = \frac{100}{1+K \quad 1+\dfrac{en\%_3}{C_3} + \dfrac{en\%_6}{C_6}} \quad [3c]$$

The ability of Equation 3 to fit the wide range of observed compositions of n-3, n-6 and n-9 among the HUFA of tissue phospholipids is illustrated in Figures 3-4, 3-5 and 3-6. For each tissue, a single set of values for the constants was selected which permitted the appropriate version of Equation 3 to fit the compositions of the n-9, n-6 or n-3 HUFA which were observed for that tissue. Figure 3-4A illustrates that as the total amount of dietary polyunsaturated fatty acid increased, the amount of 20:3n-9 maintained in plasma phospholipid HUFA decreased similarly for males and females (closed and open diamonds, respectively). The decrease was quantitatively fitted by Equation 3 (closed squares) using the values for C_6, C_3, C_o and K_s shown in panel 3-4B. These values were selected by trial and error to permit the hyperbolic equation to also fit the patterns observed for the n-6 acids (20:3 plus 20:4, Figure 3-4B) and the n-3 acids (20:5 plus 22:5, Figure 3-4C) in liver phospholipids of males and females. Differences among the metabolic selectivities of the three tissues in maintaining their tissue-specific patterns of fatty acids are reflected in the differences in the values for the constants

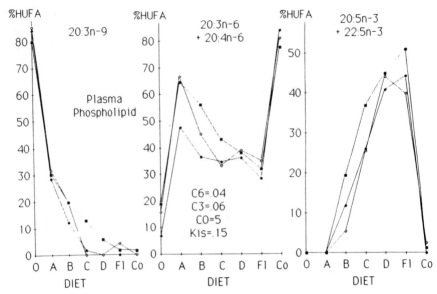

Fig. 3-4. Highly Unsaturated Fatty Acids Maintained in Phospholipids of Rat Plasma. Curves represent values for males (filled diamonds), females (open diamonds) and those predicted by the equation (filled squares) using the constants shown in B. (A) 20:3n-9 in HUFA, (B) 20:3n-6 plus 20:4n-6 in HUFA and (C) 20-5n-3 plus 22:5n-3 in HUFA.

TABLE 3-2
Summary of Fitted Constants

Component	C_6 (en%)	C_3 (en%)	C_0 (en%)	K_s (en%)	K
Liver	0.05	0.10	2.00	0.30	0.40[a]
Plasma	0.04	0.06	5.00	0.15	0.20
RBC	0.02	0.05	5.00	0.10	0.30
Average	0.036	0.07	4.00	0.18	0.30

[a]A value of 0.50 fitted results for female rats.

selected to fit the data. These differences are summarized in Table 3-2. The average values for C_6 and C_3 are less than 0.1% of the dietary calories, whereas the value for C_0 is greater than 1%.

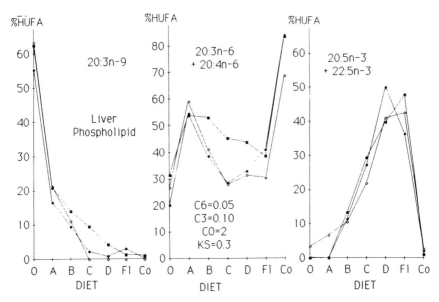

Fig. 3-5. Highly Unsaturated Fatty Acids Maintained in Phospholipids of Rat Liver. Curves represent values as described in Fig. 3-4.

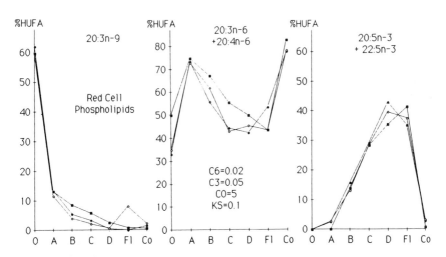

Fig. 3-6. Highly Unsaturated Fatty Acids Maintained in Phospholipids of Rat Red Blood Cells.
Curves represent values described in Fig. 3-4.

General Categories of Fatty Acids

To interpret the data in this study, we employed a hypothesis that the general metabolic properties of fatty acids could be a useful means of grouping the many different varied fatty acids that are esterified in tissue lipids. With this priority system, the categories were initially defined according to the general selectivity of the enzymes that catalyse the formation of ester bonds (SFA, UFA and HUFA) rather than to define them to some consequent physical property of the product or some eventual physiological consequence that might occur subsequently. As a result, the recognized difference between the n-3 and n-6 HUFA in the formation and function of eicosanoids (12,14) was subordinated to the finding of little *in vitro* evidence for differences of esterification selectivity between these two types of acid (15). The relative lack of evidence for any unique specificity for esterification of any of the different types of fatty acids (n-3, n-6, n-7, n-9) does not diminish the importance of the physiological consequences of their subsequent metabolism. Rather, it helps emphasize the vital importance of the initial selection of the proportions of the acids as nutritients. Once dietary selections are made, the tissue fatty acid composition tends to be defined by competitive metabolism, and the resulting physiological consequences tend to become more inescapable.

Competitive metabolic interactions among the n-3, n-6 and n-9 types of fatty acids in maintaining tissue HUFA compositions have been recognized for a long time (5,10). By describing the amounts of the different individual HUFA as a percentage of the total HUFA pool in a given tissue, the present report provides a single general algebraic relationship (e.g. Equation 3b) that quantitatively estimates the magnitude of those competitive interactions. The assignment of a single set of constants to describe the maintenance of n-3, n-6, and n-9 HUFA in each tissue also provides a way to help define tissue-specific differences. The observed similarities of these constants among different tissues probably indicates that the competitive interactions among HUFA are fairly similar in the different tissues even though the total amount of HUFA in a specific type of lipid being examined may differ appreciably among tissues. This report provides comparisons among the different fatty acids (and among different tissues) so that subsequent studies can use the quantitative steady-state information base to interpret the kinetics of tissue response to dietary changes.

A recent discussion of the fatty acid composition in human plasma lipids (3) emphasized the similarity of fatty acid compositions of plasma and adipose lipids reported for individuals from all over the world. This similarity was discussed in terms of possible similar suppplies of fatty acids in the diet of the individuals tested. In the present report, the fatty acid compositions of plasma lipids from rats can be recognized to be very similar to the world-wide averages reported for humans (3), with endogenous fatty acids (16:0, 18:0, 16:1, 18:1) constituting the majority of fatty acids in the lipids of plasma (16) and adipose (17) and with similar proportions of SFA, UFA and HUFA for rats and humans. Wide variations in the fatty acid composition of the diet were created in the present study of rats, and still the relative proportions of the endogenous fatty acids maintained in plasma and adipose lipids remained similar. The similarity of the results with rats and humans suggested that a useful alternative interpretation of the similar world-wide compositions in humans would be that (for individuals from all over the world) similar proportions of endogenous fatty acids are supplied from carbohydrate and amino acid precursors by the fatty acid synthetic system. The major dietary source of the acetate for the biosynthesis of these acids would be carbohydrates (50 to 75% of dietary calories), which may provide relatively similar proportions of endogenous fatty acids to the esterifying enzymes that synthesize the plasma and adipose lipids. In this way, similar compositions for rats and humans reflect similar general selectivities in the formation and esterification of endogenous fatty acids.

Marginal Supplies of Essential Fatty Acids

Each set of animals in this study was provided a single diet throughout the lifetime of the experiment. To ensure minimum confounding variables, the mothers of the experiment animals also were maintained on the same diet for several months prior to conception. This protocol minimized the kinetics of altered dietary compositions (which are so common with human studies) and minimized also the impact of the maternal n-6 and n-3 fatty acids that are supplied to the animals prior to delivery and weaning. Preliminary experiments produced barely discernable symptoms of essential fatty acid deficiency only after prolonged feeding of the fat-deficient diet that contained 70 percent of calories as sucrose. Diets that contained appreciable starch (with ca. 0.4 en% 18:2n-6) apparently provided the very small amounts (ca. 0.2 en%) of needed 18:2n-6. Although we had expected to see physiological signs of a deficiency of essential fatty acids with several of the diets in this study, the older literature (4,5) provides clear evidence of asymptomatic animals when they obtained at least 0.3 percent of dietary calories as

18:2n-6. Growth curves for rats with limited nutrient supply of essential fatty acids showed a hyperbolic response to dietary polyunsaturated fatty acid with a half-maximal stimulation in the range of about 0.1 percent of dietary calories as 18:2n-6 (4,5). Marginal growth conditions for rats with limited 18:2n-6 (0.2 en%) were associated with the maintenance of nearly equal amounts of 20:3n-9 and 20:4n-6 in liver lipids (4,5). Similar metabolic interactions of HUFA also occurred in humans for whom dietary 18:2n-6 at 0.5 en% produced no deficiency symptoms while maintaining plasma 20:3n-9/20:4n-6 ratios near 1 (18). In contrast, lower dietary 18:2n-6 (0.07 en%) that produced deficiency symptoms in about one-half of the babies studied maintained the plasma 20:3n-9/20:4n-6 ratios near 1.4 (19). Both results on 20:3n-9/20:4n-6 ratios and on the midpoint amount needed for growth indicate again that the general metabolic characteristics of the metabolism of HUFA and glycerolipid are similar in rats and humans. The concept that the principal role of the essential n-6 dietary acid is in maintaining an adequate amount of 20:4n-6 in tissues to serve as precursor for eicosanoid biosynthesis is supported by the similar hyperbolic response to dietary 18:2n-6 of growth and tissue 20:4n-6 of Mohrhauer and Holman (4) as discussed by Lands (20). Apparently, when adequate levels of 20:4n-6 are not maintained, adequate physiology is not maintained. Further support for this concept comes from the ability of Equation 3 to predict thrombotic occlusion times (21 as discussed in ref. 20) thromboxane formation by platelets (22,23; as discussed in ref. 20), and tumor proliferation (24; as discussed in ref. 20). The hyperbolic relationship of these physiologic events to the amounts of dietary n-3 and n-6 precursors suggests that the percent of tissue HUFA as n-6 fatty acid may be a useful index of the capacity of the tissue to form eicosanoids when stimulated.

Dietary Fat and Endogenous n-7 and n-9 Acids

The decrease in the amount of n-7 fatty acids (as a percentage of UFA) maintained in tissue lipids in response to increased fat in the diet provides a metabolic indicator of the relatively decreased influx of dietary carbohydrate which accompanied the increase in dietary lipid. Therefore, analyses of n-7 acids in plasma lipid fractions might be helpful in assessing the relative proportions of daily calories ingested as fat and carbohydrate. However, the results in this study indicate that the useful range for such an assay would most likely be with fat comprising from 0 to 20% of the daily calories. In this range, the n-7 acids as %UFA in plasma phospholipids may have the following approximate relationship to dietary fat:

$$n\text{-}7 \text{ as } \%PL\text{-}UFA = \frac{100}{1 + 1.5(1+en\%fat/5)} \qquad [4]$$

This relationship predicts that the plasma phospholipid would maintain about 40, 18, 12, 9, and 7 percent of the UFA as n-7 acids when the diets contained 0, 10, 20, 30 and 40 en% fat, respectively. Consequently, gas chromatographic analyses of the n-7 acids in plasma phospholipids would be expected to give low values that are difficult to interpret when the fat content of the diet exceeds 20% of total calories. Nevertheless, this analytical approach to estimating the percent of fat calories might be useful in estimating the compliance in dietary studies with relatively low-fat diets. Evidence that this relationship may occur in humans is found in a recent report of malabsorption (25).

The amount of 20:3n-9 (as a percentage of the HUFA) that was maintained in tissue lipids decreased in a hyperbolic response to increased polyunsaturated fat in the diet. The quantitative nature of the response confirms the results of Mohrhauer and Holman (4,5) as discussed elsewhere (20). The low value of 0.2 for K in equation 3c fits higher proportions of 20:3n-9 in plasma HUFA and indicates a corresponding lower competitive effect of the dietary en% of n-3 and n-6 fatty acids than seen with liver (i.e., K = 0.5 for females). Similarly, the value of 0.4 for K in male liver indicates a greater tendency for the n-9 derivatives to predominate in males than in females. Such a comparative difference was reported for liver phospholipids following fasting and refeeding, with a stronger entry of 18:1n-9 into the liver lecithins of males than females (26).

Synthesis, Transport and Storage of Triglycerides

Movement of fatty acids from adipose to liver triglycerides occurs rapidly via plasma NEFA (Figure 3-7), and the return flow is provided by plasma triglycerides secreted by the liver (which are then converted to plasma NEFA by lipoprotein lipase). When dietary fatty acid compositions differ greatly from that of adipose tissue, the liver would be presented with different supplies of fatty acids throughout the day as the NEFA derived from intermittent eating blends with the continual supply of plasma NEFA from adipose. The corresponding continual export of triglycerides from the liver maintains a supply of plasma triglyceride

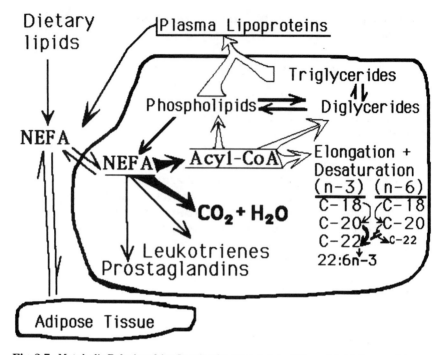

Fig. 3-7. Metabolic Relationships Involved in Maintaining Tissue Lipid Compositions.

fatty acids that will mix intermittently with dietary supplies (depending on the amount of fat in the diet) and provide a blend of fatty acids for incorporation into adipose tissue triglycerides. In the experimental protocol of this study, the tissues were given optimal opportunity to reach steady state by keeping the composition of the dietary influx relatively constant throughout the lifetime of the rats. This protocol avoided the large dietary variations commonly encountered in human nutrition, and it permitted comparisons of fatty acid composition which illustrate the basic relationships between the fatty acids of diet and tissue. The close similarities of the fatty acid composition of plasma, liver and adipose triglycerides illustrate the close metabolic interactions of these three triglyceride pools.

Recent studies (27) of the oxidation of 18:2 and 18:3 by liver mitochondria provide an explanation for the two-fold greater entry into triglycerides by 18:2n-6 compared to 18:3n-3. As the dietary polyunsaturated fatty acids enter the cell in the form of non-esterfied fatty acids

(NEFA) (see Figure 3-7) the mitochondria may convert the 18:3n-3 to acid-soluble products and CO_2 at a rate twice that for 18:2n-6 (27). This selective removal of 18:3n-3 could cause the two-fold difference in slopes noted between Figures 3-1A and 3-1B by maintaining the 18:3/18:2 ratio at one-half that provided by the diet. The overall *in vivo* selectivity in this study fits results reported for NEFA rather than the coenzyme A esters (27), and it supports the concept of a coupled action of the lipase and transferase rather than a transfer of acids for oxidative metabolism from a general pool of cellular acyl-coenzyme A esters.

Maintenance of HUFA in Phospholipids:

The general metabolic selectivities for forming rat plasma phospholipids produced a composition of about 43% SFA, 36% UFA and 20% HUFA. It seems likely that similar metabolic selectivities may also prevail in humans who have about 42% SFA, 35% UFA and 20% HUFA (calculated from data of Holman (16) and Nikkari (28)). The experimental diets in this study provided over a hundred-fold range of n-3/n-6 ratios (from 0.02 to 2.74), and the ratios for HUFA in tissue phospholipid were similar to the relative abundances of the n-3/n-6 nutrients. This similarity supports an earlier suggestion (3) that the elongation of 18-carbon n-3 and n-6 fatty acids to 20-carbon derivatives may occur with no appreciable discrimination between the two types of fatty acids.

Plasma phospholipids are primarily formed and secreted by the liver, and some selectivity in the secretion process has been reported. For example, humans, rats, dogs and oxen were all shown to maintain somewhat less stearate and arachidonate in biliary lecithin compared to plasma lecithin (29,30). Apparently, the liver may have either functionally distinct pools of lecithin or it may engage in selective secretion from a single heterogeneous pool. The lower total HUFA in phospholipids of rat plasma (ca. 20%) compared to that in liver (ca. 30%) noted in the present study also reflects a selective secretion into plasma. In this case, it was less highly unsaturated lipids than the average liver phospholipid. This difference is reflected by the differences among the fitted constants for liver and plasma in Table 3-2.

Examining the relative proportions of the n-3 HUFA provided useful insight to the metabolic selectivities. The weight percent of 22:6n-3 in plasma phospholipids was maintained at a higher average level with diets B and C than with D and F, even though the latter diets contained even greater nutrient supplies of 18:3n-3. The greater influx of 18:3n-3 from the diet may permit tissues to more rapidly synthesize 20:5 and

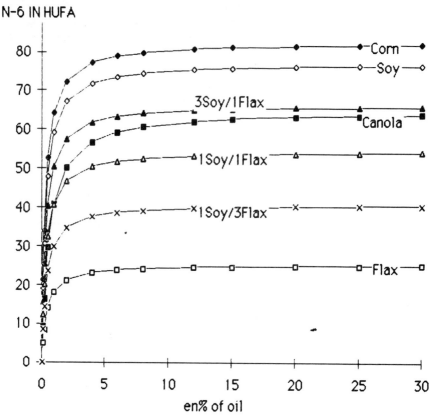

Fig. 3-8. The Effects of Food Oils.
The values for n-6 in the HUFA of phospholipids, which may relate to the capacity for biosynthesis of n-6 eicosanoids, was predicted using Equation 3b and the known compositions of the indicated dietary oils.

22:5 in amounts that could suppress the esterification of 22:6n-3 by competitive interactions. Alternatively, greater amounts of available n-3 precursor may suppress the putative Δ4 desaturase activity. Whatever the mechanism, it is important to recognize that 22:6n-3 does not respond to dietary precursors in the way that 20:5n-3 and 22:5n-3 do. The vigorous retention of 22:6n-3 when there is limited supply of n-3 precursors creates a problem in studying selective effects of dietary polyunsaturated fats on tissue HUFA. For example, our results confirm and extend the report by Iritani and Fujikawa (31) of a relatively constant sum of "polyunsaturated fatty acids with more than three double bonds" (i.e., HUFA) in phospholipids of plasma (18-20%) and liver (31-35%). However, their results were biased by the protocol of feeding for only 2 weeks, which was not long enough to develop a steady-state maintenance level for 22:6n-3. This was evident in the high values for this acid (ca. 27% of HUFA) in liver phospholipid even when no n-3 acid was in the diet for two weeks. Eight weeks on the n-3 deficient diet led to 6.7% of HUFA (31), closer to our result of about 3% following 20 weeks of the diet.

An earlier analysis (3) of the extensive data provided by Mohrhauer and Holman (4,5) emphasized that the elongation from 20- to 22-carbon HUFA appeared more facile with n-3 than n-6 acids. The present results extend the insight into factors influencing 22:6n-3 formation, showing that the elongation to 22:5n-3 proceeded with ease, but the step commonly attributed to a $\Delta 4$-desaturase may not be capable of increased flux in response to increased supplies of presursor. The competition did not appear to prevent elongation of 20:5n-3 and 22:5n-3 since both of these acids increased as dietary 18:3n-3 increased. The paradoxically lower tissue contents of 22:6n-3 with increased dietary 18:3n-3 made it difficult to fit Equation 3 to values for this fatty acid. In contrast, the sum of 20:5n-3 plus 22:5n-3 fit the same constants used in the equations to describe the maintenance levels for the n-6 and n-9 acids.

Inhibition by n-3 acids of the conversion of 20:4n-6 to 22 carbon derivatives seemed to permit very little 22-carbon n-6 HUFA being maintained in tissue phospholipids (except with the diets (0,A,Co) that contained very low amounts of 18:3n-3). The combined effects of high levels of dietary fatty acids to make 20:4n-6 the predominant n-6 HUFA results in optimal conversion of dietary 18:2n-6 into the major eicosanoid precursor. This effect may favor more vigorous formation of eicosanoids when a tissue is stimulated.

Applications of the New Information

Three important concepts have evolved from these studies:

1. Algebraic relationships can relate quantitatively the abundance of dietary polyunsaturated fatty acids with the abundance of their products in tissues.

2. The proportion of 20:4n-6 in the HUFA of tissue phospholipids may be a useful index of the capacity of a tissue to produce eicosanoids when stimulated.

3. General selectivities for the metabolism of fatty acids and glycerolipids tend to be similar for rats and humans.

People need a way to interpret the continuing possiblity that when their tissues overproduce eicosanoids, they may develop pathologies with greater frequency and severity. Expressing a high capacity to produce eicosanoids as a function of a high proportion of 20:4n-6 in tissue HUFA brings into focus the ratio of n-3/n-6 polyunsaturated fatty acids in the diet which permits tissues to maintain those high proportions of 20:4n-6 in the tissue HUFA. The very low value estimated for the constant C6 (ca. 0.07en%) that fits Equation 3 to the observed diet-tissue relationships means that the typical diet in the USA is located on the "saturated" portion of the curve (with about 70% n-6 acids in tissue HUFA). As a result, efforts to reduce the proportion of 20:4n-6 as HUFA to below 50% by merely reducing the amount of dietary n-6 acids would require difficult-to-achieve reductions. On the other hand, adding more n-3 fats to the diet might shift the proportions of n-3/n-6 HUFA more

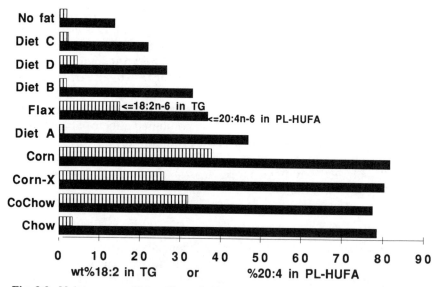

Fig. 3-9. Maintenance of Liver Fatty Acids.
Observed values for 18:2n-6 in liver triglycerides (solid bars) and 20:3n-6 plus 20:4n-6 in the HUFA liver phospholipids (hatched bars) are from this report for the upper seven diets, and from ref. 9 for Corn-X, Corn plus Chow (CoChow) and Chow.

conveniently. Equation 3 permits predictions of the probable n-6 acids in HUFA when we control the n-3/n-6 of dietary polyunsaturated fat by the use of several different food oils (Figure 3-8). The values predicted for soy-based diets fit closely to that seen for plasma phospholipids of typical Americans. Values for Japanese tend to be around 45%, and values for Eskimos tend to be much lower. As we gain understanding of our ability to control the relative content of n-6 in the tissue HUFA, it becomes increasingly important to have also some quantitative measurements of physiological responses to monitor the safety of the changes being produced. Furthermore, we need better physiological indices of which degrees of response are desirable so that we can more wisely choose the eicosanoid synthetic capacity that is desirable rather than merely accepting the one that is accidentally developed as a result of unwitting diet choices.

The term "normal" correctly conveys the statistical sense of being average or typical. However, it often is used to convey also a sense of being desirable (such as normal diets or normal behavior). An obvious concern arises when a typical value or condition is at a maximal state related to some potential risk. Then what is typical may not be desirable and what is desirable may not be typical.

An illustration of normal dietary conditions that produce near maximal conditions is seen with the standard rat chow in the USA. The 18:2n-6 in tissue triglycerides is a useful index of dietary influx of 18:2n-6. The different diets in Figure 3-9 represent a wide range of 18:2n-6 influx, and the diets supplemented with corn oil represent the extreme condition. The capacity for synthesis of n-6 eicosanoids appeared to be maximal under those conditions, in which nearly 80% of the tissue HUFA were n-6 fatty acids. The standard rat chow also fits in that extreme category even though it provides a relatively low influx of 18:2n-6. This result is probably due to little competition for the HUFA pool by the even lower influx of dietary n-3 fatty acids. The Chow diet was clearly at a maximal value of n-6 as HUFA, since adding corn oil to the it (CoChow) did not cause any significantly greater proportion of n-6 HUFA. Lower proportions of the n-6 HUFA occur when rat chow is prepared with fish meal rather than soy meal (noted in ref. 3), and the tissue eicosanoid responses may be correspondingly more moderate. We now need physiologists and clinicians to provide the insight to identify the desirable proportions of 20:4n-6 in tissue HUFA that provide the desirable degree of physiological response.

Acknowledgment

This work was supported in part by a USPHS research grant (HL-34045) and a Pfizer Biomedical Research Award.

References

1. Lands, W.E.M. and Crawford, C.G. (1975) *In: Membrane Bound Enzymes (A. Martinosi, ed.)* New York: Plenum Press, pp. 3-85.
2. Waku, K. and Lands, W.E.M. (1968) *J. Lipid Res. 9*, 12-18.
3. Lands, W.E.M. (1989) *J. Int. Med. 225, Suppl. 1*, 11-20.
4. Mohrhaurer, H. and Holman, R.T. (1963) *J. Lipid Research 4*, 151-159.
5. Mohrhauer, H. and Holman, R.T. (1963) *J. Nutr. 81*, 67-74.
6. Fulco, A.J. and Mead, J.F. (1959) *J. Biol. Chem. 234*, 1411-1416.
7. Klenk, E. and Oette, K. (1960) *Z. Physiol. Chem. 318*, 86-99.
8. Privett, O.S., Blank, M.L. and Romanus, O. (1963) *J. Lipid Res. 4*, 260-265.
9. Prasad, M.R., Culp, B. and Lands, W.E.M. (1987) *J. Biosci. 11*, 443-453.
10. Machlin, L.J. (1962) Nature: p. 868.
11. Bergstrom, S., Danielsson, S., Klenberg, D., and Samuelsson, B. (1964) *J. Biol. Chem. 239*, 4006-4408.
12. Lands, W.E.M., LeTellier, P.R., Rome, L.H., and Vanderhoek, J.Y. (1973) *Adv. in Biosci. 9*, 15-27.
13. Lands, W.E.M. (1986) *Fish and Human Health*. Academic Press, Orlando, FL. pp. 1-186.
14. Needleman, P., Raz, A., Minkes, M., Ferrendelli, J.A., and Sprecher, H. (1979) *Proc. Nat. Acad. Sci. USA 76*, 944-948.
15. Lands, W.E.M., Inoue, M., Sugiura, Y., and Okuyama, H. (1982) *J. Biol. Chem. 257*, 14968-14972.
16. Holman, R.T., Smythe, L., and Johnson, S. (1979) *Am. J. Clin. Nutr. 32*, 2390-2399.
17. Berry, E.M., and Hirsch, J. (1986) *Am. J. Clin. Nutr. 44*, 336-340.
18. Combes, M.A., Pratt, E.L., and Wiese, H.F. (1962) *Pediatrics 30*, 136-144.
19. Hansen, A.E., Wiese, H.F., Boelsche, A.N., Haggard, M.E., Adam, D.J.D., and Davis, H. (1963) *Pediatrics 31*, 171-192.
20. Lands, W.E.M. (1990) *In II International Conference on the Health Effects of Omega 3 Polyunsaturated Fatty Acids in Seafoods* (eds. A. Simopoulos, R.E. Kifer, R.R. Martin and S.E. Barlow) Karges, Basel in press.
21. Hornstra G: *Dietary fats and arterial thrombosis*: Ph.D. thesis. 1980; Univ. Limburg, Maastricht.
22. Hwang, D.H., Boudreau, M., and Chanmugam, P. (1988) *J. Nutr. 118*, 427-437.
23. Hwang, D.H., and Carroll, A.E. (1980) *Am. J. Clin. Nutr. 33*, 590-597.
24. Ip, C., Carter, C.A., and Ip, M.M. (1985) *Cancer Res. 45*, 1997-2001.
25. Siguel, E.N., Chee, K.M., Gong, J., and Schaefer, E.J. (1987) *Clin. Chem. 33*,

33, 1869-1873.
26. Lands, W.E.M., Hart, P. (1966) *J. Am. Oil Chem. Soc. 43*, 290-295.
27. Clouet, P., Niot, I., and Bezard, J. (1989) *Biochem J. 263*, 867-873.
28. Nikkari, T., Salo, M., Maatela, J., and Aromaa, A. (1983) *Atherosclerosis 49*, 139-148.
29. Balint, J.A., Kyriakides, E.C., Spitzer, H.L., and E.S. Morrison (1965) *J. Lipid Res. 6*, 96-99.
30. Balint, J.A., Beeler, D.A., Treble, D.H., and Spitzer, H.L. (1967) *J. Lipid Res. 8*, 486-493.
31. Iritani, N. and Fujikawa, S. (1982) *J. Nutr. Sci. Vitaminol.28*, 621-629.

Chapter Four

Are N-3 Polyunsaturated Fatty Acids Essential for Growth and Development?

Susan E. Carlson, Ph.D.

>The Newborn Center
>Department of Pediatrics and Obstetrics and Gynecology
>853 Jefferson Avenue
>The University of Tennessee
>Memphis, TN 38103

There is little doubt that omega-3 fatty acids are essential for growth and development. The evidence for this statement will be reveiwed briefly in this manuscript and has been reviewed extensively elsewhere (1). Recognition of the importance of n-3 fatty acids in developing mammals logically leads however, to questions about n-3 sufficiency in vulnerable humans, such as the very low birth weight infant. The majority of this article will deal with our current understanding of, and unanswered questions related to, n-3 fatty acids in the developing premature newborn.

It is a truism that all advances in knowledge build upon past discoveries. A number of pioneers in the area of n-3 fatty acid metabolism must be acknowledged: O'Brien et al. (2), Sinclair and Crawford (3) and Anderson and coworkers (4) determined the importance of n-3 fatty acids as structural lipids in neural and retinal phospholipids. Clandinin et al. (5) and Martinez and coworkers (6) have provided information about the normal timing of n-3 and n-6 accumulation during development of the human infant. Sinclair and Crawford (7) demonstrated the importance of preformed 20 and 22 carbon n-6 and n-3 fatty acids in neural accumulation. Galli and coworkers (8) showed that manipulation of the ratio of linoleic and linolenic acid could be employed to create very low levels of membrane docosahexaenoic acid (DHA, 22:6n-3). And finally, Lamptey and Walker (9), Benolken et al. (10), and Wheeler and coworkers (11) first demonstrated the functional importance of n-3 fatty acids in learning and retinal physiology, respectively.

More recently, Connor, Neuringer and their coworkers and Yamamoto and coworkers have expanded upon these biochemical and functional studies with more sophisticated techniques in the rhesus monkey and rat. Uauy and coworkers and Carlson et al. have borrowed these techniques and others for studies of premature human infants. Innis and coworkers (12) have contributed valuable data using the suckling newborn pig as a model for the effects of diet upon accumulation of n-6 and n-3 fatty acids in the brain and retina.

Functional Effects Associated With n-3 Deficiency

Studies of n-3 deficiency in developing animals have employed dietary fats with high ratios of linoleic (n-6) to linolenic (n-3) acid. In n-3 deficiency, DHA, the predominant neural and retinal n-3 fatty acid is replaced by docosapentaenoate (DPA, 22:5n-6) in an essentially equimolar fashion. Rats fed n-3 deficient diets for several generations have been employed for studies of discriminant learning (9, 13-15) and retinal physiology (14), while rhesus monkeys have been used to study both visual acuity and retinal physiology (16,17).

Lamptey and Walker (9) first reported poorer discriminant learning in n-3 deficient rats compared to controls fed a good source of linolenic acid (soybean oil). This was confirmed more than 10 years later by Yamamoto and coworkers (13,14) who determined the number of trials required by rats to learn that food pellets were available only at a specific light intensity. Almost twice as many trials were required by n-3 deficient rats compared to controls. In yet another study of exploratory behavior, learning time was also increased in n-3 deficient rats (15).

The rat was also the first species in which retinal physiology was studied in response to depletion and repletion of n-3 and n-6 fatty acids (10,11). Retinal function can be estimated by its electro-physiological response to light. Benolken et al. (10) and Wheeler and coworkers (11) found that diets deficient in n-6 and n-3 fatty acids reduced the electroretinogram a-wave and that linolenic compared to linoleic acid was more effective in improving the a-wave response after depletion. More recently, reductions in both a- and b-wave amplitudes were reported in rodents depleted by feeding a high linoleic to linolenic acid ratio (14). Other investigators have not found a- and b-wave changes with n-3 deficiency (18,19) perhaps due to differences in stimulus duration, interval or intensity.

Neuringer, Connor and coworkers have studied n-3 deficiency in the rhesus monkey. As in rodent studies, n-3 deficiency was produced by feeding fats with low concentrations of linolenic compared to linoleic acid during pregnancy. Unlike rodent studies, only first generation, n-3 deficient infant monkeys have been studied. Monkey infants were born with about half the amount of DHA in neural phospholipids as the n-3 sufficient controls (16). Retinal DHA was also much lower than in controls. Generally, infants were continued on an n-3 deficient diet following delivery. Electroretinogram peak latencies were observed in both retinal rods and cones, and the time required for retinal recovery of the dark adapted retina of n-3 deficient infants was increased (17). Peak latencies and increased recovery times continued to occur even after the DHA content of the membranes was repleted with marine oil (20, 21) evidence for a critical epoch of DHA accumulation in the retina. After normal intrauterine accretion of n-3, monkey infants produced similar latencies in electro-retinogram recovery times (22) although at birth the retina of monkeys is more mature than that of term human infants.

In addition to differences in retinal physiology, Neuringer et al. (16) have reported delayed visual acuity development in n-3 deficient monkey infants using the forced-choice-preferential-looking technique to measure visual acuity. The mechanism by which DHA functions in visual acuity and learning is not well understood. A recent review discusses some of the possible functions of DHA at the cellular level (1).

N-3 Fatty Acids and the Developing Premature Infant

Very Long Chain n-3 and n-6 Fatty Acids Following Birth

Following premature birth, both DHA and AA decline in red blood cell phospholipids of infants nourished intravenously or with standard infant formulas (23, 24). In our studies, we have found only 2 factors which predict red blood cell DHA following premature birth: postnatal age ($r2 = 0.239$, $p < 0.0001$) and birth order ($r2 = 0.12$, $p < 0.005$)(25). Both negatively affect phospholipid DHA suggesting that DHA accumulated via new synthesis does not keep up with that supplied to the infant in utero, and that repeated pregnancies adversely affect infants' DHA status. Human milk contains both arachidonic (AA) and docosahexaenoic (DHA) acids, and human milk-fed infants have higher concentrations of both in red blood cell phospholipids compared to infants fed formula (23, 26, 27).

Is Exogenous DHA Important for the Preterm Infant?

Are DHA and AA conditionally essential nutrients for preterm infants? In order to answer this question, phospholipid DHA and AA must be maintained in a standard range for a defined period of time during development. For DHA, we have arbitrarily defined a range intermediate between that which we find in the last intrauterine trimester and in the human-milk-fed term infant. In our studies, we have provided dietary DHA but not AA for several scientific and practical reasons: 1.) Physiological declines in red blood cell (28), neural and hepatic (29) phospholipid AA, but not DHA occur during the last intrauterine trimester. 2.) Compared to human-milk-fed infants, those fed formula have larger reductions in red blood cell phospholipid DHA than AA (23,30). 3.) The red blood cell DHA reflects neural accumulation in developing animals (31,32), but the same does not appear to be true of AA (32). 4.) The retinal and neural accumulation of DHA and AA in the last intrauterine trimester suggests a greater need for DHA than AA accumulation (5,33). 5.) Animal studies have targeted failure to accumulate neural and retinal DHA but not AA as a risk factor for poorer visual acuity, retinal function and discriminant learning. Finally, 6.) marine sources have been available to provide DHA, but good alternatives for AA supplementation have not been available with which to test the hypothesis that poor AA accumulation limits development in some preterm infants.

Declines in red blood cell and plasma DHA can be prevented with very small amounts of dietary marine oil (24,34). When marine oil is microdispersed in formula, even smaller amounts are required to maintain red blood cell phospholipids in a range intermediate between phospholipids of human-milk-fed term infants and cord blood (30,34). Preterm infants have been fed formula with or without marine oil. Visual acuity measured by the Teller Acuity Card procedure (Vistech Consultants, Inc., Dayton, OH) was enhanced by n-3 supplementation in the first 6 mos of infancy (35,36). Uauy and coworkers (37) have reported poorer early electroretinogram responses in preterm infants receiving high ratios of linoleic to linolenic acid compared to infants fed human milk, marine oil-containing formula or a low ratio of linoleic to linolenic acid. At 57 wks postconception, these electroretinogram differences were no longer apparent, but the visual evoked potential (VEP) acuity was significantly better in those who had received dietary DHA (either human milk and/or a marine oil-containing formula (38).

Speculation About the Importance of Endogenous DHA and AA

Although preterm infants apparently have a limited ability to synthesize adequate amounts of DHA to support normal retinal development in the first half of infancy, they clearly make DHA: Plasma DHA does not fall as low in these infants (25) as in monkeys fed very low levels of linolenic acid (16). That some preterm infants have more endogenous DHA in infancy is also clear from the wide range of DHA found in plasma phospholipids of preterm infants receiving the same formula without either DHA or AA (25). Whether or not these differences in endogenous n-6 and n-3 fatty acids are due to differences in synthesis is not clear, but this is a very real possibility since plasma DHA is highly related to membrane (red blood cell) DHA throughout infancy in these babies (unpublished results). Higher endogenous DHA was associated with better acuity since among infants who did not receive DHA there was a positive relationship between red blood cell DHA and acuity (36). In addition, red blood cell phospholipid DHA entered in the multiple regression analysis as a continuous variable correlated better with acuity than did the type of formula (n-3 supplemented or control) even though the type of formula was the best predictor of red blood cell phospholipid DHA (35). These observations suggest that both endogenous and exogenous DHA positively influence acuity in the first half of infancy.

Recently we have observed that endogenous DHA and AA are highly correlated in individual infants, although the quantity of each in plasma phospholipids varies 3-4 fold within each dietary group (39). These data are further support for the suggestion that preterm infants have a highly variable ability to elongate and desturate 18 carbon PUFA. This ability is significantly and positively correlated with both growth and performance on early measures of cognitive performance. The quantity of plasma phospholipid AA was significantly related to growth and to performance on early cognitive tests (the Fagan Infantest, Cleveland, OH and the Bayley Mental and Psychomotor Developmental Indices) (39,40).

While our initial analysis of the data suggest that the ability to elongate and desaturate 18 carbon PUFA may be a marker for some other variable which directly impacts upon growth and cognition in infancy, it is not possible to rule out AA as the ultimate compound of importance without further prospective study. In the meantime, the appropriateness of fish oil as a source of preformed DHA for premature infants needs to be evaluated since marine oil-supplemented formula has a significant negative effect upon plasma AA in individual infants, even though DHA and AA are highly correlated in supplemented infants as a group.

In summary, premature infants appear to be at risk for too little accumulation of both DHA (n-3) and AA (n-6) during the first half of infancy. Poorer accumulation of DHA correlates with less than optimal development of visual acuity by two independent measures at 57 wks postconception 35,36,38). Furthermore, since dietary DHA has been provided and phospholipid DHA has been determined in individual control and supplemented infants, it has been possible to observe positive, independent effects of both exogenous and endogenous DHA on acuity.

On the other hand, AA accumulation in control infants correlated positively with more desirable growth and performance on early tests of cognition. Since exogenous AA was not provided it has not been possible to distinguish between a direct effect of endogenous AA on these outcomes in contrast to an indirect one in which AA is a marker for some other critical variable. The fact that marine oil-supplementation negatively affected endogenous AA without appearing to affect growth or development is strong suggestive evidence that another variable is involved.

Only prospective studies of AA supplementation, with analysis of phospholipid AA, growth and cognition following the model of DHA supplementation-function studies, will determine if AA is a limiting factor for optimal growth and development in some preterm infants. In the meantime, since marine oil does have a direct effect on endogenous AA, the possibility remains that marine oil feeding may increase risk of poor growth and development outcomes in that group of infants with the poorest ability to elongate and desaturate 18 carbon PUFA. Until the actual role of AA is determined it is not appropriate to supplement preterm infants with any DHA-containing formula which significantly reduces plasma and red blood cell AA. Likewise, a strong argument could be made against supplementation of preterm infants with AA pending randomized, controlled trials which measure functional outcomes as there is a real danger of masking marginal deficiencies of some other nutrient(s) which may mask poor growth and developmental outcomes in some of these infants.

References

1. Salem, Jr., N., In New Protective Roles for Selected Nutrients, Current Topics in Nutrition and Disease (eds. Spillar, G.A. and Scala, J., New York, Alan R. Liss, Inc., 1989, vol. 22, pp. 188-190.
2. O'Brien, J.S., Fillerup, D.L., and Mean, J.F. (1964) J. Lipid Res. 5, 329-330.
3. Sinclair, A.J. and Crawford, M.S. (1972) J. Neurochem. 19, 1753-1758.
4. Anderson, R.E., Maude, M.B., and Zimmerman, W. (1975) Vision Res. 15, 1087-1090.
5. Clandinin, M.T., Chappell, J.E., Leong, S., et al. (1980) Early Hum. Dev. 4,

121-129.
6. Martinez, M. et al. (1990) Proceedings of the II International Conference on the Health Effects of Omega-3 Polyunsaturated Fatty Acids in Seafoods, Washington, D.C. (in press).
7. Sinclair, A.J., and Crawford, M.A. (1972) FEBS Lett. 26, 127-129.
8. Galli, C., Trzeciak, H.I., and Paoletti, R. (1971) Biochim. Biophys. Acta 248, 449-454.
9. Lamptey, M.S., and Walker, B.L. (1976) J. Nutr. 106, 86-93.
10. Benolken, R.M., Anderson, R.E., and Wheeler, T.G. (1973) Science 182, 1253-1254.
11. Wheeler, T.G., Benolken, R.M., and Anderson, R.E. (1975) Science 188, 1312-1314.
12. Hrboticky, N., MacKinnon, M.J., and Innis, S.M. (1990) Am. J. Clin. Nutr. 51, 173-182.
13. Yamamoto, N., Saitoh, M., Moriuchi, A., et al. (1987) J. Lipid Res. 28, 144-151.
14. Okuyama, H., Saitoh, M., Naito, Y. et al. (1987) Proceedings of the AOCS Short Course on Polyunsaturated Fatty Acids and Eicosanoids. Champaign, IL, American Oil Chemists Society, pp 296-300.
15. Enslen, M., Nouvelot, A., and Milon, H. (1987) Ibid., pp 495-497.
16. Neuringer, M., Connor, W.E., Van Petten, C., et al. (1984) J. Clin. Invest. 73, 272-276.
17. Neuringer, M., Connor, W.E., and Luck, S.L. (1985) Am. J. Clin. Nutr. 43, 706.
18. Cho, E.S., Kolder, H.E., Wertz, P.E., et al. (1985) XIII International Congress of Nutrition, Brighton, US, p. 104.
19. Leat, W.M.F., Curtis, R., Millichamp, N.J., et al. (1986) Ann. Nutr. Metab. 30, 166-174.
20. Connor, W.E., Neuringer, M., and Lin, D. (1985) Clin. Res. 33, 598A.
21. Neuringer, M., Connor, W.E., Luck, S.J. (1985) Invest. Ophthalmol. Vis. Sci. 26 (suppl. 3), 31.
22. Neuringer, M., Connor, W.E., Daigle, D., et al. (1988) Invest. Ophthalmol. vis. Sci. 29 (suppl. 3), 145.
23. Carlson, S.E., Rhodes, P.G., Ferguson, M.G. (1986) Docosahexaenoic acid status of preterm infants at birth and following feeding with human milk or formula. Am. J. Clin. Nutr. 44, 798-804.
24. Carlson, S.E., Rhodes, P.G., Rao, V.S., and Goldgar, D.E. (1987) Ped. Res. 21, 507-510.
25. Carlson, S.E., and Salem, Jr., N. (1990) in Proceedings of the II International Conference on the Health Effects of Omega 3 Polyunsaturated Fatty Acids in Seafoods (eds. Simopoulos, A.P., Bradlow, S., Kifer, R.R. and Martin, R.E.) Basel, Karger Press (in press).
26. Sanders, T.A.B. and Naismith, D.J. (1979) Br. J. Nutr. 41, 619-623.
27. Putnam, J.C., Carlson, S.E., Devoe, P.W., and Barness, L.A. (1982) Am. J.

Clin. Nutr. 36, 106-114.
28. Carlson, S.E. (1990) In Neonatal and Fetal Medicine: Physiology and Pathophysiology (eds. Fox, W.W. and Polin, R.A.) Philadelphia, W.B. Sanders (in press).
29. Martinez, M., and Ballabriga, A. (1987) Lipids 22, 133-138.
30. Peeples, J., Carlson, S., Cooke, R., and Werkman, S. (1989) FASEB Journal 3, A1056.
31. Carlson, S.E., Carver, J.D., and House, S.G.(1986) J. Nutr. 16, 718-725.
32. Hrboticky, N., MacKinnon, M.J., and Innis, S.M. (1990) Am. J. Clin. Nutr. 51, 173-182.
33. Martinez, M., Ballabriga, A., and Gil-Gibernou, J.J. (1988) Neurosci. Res. 20, 484-490.
34. Liu, C-C. F., Carlson, S.E., Rhodes, P.G., Rao, V.S., and Meydrech, E.F. (1987) Ped. Res. 22, 292-296.
35. Carlson, S., Cooke, R., Werkman, S., and Peeples, J. (1989) FASEB Journal 3, A1056.
36. Carlson, S.E., Cooke, R.J., Peeples, J.M., Werkman, S.H., and Tolley, E.A. (1989) Ped. Res. 25, 285A.
37. Uauy, R., Birch, D., Birch, E., and Tyson, J. (1989) FASEB Journal 3, A1247.
38. Uauy, R., Birch, D., Birch, E., and Hoffman, D.R. (1990) in the Proceedings of the II International Conference on the Health Effects of Omega-3 Polyunsaturated Fatty Acids in Seafoods (eds. Simopoulos, A.P., Bradlow, S., Kifer, R.R., and Martin, R.E.), Basel: Karger Press (in press).
39. Carlson, S.E. (1990) In "Effects of diet on metabolism of lipids and polyunsaturated fatty acids," eds. Koletzko, B. and van Biervliet, J.M., in Recent Advances in Infant Feeding, Stuttgart, Thieme Verlag, in press.
40. Carlson S.E., Werkman, S.H., Peeples, J.M., Cooke, R.J., and Tolley, E.A. (1990) Proceedings of the II International Conference on the Health Effects of Omega-3 Polyunsaturated Fatty Acids in Seafoods, Basel, Karger Press (in press).

Chapter Five

Dietary Fatty Acids, Serum Cholesterol and Coronary Heart Disease

D. M. Hegsted

New England Regional Primate Research Center
Harvard Medical School
Southboro, MA 01772

We need not spend much time on the relationship between serum cholesterol and coronary heart disease (CHD) since it is generally accepted that an elevated serum cholesterol is an important risk factor of CHD. Probably the most convincing evidence came from the Framingham study. After a very few years they could identify 3 important factors related to heart attacks—serum cholesterol level, blood pressure, and an abnormal ECG. The "risk factors" appeared to be additive. The relationship of serum cholesterol and blood pressure were continous, i.e. each increase was associated with some increase in risk. It is important to note that a clear cut case for these risk factors became apparent long before the effects of smoking, obesity, lack of exercise, etc. The importance of serum cholesterol levels has been strengthened over the years of this study (Table 5-1) (1).

It had long been known, of course, that very high serum cholesterol levels were associated with atherosclerosis; that you could produce

TABLE 5-1

CHD Incidence in Framingham Men 10 and 20 Years After Examination Three by Quintile of Serum Cholesterol (1)

Quintile of serum Cholesterol	Ten Year Incidence		Twenty Year Incidence	
	Number	Rate/100	Number	Rate/100
1 (114-193)	2	1.0	18	8.6
2 (194-213)	11	5.3	32	15.3
3 (214-230)	14	6.7	46	22.0
4 (231-255)	26	12.4	56	26.8
5 (256-514)	32	15.3	64	30.6

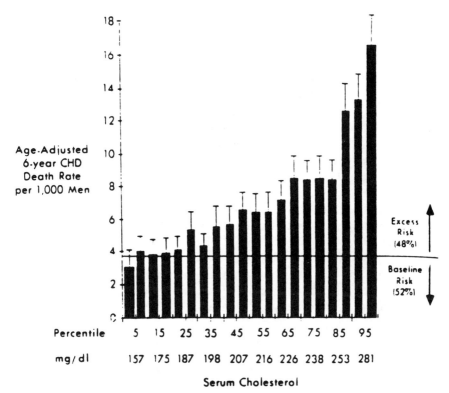

Fig. 5-1. Age-adjusted 6-year death rate per 1000 men screened for MRFIT according to serum cholesterol level (2).

atherosclerosis in rabbits by feeding cholesterol; and that whereas atherosclerosis was common—nearly universal—in our population, atherosclerosis and heart attacks were rare in some countries. This did not attract much attention until after World War II when there was evidence that CHD decreased in some European countries and then increased after the war. This clearly indicated that this disease was not simply due to aging or genetics and might be preventable. This stimulated research of all kinds including the epidemiology of the chronic diseases.

It should be noted that after the War the nutritional deficiency diseases had almost disappeared and the infectious diseases were being brought under control. The chronic diseases, like CHD and cancer, inevitably became the primary causes of death in the more affluent countries.

The more recent data which demonstrate the relationship between serum cholesterol and CHD mortality comes from the 361 thousand men who were screen for the Multiple Risk Factor Intervention Trial (MRFIT) (2) (Fig. 5-1). These were men who were between the ages of 35 and 57 years and who were followed for 6 years. I would call your attention to the fact that, even with a sample this large, the mortality was the same for men with serum cholesterol levels between 230 and 250 mg/dl and then a very large increase at 255 mg/dl. This is, no doubt, happenstancial but if data were only available from these groups, it might be concluded that serum cholesterol was not related to risk. It seems clear that risk rises continuously and there appear to be no "cut-off" points. Any decision to call one group "high risk" and another "low risk" is purely arbitrary.

Autopsy studies in a number of large studies confirm the general relationship between elevated serum cholesterol, more atherosclerosis and heart disease. Although it is difficult to estimate the average serum cholesterol levels in countries, the data indicate that they are related to CHD rates (3).

There have now been a number of trials with drugs and diets which show a reduction in serum cholesterol associated with reduced numbers of heart attacks (4). Changes in diet, serum cholesterol levels and CHD in immigrant populations have provided convincing evidence that diet plays a major role. Hence, the data of various kinds are quite consistent in showing that elevated serum cholesterol is causally related to risk of CHD.

It is true, of course, that the situation has become somewhat more complicated by the evidence that elevated levels of high density lipoproteins (HDL) are associated with reduced risk of CHD and that it is really the low density lipoproteins (LDL) that is the "bad" cholesterol. I will have more to say about this later. However, most of the circulating cholesterol is contained in LDL so this evidence does not refute the relationship between elevated serum cholesterol and risk of CHD.

On the other, Kannel and Gordon (1) state that 1) serum cholesterol is not a very strong risk factor compared, for example, to smoking and lung cancer; 2) CHD is a multifactorial disease and the effects of serum cholesterol are modified by other risk factors; 3) Coronary atherosclerosis undoubtedly reflects a person's lifetime history and not recent events which may be measured; and 4) Serum cholesterol is not a pure risk factor since it represents a number of different lipoproteins. I would emphasize, however, that one of the important reasons serum cholesterol is not as predictive as one might hope, is that the serum cholesterol level of an individual is quite variable. For unexplained reasons, a single or a few measurements does not characterize the individual very well (5). It is the average level over long periods that is important. Serum cholesterol measurements made in the same men in 1947 and 1979 (6) show a significant correlation but it is not very impressive. It is difficult to determine the average cholesterol over time which is the important parameter.

Dietary Fat and Serum Cholesterol

My major purpose today is to discuss the evidence relating diet, especially dietary fat, to serum cholesterol. It became clear in the 1950s that serum cholesterol levels could be changed markedly by the type of dietary fat. The studies of Keys et al. (7) were the first to provide an estimate to the quantitative effect of the various classes of fatty acids on serum cholesterol. We (8) (Figure 5-2) published similar data in 1965. Keys et al. compared 30 different diets; we compared 36. In both studies the results were evaluated by regression analysis relating change in serum cholesterol (mg/dl) to change in intake of saturated, monounsaturated and polyunsaturated fatty acids (% of calories). We also included change in dietary cholesterol in the calculations. Although the quantitative estimates were somewhat different, the two studies were consistent in concluding that the saturated fatty acids elevated and that polyunsaturated fatty acids lowered serum cholesterol and that the saturated fatty acids had the greatest effect. In neither study could a specific effect of the monounsaturated fatty acids be demonstrated. Although Keys stated that dietary cholesterol was of no importance, he later modified his conclusion.

These papers provided the primary basis for the various dietary recommendations, such as those of the American Heart Association, that Americans should reduce their consumption of fat, especially saturated fat and cholesterol, and modify the composition of the fat to increase the polyunsaturated content.

Since that time there have been many papers published on the effects of modifying dietary fat on serum cholesterol levels. The question is how well does the data now available confirm or deny the conclusions of Keys et al. and Hegsted et al. We (Hegsted, Ausman, Johnson, Dallal, unpublished) have reviewed the available data and find published data on 227

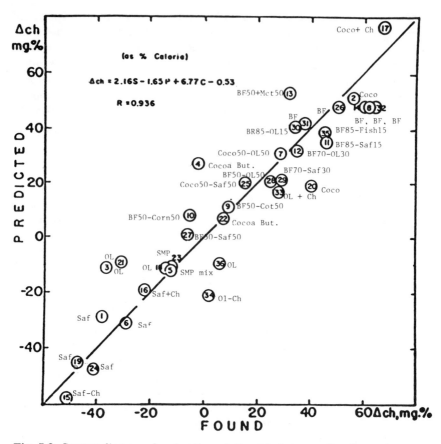

Fig. 5-2. Scatter diagram showing the relationship between the change in serum cholesterol found and those predicted by the regression equation. Modified from (8).

changes in dietary fat and the resultant change in serum cholesterol. There are quite a few papers which could not be included because the description of the diet was inadequate. We also excluded all papers where "formula diets" were used, as well as those in which the fats were greatly modified, as by excessive hydrogenation or re-esterification. The data have been examined by regression analysis, as was done by Keys et al. and Hegsted et al. to evaluate the effects of changes in saturated, monounsaturated and polyunsaturated fatty acids (% of calories) and dietary cholesterol (mg/1000) on the change in serum cholesterol (mg/dl).

The papers were divided into those we called "metabolic studies" and those we labelled "field trials". The metabolic studies were those in which specific diets were prepared and fed to the subjects although often not under strictly metabolic ward conditions. In the field trials the diet was modified by instruction. Presumably the metabolic studies were better controlled but these have usually been conducted with rather small groups of subjects while the field trials usually were with rather large groups. Since individuals do vary in their response to diet, the larger trials might be more representative than those from the metabolic trials.

Most of the data come from metabolic studies. The conclusions from these are quite consistent with the prior conclusions. That is, the saturated fatty acids elevate serum cholesterol and are the primary determinants of serum cholesterol levels. The changes in saturated fatty acids alone account for about 75% of the variance in the observed serum cholesterol changes. However, both the polyunsaurated fatty acids and dietary cholesterol have highly significant effects (p=0.001) with polyunsaturated fatty acids lowering and dietary cholesterol elevating serum cholesterol. We can find no evidence that modification of the intake of the mounsaturated fatty acids changes serum cholesterol.

Our conclusions differ somewhat from those of Keys et al. and Hegsted et al. in that we find two interactions that are statistically significant. These are the product of the change in saturated fatty acids and change in dietary cholesterol (p=0.012) and the product of the change in saturated and polyunsaturated fatty acids (p=0.002). Thus, although the saturated fatty acids elevate serum cholesterol and are 2 to 3 times as potent as are the polyunsaturated fatty acids in lowering serum cholesterol, their effects are partly interdependent and the same is true of the saturated fatty acids and dietary cholesterol. Key et al. concluded that the saturates were twice as active as the polyunsaturates. This is a reasonable estimate but one cannot expect that the quantitative effects of the saturated, polyunsaturated and dietary cholesterol will always be the same because their effects are somewhat interdependent. These kinds of modest interactions will, of course, rarely be demonstrated in relatively small studies.

Another important conclusion is that although the best predictive equation accounts for about 83% of the total variance, the standard error around the regression line is rather large, about 12 mg/dl. This means that the same or very similar dietary comparisons may yield changes in serum cholesterol which differ by as much as 50 mg/dl (2 s.e. on either side of the line) even when the data are derived from apparently well controlled studies with adequate numbers in the groups. This must mean either that there are important determinants of serum cholesterol other than the fatty acids and serum cholesterol or that the mean change in serum cholesterol, even under apparently good experimental control, is not a very reliable or reproducibly estimate. I believe the latter is the explanation.

In our own studies (8) (Fig. 5-2), the same basal diet was used as a base of comparison throughout. Thus, it is unlikely that dietary factors other than those in the fats affected the results very much although the standard error in our studies was of the same magnitude as those found in the combined data. In practically all of the studies, one fat was replaced by another. So we do not argue that other factors may not affect serum cholesterol levels; we only believe that since we are looking at change in serum cholesterol after a change in dietary fat composition, it is unlikely that factors other than those in the oils tested had a substantial effect.

Everyone finds rather large differences in the way individuals respond to the same diet and the literature is full of the words, hypo- and hyper-responders. There appears, however, to be only one study which has attempted to evaluate the reproducibility of these responses and the results are not encouraging. Katan et al. (9) fed the same individuals the same diets a year or so apart. There is obviously some correlation between the two responses, confirming the fact that individuals do respond differently, but the correlation was poor. The correlation coefficient was of the order of 0.6 which means that only 36% of the variance could be explained by the the similarity of reponse. What happens at one time, is apparently, not a very good indication of what may happen the next. If individual responses are not reproducible, groups responses must also be variable. Unfortunately, we find no adequate examples in the literature comparing the effects of the same dietary changes in groups at different times or comparing the same dietary change in different groups.

If these conclusions are correct, it follows that comparisons of 2 or 3 dietary fats or oils, as are reported in most papers, can never refute the general conclusions based upon the total data now available. An example may be instructive. Mensink and Katan (11) recently reported that an oil high in monounsaturated fatty acids yielded the same cholesterol reduction as an oil high in polyunsaturated fatty acid. The minimal power of such a study can be demonstrated by comparing the data-set of Hegsted et al. (8) with and without the inclusion of the data provided by Mensink and Katan. The data of Hegsted et al. (8) recalculated to include dietary cholesterol expressed as mg/1000 calories yields the equation:

$$\Delta sc = 2.16 \Delta S - 1.65 \Delta P + 0.168 \Delta C + 0.857 \quad R = 0.934$$

If one adds the data provided by Mensink and Katan and recalculated the equation, one obtains:

$$\Delta sc = 2.20 \Delta S - 1.62 \Delta P + 0.168 \Delta C + 0.554 \quad R = 0.937$$

Thus, these few additional data do not change the general predictive equation in any significant way. Indeed, the correlation coefficient is slightly improved. The same conclusion will be reached if one adds these few points to the data of Keys et al.

Thus, the real merit of the studies of Keys et al. (7) and our own (8), as opposed to all of those since that time, is that a sufficient number of diets were compared to allow the definition of the general effects. I believe that it is never safe to generalize from comparisons of a few oils or diets and such studies cannot challenge the conclusion from the mass of data now available.

Long-term Dietary Effects

Practically all experimental data have been obtained from relatively short-term studies of a few weeks. Is it possible that people adapt to diets and the experimental findings may be invalid over time? This possibility is well illustrated by data on "carbohydrate-induced hypertriglyceridemia" which many people have reported when low fat diets are fed. Figure 5-3 shows the data of Antonis and Bersohn (11). The high triglyceride levels returned to normal but this required weeks to months. This adaptation to low fat diets must occur since populations consuming low fat diets do not have unusually high triglyceride levels.

The only very long-term data come from descriptions of the serum cholesterol and diet of groups consuming their "usual" diet. Although our evaluation is not complete, it appears that the published data show that, as expected, serum cholesterol is proportional with the saturated fatty acid content of their "usual diet". However, we were surprised that we could not show a "cholesterol-lowering" effect of the polyunsaturated fatty acids. This appears to be due to the groups whose diets are very low in fat (Japanese, Koreans, Guatemalans, Mexican Indians). If these

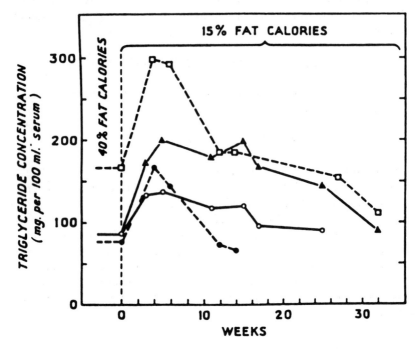

Fig. 5-3. Serum triglyceride levels in White (———) and Bantu (----) subjects when changed to a low fat diet. Subjects were arbitrarily divided into those with relatively high and low triglyceride levels (12).

data are removed from the data set, then the multiple regression shows, as expected, a positive coefficient for the saturated fatty acids and a negative coefficient for the polyunsaturated fatty acids. That is, polyunsaturated fatty acids only lower cholesterol when the serum cholesterol levels are elevated, at least to some degree.

We can rationalize this finding in that if serum cholesterol levels are already near minimal levels, its unlikely that one can show a cholesterol-lowering effect of anything. In fact, there are good data (12) showing that the cholesterol-lowering effect of polyunsaturated oils is rather closely related to original serum cholesterol levels. Finally, the data would appear to be consistent with the conclusion of Dietschy and his group (13). In studies with hamsters, they conclude that saturated fatty acids and dietary cholesterol suppress lipoprotein receptors. Polyunsaturated fatty acids stimulated the receptors but this could only be shown after they were suppressed by feeding cholesterol and saturated fat.

Hence, the over-all conclusions from rather abundant data from both experimental and epidemiologic studies, are consistent in showing that saturated fatty acids elevate serum cholesterol and are the primary dietary factor while the polyunsaturated fatty acids lower serum cholesterol. The latter appears to be true only if the total dietary fat is above 15% of calories which is the area of primary interest. The effects of these are not entirely independent nor is the effect of dietary cholesterol. The data fail to demonstrate any specific role for the monounsaturated fatty acids.

Formula Diets and Monounsaturates

How then do we explain the data of Mattson and Grundy (14) who found that the mono- and polyunsaturated fatty acids had comparable effects? We believe this was due to the dietary conditions that they used. Figure 5-4 summarizes the data of Ahrens et al. (15) published in 1957. These authors studied individual patients, most of whom were quite hyper-cholesterolemic so the data cannot be compared to that obtained with groups of subjects. These authors utilized "formula diets" containing the oil being tested. Each subject received the formula diet containing corn oil to provide a base for comparison. The figure shows that minimal cholesterol levels were obtained with oils with an Iodine Number of about 90, about the value for olive oil which is composed primarily of oleic acid. More highly unsaturated oils, like corn and safflower oil did not reduce the serum cholesterol further. It appears to use that all of the reported studies in which formula diets have been used (16-19) have produced similar results, i.e. no difference in the effects of oils high in the mono- and polysaturated oils, which is quite different from that found when diets composed of ordinary foods are used. Our conclusion is that there is something unusual—they either contain something or lack something—that affects the response to polyunsaturated fatty acids. We think that the results obtained under such conditions cannot be legitimately extrapolated to other conditions.

We should recognize a general weakness of the evaluation of the data available by regression analysis. In all of the studies where one fat is substituted for another, there are substantial correlations between the various parameters. It is clear that if the amount of fat in the diet is maintained more or less constant, you cannot modify one variable at a time. If you substitute a polyunsaturated fat for a saturated fat, the

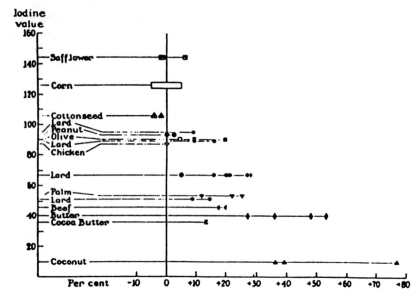

Fig. 5-4. Relationship between serum cholesterol levels in individual patients and Iodine Number (degree of unsaturation) of the oil in the formula diet. Data are expressed as the percentage difference from baseline values obtained with a formula diet containing corn oil (15).

TABLE 5-2

Correlations between Saturated Fatty Acid Intakes and Other Dietary Fat Constituents

Data Set	P	M	C	SC
Metabolic Studies	-.58	.20	.44	.86
Field Trials	-.59	.69	.39	.91
Total Data	-.59	.30	.43	.87
Keys et al.	-.31	.46	—	.90
Hegsted et al.	-.58	-.26	.31	.85

saturated fatty acids fall and the polyunsaturated fatty acids rise and, usually, the level of the monounsaturated fatty acids changes as well. Table 5-2 shows the inter-correlations in some of the data sets. The question is how well can regression analysis distinguish between the

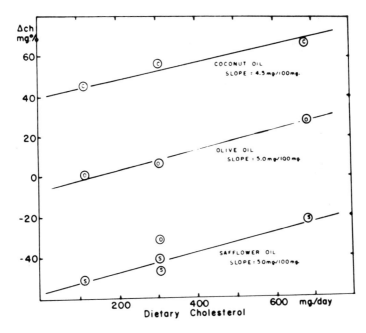

Fig. 5-5. Change in serum cholesterol from basal levels induced by three different fats fed with three levels of dietary cholesterol from egg (8).

TABLE 5-3
CHD Patients Consuming Low Animal Fat Diets with Additional Doses of Olive & Corn Oil

Group	Period (months)	Consumed gm/day	Serum Cholesterol Change, mg/dl
Control	0-12		+2.4
Control	12-24		-5.4
Olive Oil	0-12	63	+7.8
Olive Oil	12-24	49	+1.6
Corn Oil	0-12	69	-27.9
Corn Oil	12-24	57	-25.1

Data from Rose et al. (20)

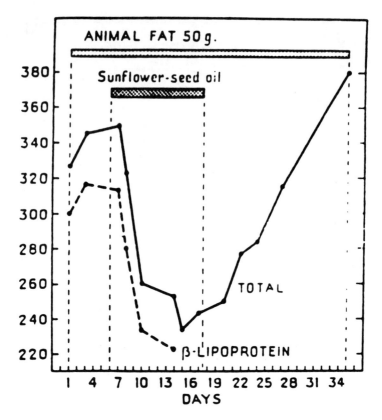

Fig. 5-6. Serum cholesterol and beta-lipoprotein response in a single patient supplemented with 100 grams of sunflowerseed oil (21).

effects of the specific fatty acids when the inter-correlations are relatively high? I doubt if there is an entirely adequate explanation. Presumably an ideal study would be one in which all the variables were randomly distributed with little or no inter-correlations. I don't know whether this could be designed but it would be a very large study and it is not likely to be achieved.

There are, however, a number of studies which indicate that the monounsaturate and polyunsaturated fatty acids do not have similar effects on serum cholesterol. Figure 5-5 is taken from our paper (8) and compares the effects of coconut, olive and safflower oils, each fed at three levels of dietary cholesterol (egg). The first time we fed olive oil at the lower cholesterol intake, we found an unusually large effect which seemed inconsistent and we questioned the data. When this was repeated, the result seemed consistent with the other data.

I would call your attention to the study reported by Rose et al. (20) (Table 5-3). In this study patients with cardiovascular disease were advised to consume a diet low in animal fats and then to dose themselves with either olive oil or corn oil. The table summarizes results of those who completed the two year study. Although they did not monitor the rest of the diets, it seems quite clear that corn oil did lower serum cholesterol while olive oil did not.

I would also note the data from the single patients reported by Bronte-Stewart et al. (21) (Fig. 5-6). This patient's diet contained 50 grams of fat, mostly of animal origin. When 100 grams of sunflowerseed oil was added there was precipitous fall in the serum cholesterol and beta-lipoprotein. This cannot be due to a decrease in saturated fatty acids. I suggest that with studies of the design suggested here we could feed several levels of an oil and develop dose-response curves of serum cholesterol to that oil. Using different basal diets we should be able to determine whether the response depends upon the fat in the basal diet.

Saturated Fatty Acids

There are substantial reasons to believe that not all of the saturated fatty acids are equally hypercholesterolemic, especially stearic acid (8,22,23). I want to call your attention to a few issues. The first is that we can never prove a negative. We cannot prove that stearate has no effect. Secondly, that if we decide that stearate should not be included with the saturated fatty acids, the whole field will have to be re-evaluated. For example, the original equation developed by Keys et al. (7) was:

$$SC = 2.74\ S - 1.31\ P.$$

It is certain that if the size of S is lowered by removing stearic acid, the coefficient of S will have to increase. The cholesterol- elevating effects of S would have to be accounted for by a smaller value of S. It is possible that the whole equation might change. Indeed, we might note that after Keys (24) decided that dietary cholesterol ought to be included in the equation, he simply added his estimate of the effect to the above equation. This is not appropriate. If dietary cholesterol had been included in the original estimation, the size of the coefficient of S would have been

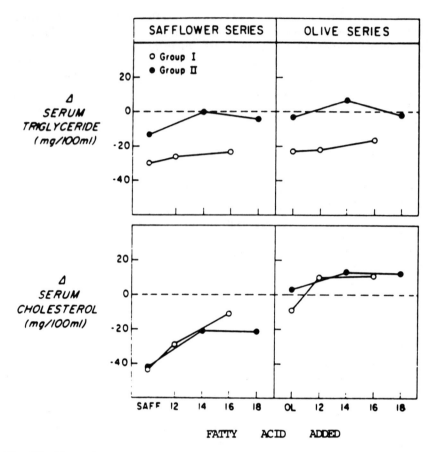

Fig. 5-7. Change in serum triglyceride and cholesterol levels from baseline induced by safflower and olive oils transesterified with saturated fatty acids of varying chain length (25).

smaller because the dietary content of the saturated fatty acids and dietary cholesterol are rather highly correlated.

Finally, Figure 5-7 is from the paper of McGandy et al. (25). We wished to evaluate the effects of the various saturated fatty acids. Since tristearin and tripalmtin are poorly absorbed Proctor and Gamble prepared olive and safflower oils which had been trans-esterified with the different saturated fatty acids. It appears from these data that there are no or only minor differences in the effects of the acids of varying chain length. This is obviously inconsistent with the other data indicating that steric acid has less effect that the other saturated fatty acids. I believe that the only way one can rationalize the two different findings is by assuming that triglyceride structure has a significant effect. I suppose that in most oils, stearic acid will be in the 1,3 position but should be equally distributed in the transesterified oils. In any event, I believe it is too early to decide that stearic acid is without effect on serum cholesterol. Indeed, we have little data, as yet, which adequately demonstrates the relative potency of the other saturated fatty acids.

Polyunsaturated Fatty Acids and HDL

There has been concern expressed about the possibility that polyunsaturated fats may lower HDL and that this is an undesirable effect. This response appears to have been shown when the diets were extreme, i.e. the fat was almost entirely corn oil or some other polyunsaturated fat, but not with reasonable levels of intake. Also, it is important to note that low fat diets—diets that clearly protect against CHD—also lower HDL levels. Our real concern should be the ratio of LDL to HDL rather than absolute levels. I believe that unsaturated oils always improve the ratio even if HDL levels fall slightly.

TABLE 5-4
Adipose Tissue Fatty Acids, %(30)

Acid	N. Karelia	SW Finland	Scotland	Italy
14:0	4.5	4.5	3.6	1.9
16:0	27.0	26.3	26.3	20.4
18:0	7.0	7.4	6.4	3.6
18:1	45.0	45.0	46.4	54.3
18:2	7.4	8.1	8.8	13.5
18:3	0.8	0.8	0.8	0.8
Serum Cholesterol, mg/dl	257	247	223	207

TABLE 5-5
Plasma Triglyceride Fatty Acids, % (28)

Fatty Acid	Patients	Controls
14:0	1.5	1.7
16:0	31.2	24.0
18:0	4.8	5.5
18:1	42.5	40.2
18:2	11.9	18.5
18:3	1.2	1.9

Finally, I believe it is important to note that we now have few reports on the linoleic acid content of adipose tissue and serum triglycerides in CHD cases and controls (26-31). Table 5-4 and 5-5 summarize some of the data. The cases of CHD have lower levels of linoleic acid and it appears that there has been a rise in the adipose tissue content of linoleic acid as CHD has fallen in the U.S. We do not know how well the linoleic acid content of adipose tissue reflects dietary intake but it may be that it is a better indicator of the usual diet that the dietary intake data. These kinds of data lend credence to the likelihood that high levels of intake of linoleic has a beneficial effect. It is of interest that the Italians, who have relatively little CHD, have fairly high levels of linoleic acid although the diet is not thought to be especially rich in this fatty acids.

We are inclined to think of the fatty acids only in relation to serum lipids but we now know that they affect thrombosis and probably blood pressure. We should not take to parochial a view since the field is always changing. I will hazard a guess that relatively high intakes of linoleic acid have beneficial effects not reflected in the serum lipids and lipoproteins.

References

1. Kannel, W.B., and Gordon, T. (1982) Lancet 2, 374-375.
2. Martin, M.J., Hulley, S.B., Browner, W.S., Kuller, L.H., and Wentworth, D. (1986) Lancet 2, 933-936.
3. Simons, L.A. (1986) Am. J. Card. 57, 5G-10G.
4. Castelli, W.P. (1988) Internat Lipid Forum 1, 1-8.
5. Hegsted, D.M., and Nicolosi, R.J. (1987) Proc. Natl. Acad. Sci. USA 84, 6259-6261.
6. Gillum, R.F., Taylor, H.L., Brozek, J., Anderson, J.T., and Blackburn, H. (1982) J. Chron. Dis. 35, 635-641.

7. Keys, A., Anderson, J.T., and Grande, F. (1957) Lancet 2, 959-966.
8. Hegsted, D.M., McGandy, R.B., Myers, M.L., and Stare, F.J. (1865) Am. J. Clin. Nutr. 17, 281-295.
9. Katan, M.B., Berns, M.A.M., Glatz, J.F.C., Nobels, A., and de Vries, J.H.M. (1988) J. Lipid Res. 29, 883-892.
10. Mensink, R.P., and Katan, M.B. (1989) New Eng. J. Med. 321, 436-441.
11. Antonis, A., and Bersohn, I. (19) Lancet; 1, 3-7.
12. Keys, A., Anderson, J.T., and Grande, F. (1959) Circulation 19, 201-214.
13. Spady, D.K., and Dietschy, J. (1985) Proc. Natl. Acad. Sci. USA. 82, 4526-4530.
14. Mattson, F.H., and Grundy, S.M. (1985) J. Lipid Res. 26, 194-202.
15. Ahrens, E.H., Hirsh, J., Insull, W., Tsaltas, T.T., Bloomdtrand, R., and Peterson, M.L. (1957) Lancet 1, 943-953.
16. Hashim, S.A., Clancy, R.E., Hegsted, D.M., and Stare, F.J. (1959) Am. J. Clin. Nutr. 7, 30-34.
17. McOsker, D.E., Mattson, F.H., Sweringen, H.B., and Kligman, A.M. (1962) J.A.M.A. 180, 380-385.
18. Erickson, B.A., Coots, R.H., Mattson, F.H., and Kligman, A.M. (1964) J. Clin. invest. 43, 2017-2025.
19. Becker, N., Illingworth, D.R., Alaupovic, P., Connor, W.E., and Sundbery, E.E. Am. J. Clin. Nutr. 37, 355-360.
20. Rose, G.A., Thomson, W.B., and Williams, R.T. (1965) Brit. Med. J. 1, 1531-1533.
21. Bronte-Stewart, B., Antonis, A., Eales, L., and Brock, J.F. (1956) Lancet 1, 521-527.
22. Grande, F., Anderson, J.T., Taylor, H.L., Keys, A., and Frantz, I.D. (1970) Am. J. Clin. Nutr. 9, 1184-1193.
23. Bonanome, A., and Grundy, S.M. (1988) N. Eng. J. Med. 318, 1244-1248.
24. Anderson, J.T., Grande, F., Chlouveraskis, C., Proja, M., and Keys, A., Fed. Proc. 21, 100-102.
25. McGandy, R.B., Hegsted, D.M., and Myers, M.L. (1970) Am. J. Clin. Nutr. 23, 1288-1298.
26. Logan, R.L., Riemersma, R.A., Thomson, M., and Oliver, M.F. (1978) Lancet 1, 949-955.
27. Katan, M.B., and Beynan, A.C. (1981) Lancet 2, 371.
28. Simpson, H.C.R., Barker, K., Cassels, E., and Mann, J.I. (1982) Brit. Med. J. 285, 683-684.
29. Wood, D.A., Butler, S., Riemersma, R.A., Thomson, M., and Oliver, M.F. (1984) Lancet 2, 117-121.

30. Riemersma, R.A., Wood, D.A., Butler, S., Elton, R.A., Oliver, M., Salo, M., Nikkari, T., Vartianen, E., Puska, P., Gey, F., Rubba, P., Mancini, M., and Fidanza, F. (1986) Brit. Med. J. 292, 1423-1427.
31. Wood, D.A., Riemersma, R.A., Butler, S., Thomson, M., MacIntyre, C., and Oliver, M.F. (1987) Lancet 1, 177-183.

Chapter Six

Effects of Dietary Fatty Acids on Cholesterol, Triglyceride and Lipoprotein Distribution

William S. Harris, Ph.D.

Lipid Laboratory
University of Kansas Medical Center
3800 Cambridge
Kansas City, KS 66103

A short discussion of the effects of dietary fatty acids on cholesterol, triglyceride and lipoprotein distributions must, of necessity, focus on a few selected topics as the literature in this area is vast. In this paper, I will address three somewhat unrelated questions. First, the issue of quantity vs. quality of dietary fat, does polyunsaturated fat lower HDL and, finally, what are the effects of fish oils on lipids?

Does the Amount of Dietary Fat Affect Lipids and Lipoproteins?

This question has been addressed in a variety of ways. Epidemiologically, in the Seven Countries Study by Keys and associates (1), there was a high correlation between saturated fat intake and serum chloesterol levels (r=0.89), but the relationship between total fat was weak. For example, the serum cholesterol levels were equivalent in Montegiorgio, Italy (25% fat) and Crete (40% fat). In these two locations, saturated fat intakes were equivalent. Cholesterol levels were actually lower in Crete (40% fat) than in West Finland (35% fat). Saturated fat levels were

TABLE 6-1
Effects of Dietary Fat Levels on LDL-C and HDL-C

Fat(%en)	S/M/P	LDL-C	HDL-C
40%	(17/18/5)	153±10	38±3
30%	(10/10/10)	118±8*	39±3
20%	(7/7/7)	114±8*	33±3

Grundy et al JAMA 256:2351, 1986 *p<0.05

higher in Finland. Thus, saturated fat and not total fat levels appeared to determine serum cholesterol levels.

Experimentally, Grundy et al. (2) reported that using metabolically controlled diets of varying fat contents in normal volunteers for 4 weeks, there was a decrease in LDL levels going from 40% of calories to 30% (Table 6-1). However, this was accompanied by a large decrease in saturated fat and a doubling of the polyunsaturated fat intake. The changes seen were most likely due to the changes in fat quality vs. quantity. Decreasing from 30% to 20% of calories had no further effect on LDL-C levels, but HDL-C levels did fall on the low fat diet. Thus, here again, total fat had less of an impact than the nature of the fat.

In a recent review of this topic, Kris-Etherton et al. (3) concluded, "The data summarized demonstrate that fat quality has a more significant effect on the plasma lipid response than does fat quantity. Lowering the total fat content of the diet facilitates the reduction of dietary saturated FAs. Substituting unsaturated FAs for saturated FAs without changing the quantity of fat in the diet effectively modifies plasma lipid levels." In another review, Nichaman and Hamm (4) concurred, "There does not appear to be a strong lipid lowering effect of low-fat diets that is independent of their fatty acid composition."

Do Polyunsaturated Fatty Acids Lower HDL?

Since lowering saturated fat is clearly more important than lowering total fat, the question arises, what should be substituted for saturated fat? Monounsaturated fats or polyunsaturated fats? Some have favored monounsaturated oils because polyunsaturated fats have been reported to lower HDL-C levels. This is a complicated area with extensive literature, all of which cannot be addressed here. I will only offer a suggestion that, when polyunsaturated fats are consumed in amounts similar to those found in the usual American diet, (and in nationally-endorsed, recommended diets) they really have very little impact on HDL-C levels. This can be seen from three studies addressing this question; Vega (5), McDonald (6) and Mensink (7) all fed whole-food diets to normal volunteers and compared control diets to diets high in polyunsaturated FAs (Table 6-2). All diets provided between 37% and 40% of calories as fat, but varied widely in fatty acid composition. For reference, the NCEP guidelines suggest that no more than 10% of calories come from saturated fat and the same for polyunsaturated. Vega et al. (5) fed a very low polyunsaturated control diet (1%) and a very high polyunsaturated test diet (30%). Control saturated fat intakes were typical of the

TABLE 6-2
Do Polyunsaturated Fatty Acids Lower HDL?

Author	Diet	%Fat	%Sat	%Poly	HDL-C	Change
Vega et al.	Control	40	14	1	51	-8
	Poly	40	4	30	43	
McDonald et al.	Control	36	14	7	53	-4
	Poly	36	7	22	49	
Mensink et al.	Control	37	19	5	54	-2
	Poly	37	13	13	52	
NCEP Guidelines		30	10	10		

American diet, but the saturated fat content of the polyunsaturated diet was extraordinarily low (4%). These two diets produced HDL-C levels which differed by 8 mg/dL (16% decrease). Was this decline due to the change in saturated fat or polyunsaturated fat?

McDonald et al. (6) fed a more reasonable control diet (14% saturated, 7% polyunsaturated), but they still cut the saturated fat in half and tripled the polyunsaturated content in the high polyunsaturated diet. These two diets were less extreme than those used by Vega, and HDL-C levels differed by only 4 mg/dL.

Finally, Mensink and associates (7) fed diets which were even more typical, and more practical, although the polyunsaturated fat content was still higher than recommended. The difference in HDL-C levels between these two groups was trivial (2 mg/dL). These studies suggest that using polyunsaturated oils in the context of a practical, prudent diet would not cause a significant reduction in HDL-C levels. Therefore, in my view, consumers should be encouraged to substitute either monounsaturated or polyunsaturated rich oils for saturated fats—the effects should be the same on LDL, and HDL levels should not suffer for using the latter.

Fish Oils and Lipoprotein Levels—Why The Disparate Findings?

Turning to the last topic, I'd like to review for you the effects of fish oils on lipid and lipoprotein levels. Fish oils are unique polyunsaturated fats since they are rich in the n-3 or omega-3 FAs (EPA and DHA) as opposed to those of the n-6 family such as linoleic acid characterize vegetable oils.

The n-3 fatty acids have a wide variety of metabolic effects. They have been reported to be anti-atherogenic (8), and anti-hypertensive (9), anti-inflammatory (10), and possibly anti-neoplastic (11), but the first and most widely recognized effects of these fatty acids was on serum lipid levels (12,13).

The story began in the 1970s when a group of Danish scientists investigated a group of Greenland eskimos who appeared to be "immune" to coronary disease. Despite a relatively high fat, high cholesterol diet, these eskimos had lower serum cholesterol levels than their westernized counterparts (14). Further investigations revealed that there was a predominance of n-3 fatty acids in their diet. Dyerberg and Bang hypotheorized that it was these n-3 FAs that were responsible for both the reduced blood lipids and the low incidence of myocardial infarction.

At this time, there was little clinical data to support this hypothesis. Therefore, in 1978 at the University of Oregon we began to examine the effects of fish oils on lipoprotein levels in normal volunteers. We were interested to see if in a metabolic ward study, normal Americans would also experience the lipid lowering effects of n-3 fatty acids.

We found that cholesterol levels were in fact reduced by the fish oil, but they were also decreased by an equivalent amount of vegetable oil (15). What was unique about the fish oil was its triglyceride lowering effect. This effect had been seen nearly 20 years earlier by at least four groups (13) but since cholesterol was the focus of the studies and, as so often happens in science, there was no theoretical framework in which to place the triglyceride lowering effects, so they were largely overlooked and forgotten.

Our original interpretation of our results was that gram for gram, w3 FAs were more hypocholesterolemic than W6 FAs. In retrospect, I now believe that another explanation is more likely. In those experiments the saturated fat content was not held constant and was lower during the fish oil diet and the vegetable oil diet than during the control diet. It is likely that the reduction in cholesterol levels was not the result of increased intake of polyunsaturated fatty acids, but of the decrease saturated fatty acid intake.

In a second study from Oregon, we addressed the effects of fish oil on plasma lipids in hypertriglyceridemic patients (16). In that study, LDL levels of our patients with type IIb hyperlipidemia decreased on the fish oil and vegetable oil diet. When I reviewed all of the studies using fish oils in hyperlipidemic patients two years ago, this was the only study, out of a total of 19, in which LDL cholesterol decreased in patients fed with fish oil, and it was the only trial in which saturated fat intakes were lower on the fish oil treatment period (13).

In retrospect, it is regretable that these early studies were used by major supplement manufactures to promote fish oils as cholesterol lowering agents. As further evidence accumulated from around the world that fish oil supplements alone did not lower cholessterol (17), a tremendous amount of confusion was generated which has yet to be fully resolved and understood. From my perspective, fish oils are not hypocholesterolic treatments, but they are effective in the treatment of hypertriglyceridemia. Typical reductions in triglyceride levels range from 20% in normals to 40-60% in patients with elevated triglyceride levels. Thus, fish oils can be as effective as the fibrate drugs in reducing triglyceride levels. However, like these drugs, LDL levels may not only fail to decrease, but may also increase. In patients with combined hyperlipidemia (IIb) a rise of 8-12% is not uncommon, and in patients with isolated hypertriglyceridemia the increase may be 20-30%.

One would naturally wonder whether fish oils might, therefore, be "bad" for people. At present, we do not have a firm answer to this question. These are some points we should consider, however.

First, in several animal trials, fish oil has been shown to retard the development of coronary artery disease. Weiner et al. (18) were first to report this effect in swine. The point I want to make here is that fish oil exerted this protective effect even in the face of generally higher LDL levels. Others have reported that fish oil exerts this effect even in normolipidemic swine (19). In monkeys, fish oil is also protective (10), but in this model, diets were lower in saturated fat and LDL levels were reduced, but HDL levels were markedly reduced, and the ratio of LDL/HDL was unfavorably impacted, nevertheless, less disease was reported.

There have been four published reports on the effects of fish oil on the rate of restenosis after PTCA in patients (21-24). Two studies found beneficial effects (21,22), the other two found no effect (23,24). Larger trials are currently underway to help resolve this question. The point here is that in the positive effect study of Dehmer et al. (21), the group receiving fish oil tended to experience increases in LDL levels, while the control group did not. Once again, evidence that one can reduce arterial disease without decreasing LDL.

A recent report from Wales provided the strongest data to date that fish oil can reduce mortality coronary disease in patients who had survived myocardial infarction (8). Two thousand such patients were randomly allocated to either receive or *not* receive advice to increase their intake of oily fish (they were also allowed to take fish oil capsules if they did not like fish). Their estimated intake of eicosapentaenoic acid was about 800 mg/day over the ensuing two years. After which time, those who had received the fish advice had about a 30% lower overall death rate, almost entirely due to reduced coronary mortality. The authors noted that the fish oil did not lower cholesterol levels.

Finally, it should be noted that those patients who appeared to receive the most benefit from the drug, gemfibrozil, in the Helsinki Heart Study (25) were the ones with elevated VLDL levels, not LDL levels. Since fish oil and gemfibrozil have similar effects on the plasma lipid profile, the Helsinki data also suggests that alterations in non-LDL cholesterol levels may beneficially impact coronary artery disease rates.

Therefore, does a fish oil induced 15% rise in LDL cholesterol (which would also be accompanied by a fall in VLDL levels) produce an increase in coronary risk? There is data to suggest that it might not (26,27), nevertheless, I believe we must remain cautious and carefully monitor any hypertriglyceridemic patients taking fish oils and use low doses until these questions can be more fully explored.

If fish oil does not favorably impact LDL levels and has a relatively small effect on HDL levels, do fish oil induced changes in lipoprotein metabolism play any role in their apparent protective effect in coronary disease? With this question, I will move to my final topic—how do fish oils impact levels of postprandial lipoproteins?

Postprandial lipoproteins are those lipid filled particles which carry fats from the intestine to the tissues of the body. They consist almost entirely of triglycerides and persist in the circulation for up to 8 hours after a meal. Since it is not uncommon for Americans to eat appreciable amounts of fat at breakfast, lunch and dinner, chylomicron particles can be found in the blood for up to 20 out of every 24 hours. And yet, when blood samples are taken for lipid analysis, these paricles are usually completely gone. It has been hypothesized, and there is considerable data to support the idea that partially metabolized remnants of chylmicrons may be atherogenic (28). Hence, interventions which reduce levels of these particles may be beneficial.

With that in mind, we conducted fat tolerance studies in our salmon oil fed subjects in Oregon and found that fat tolerance was markedly improved during the fish oil period (29). We pursued this observation in subsequent studies and learned that the reduction in postprandial triglyceride levels was not seen when subjects were not fed fish oil chronically; i.e., a fish oil test meal appeared to be absorbed and cleared at the same rate as a control meal containing typical dietary fats (30). This naturally led us to test the hypothesis that a chronic intake of n-3 fatty acids produced a fundamental change in the way that dietary fats are handled. In this study, we fed a control background diet and then gave fish oil and control test meals. We also fed a fish oil background diet with the same two tests meals given at the end. We found that postprandial lipid levels were lower on the fish oil background diet than on the control diet regardless of the nature of the fat in the test diet. This study was largely confirmed by Weintraub et al. (31) who used a vitamin A load test to assess chylomicrons remnant levels. Therefore, by as yet unknown mechanisms, dietary n-3 fatty acids appear to reduce the levels of postprandial particles, and may, by this mechanism have a beneficial effect on cardiovascular disease.

Acknowledgments

The following investigators made significant contributions to the studies discussed here, and their collaboration was greatly appreciated. William E. Connor, D. Roger Illingworth, Martha McMurray, and Carlos A. Dujovne.

References

1. Keys, A. (1975) Atherosclerosis 22, 149.
2. Grundy, S.M., Nix, D., Whelan, M.F., and Franklin, L. (1986) JAMA 256, 2351-2355.
3. Kris-Etherton, P.M., Krummel, D., Russell, M.E., Dreon, D., Mackey, S., Borchers, J., and Wood, P.D. (1988) J. Am. Diet. Assoc. 88, 1373-1400.
4. Nichaman, M.Z., and Hamm, P. (1987) Am. J. Clin. Nutr. 45, 1155.
5. Vega, G.L. Groszek, E., Wolf, R., and Grundy, S.M. (1982) J. Lipd Res. 23, 811-822.
6. McDonald, B.E., Gerrard, J.M., Bruce, V.M., and Corner, E.J. (1989) Am. J. Clin. Nutr. 50, 1382-1388.
7. Mensink, R.P., and Katan, M.B. (1989) N. Engl. J. Med. 321, 436-441.
8. Burr, M.L., Fehily, A.M., Gilbert, J.F., Rogers, S., Holliday, R.M., Sweetnam, P.M., Elwood, P.C., and Deadman, N.M. (1989) Lancet 2, 757-761.
9. Knapp, H.R., and FitzGerald, G.A. (1989) N. Engl. J. Med. 16, 1037-1043.
10. Lee, T.H., Hoover, R.L., Williams, J.D., et al. (1985) N. Engl. J. Med. 312, 1217-1224.
11. O'Connor, T.P., Roebuck, B.D., Peterson, F.J., Lokesh, B., Kinsella, J.E., and Campbell, T.C. (1989) J. Natl. Cancer Inst. 81, 858-863.
12. Goodnight, S.H., Harris, W.S., Connor, W.E., and Illingworth, D.R. (1982) Arteriosclerosis 2, 87-113.

13. Harris, W.S. (1989) J. Lipid Res. 30, 785-807.
14. Dyerberg, J. (1986) Nutr. Rev. 44, 125-134.
15. Harris, W.S., Connor, W.E., and McMurry, M.P. (1983) Metabolism 32, 179-184.
16. Phillipson, B.E., Rothrock, D.W., Connor, W.E., Harris, W.S., and Illingworth, D.R. (1985) N. Engl. J. Med. 312, 1210-1216.
17. Harris, W.S., Dujovne, C.A., Zucker, M.L., and Johnson, B.E. (1988) Ann. Intern. Med. 109, 465-470.
18. Weiner, B.H., Ockene, I.S., Levine, P.H., et al. (1986) N. Engl. J. Med. 315, 841-846.
19. Hartog, J.M., Lamers, J.M.J., Essed, C.E., Schalkwijk, W.P., and Verdouw, P.D., (1989) Atherosclerosis 76, 79-88.
20. Davis, H.R., Bridenstine, R.T., Vesselinovitch, D., and Wissler, R.W. (1987) 7, 441-449.
21. Dehmer, G.J., Popma, J.J., van den Berg, E.K., Eichorn, E.J., Prewitt, J.B., Campbell, W.B., Jennings, L., Willerson, J.T., and Schmitz, J.M. (1988) N. Engl. J. Med. 319, 733-740.
22. Milner, M.R., Gallino, R.A., Leffingwell, A., Pichard, A.D., Rosenberg, J., and Lindsay, J. (1988) Circulation 78, Supp. II-634, 2527A.
23. Grigg, L.E., Kay, T., Manolas, E.G., Hunt, D., and Valentine, P.A. (1987) Circulation, 76, Supp. IV-214, 0850A.
24. Reis, G.J., Sipperly, M.E., Boucher, T.M., McCabe, C.H., Baim, D.S., Grossman, W., and Pasternak, R.C. (1988) Circulation, 78, Supp. II-291, 1159A.
25. Frick, M.H., Elo, O., Haapa, K., et al. (1987) N. Engl. J. Med. 317, 1237-1245.
26. Von Schacky, C. (1988) Ann. Intern. Med. 107, 890-899.
27. Leaf, A., and Weber, P.C. (1988) N. Engl. J. Med. 318, 549-557.
28. Zilversmit, D.B. (1979) Circulation 3, 473-485.
29. Harris, W.S., and Connor, W.E. (1980) Trans. Assoc. Am. Physic. 93, 148-154.
30. Harris, W.S., Connor, W.E., Alam, N., and Illingworth, D.R. (1988) J. Lipid Res. 29, 1451-1460.
31. Weintraub, M.S., Zechner, R., Brown, A., Eisenberg, S., and Breslow J.L. (1988) J. Clin. Invest. 82, 1884-1893.

Chapter Seven

Effect of Dietary Fat Saturation on Low Density Lipoprotein Metabolism

Robert J. Nicolosi[a], Arthur F. Stucchi[a] and Joseph Loscalzo[b]

[a]Department of Clinical Sciences
University of Lowell
Lowell, MA 01854

[b]Department of Medicine
Brigham and Women's Hospital and Harvard Medical School
Boston, MA 01854

Among the ingredients in the diet, the type of fatty acids, especially saturated fatty acids are considered to be the major contributor to hypercholesterolemia, an established risk factor of coronary heart disease (CHD). Both experimental animal and human studies have demonstrated elevations in serum cholesterol levels following increased saturated fat intake and these observations coupled with the epidemiological evidence of increased risk of CHD in populations consuming excessive amounts of saturated fatty acids explains the emphasis on the reduction of saturated fat by most health agencies.

Saturated and Omega 6 Polyunsaturated Fatty Acids

The mechanism(s) whereby saturated fatty acids, especially those of chain length C12-16 raise serum cholesterol levels has been and is currently being intensely investigated. For example, in earlier studies in which diets enriched in saturated fatty acids (SATS) were replaced by those enriched in polyunsaturated fatty acids (PUFA), the observed reductions in LDL cholesterol were associated with increased fractional catabolic rate (FCR) (1,2) or decreased production rate (3), although more recent studies in hamsters (4) and our investigations in monkeys (5) would indicated that the PUFA-induced increases in FCR of LDL may be more important. In fact, we have previously suggested that it is possible that the reported decreases in production rate or conversion of VLDL to LDL apo B may be secondary to an increase in LDL receptor uptake of LDL precursors, i.e. VLDL and VLDL remnants, thus reducing

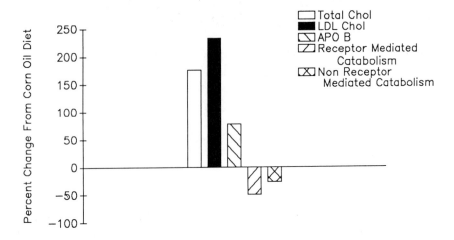

Fig. 7-1. Bar graph showing the percent increase of coconut oil fed monkeys compared to the corn oil group for total cholesterol, LDL cholesterol, and apo B and the percent decrease in receptor and nonreceptor mediated catabolism of LDL of the coconut oil fed monkeys compared to the corn oil fed monkeys.

their conversion to LDL (5). The major pathway of LDL catabolism is receptor-mediated and is influenced by both the type of dietary fatty acids and the level of dietary cholesterol. Thus Spady and Dietschy (4) showed that feeding dietary cholesterol alone to hamsters can suppress LDL uptake by LDL receptors. This decrease in LDL receptor uptake by dietary cholesterol is consistent with the decrease in mRNA levels for the LDL receptor observed in nonhuman primates fed dietary fat and cholesterol (6). However, Spady and Dietschy (7) demonstrated that the regulation of the LDL receptor by dietary cholesterol can be influenced by the accompanying type of dietary fat with saturated triglycerides down-regulating LDL receptor activity compared to unsaturated triglycerides. Along these lines, Ibrahim and McNamara (8) demonstrated decreased binding of LDL to isolated hepatocytes in SAT-fed compared to PUFA-fed guinea pigs. The ability of unsaturated fatty acids to attenuate the suppression of LDL receptor activity by SATS is also supported by the findings of increased mRNA levels for the LDL receptor in unsaturated fat-fed monkeys implying an increase in LDL receptor synthesis (9). In our non-human primate studies (5), we reported that the striking

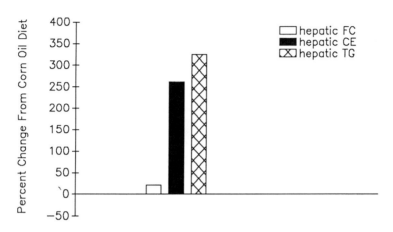

Fig. 7-2. Bar graph showing the percent increase compared to the corn oil group of coconut oil fed monkeys in hepatic free cholesterol, cholesteryl ester and triglycerides.

increase in LDL cholesterol and apo B in SAT-fed vs PUFA-fed monkeys was associated with a 50% decrease in LDL receptor activity (Fig. 7-1). Moreover, we reported that this decrease in LDL receptor activity in SAT-fed monkeys was significantly correlated with increased accumulation of hepatic cholesteryl esters and triglycerides (Fig. 7-2), which were enriched in saturated fatty acids. Thus, we proposed that these hepatic lipids enriched in saturated fatty acids can induce changes in cellular membrane lipids that could influence receptor-mediated uptake of lipoproteins. The fatty acid effects on LDL receptor activity were further investigated by evaluating the degree of LDL degradation by peripheral mononuclear cells isolated from the same cohort of SAT and PUFA-fed monkeys (10). Results from these *in vitro* studies paralleled the whole animal LDL catabolism investigations i.e., cellular LDL degradation by mononuclear cells from SAT-fed monkeys were significantly reduced (82%) compared to corn oil (Fig. 7-3). This reduction in LDL catabolism was associated with decreased enrichment of cellular PUFA and increased fluorescence polarization or decreased membrane fluidity in the mononuclear cells of SAT-fed monkeys (Fig. 7-3). While the manner in which these membrane fatty acid changes can influence LDL receptor

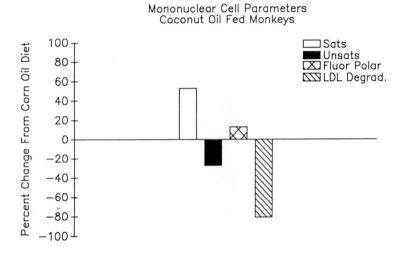

Fig. 7-3. Bar graph showing the percent increase of saturated fatty acid enrichment and fluorescence polarization of mononuclear cells of coconut oil fed monkeys and the percent decrease in unsaturated fatty acid enrichment and LDL degradation compared to mononuclear cells from corn oil fed monkeys.

activity is not known, we hypothesized that (1) changes in membrane fluidity can alter LDL receptor conformation and thus ligand affinity and/or (2) that the LDL receptor phospholipid matrix may have a specific fatty acid requirement for optimum function. The sensitivity of plasma membranes to the fatty acid-induced changes on LDL metabolism of peripheral mononuclear cells as well as monocyte cell lines has been further supported by additional studies from Loscalzo et al. (11) and Kuo et al. (12). Thus, these results suggest that dietary fatty acids along with intracellular pools of cholesterol can influence LDL metabolism.

Omega 3 Polyunsaturated Fatty Acids

There have been few findings on the effect of omega-3 PUFA on LDL metabolism. Studies in humans by Illingworth et al. (13) demonstrated that omega-3 fatty acids inhibited LDL synthesis without influencing catabolic rates. Wong and Nestel (14) found that HepG2 cells incubated in the presence of omega-3 fatty acids bound less LDL implying a decrease in LDL receptor activity. On the otherhand, Ventura et al. (15) demonstrated that receptor-mediated removal of LDL was clearly enhanced in fish-oil fed rats. Our own preliminary reported-findings in monkeys fed menhaden oil compared to SAT-feeding also noted upregulation of LDL receptor activity both *in vivo* (16) and *in vitro* (17). Thus, depending on the study, one can demonstrate either up or down regulation of LDL receptor activity with fish oil feeding indicating that much more work needs to be done in this area.

Monounsaturated Fatty Acids

While there is little argument among scientists regarding the beneficial aspects of reducing saturated fat content in the diet, there is considerable controversy concerning the type of nutrient which should replace the saturated fatty acids. Earlier studies by Hegsted et al. (18) and Keys et al. (19) found that replacing dietary saturated fatty acids with omega-6 polyunsaturated fatty acids, especially linoleic acid resulted in greater reductions of total serum cholesterol than monounsaturated fatty acids (MUFA) such as oleic acid. More recent studies in humans by Mattson and Grundy (20), Mensink and Katan (21), McDonald et al. (22) and Sirtori et al. (23) have demonstrated that replacement of dietary saturated fatty acids by MUFA resulted in reductions of LDL cholesterol that were equal to (20,22), less than (23) or greater than (21) those associated with PUFA intake. One study showed that enrichment of the American Heart Association Step 1 diet with MUFA did not add any additional benefit (24). These inconsistencies underscore the importance of much-needed further investigation. The mechanism as to how MUFA-containing diets lower LDL cholesterol when replacing SATS is not known, although Grundy (25) has postulated that the effects of MUFA are not direct but probably act to attenuate the LDL receptor suppressive effect of saturated fatty acids. However, one study *in vitro* by Kuo et al. (12) and our own preliminarily-reported studies in hamsters (26) suggest that some of these vegetable oils may have direct effects on lowering LDL independent of replacing saturated fatty acids.

References

1. Portman, O.W., Alexander, M., Tanaka, N., Saltys, P., (1976) Biochim Biophys Acta 198:55.
2. Shepherd, J., Packard, C.J., Grundy, S.M., Yeshurin, D., Gotto, A.M., Taunton, O.D., (1980) J Lipid Res 21:91.

3. Turner, J.D., Le, A.N., Brown, V.W., (1981) Am J. Physiol 241:E57.
4. Spady, D.K., Dietschy, J.M., (1988) J Clin Invest 81:300.
5. Nicolosi, R.J., Stucchi, A.F., Kowala, M.C., Hennessy, L.K., Hegsted, D.M., Schaefer, E.J., (1990) Arteriosclerosis 10:119.
6. Fox, J.C., McGill Jr., H.C., Carey, K.D., Getz, G.S., (1987) J Biol Chem 262:7014.
7. Spady, D.K., Dietschy, J.M., (1985) Proc Natl Acad Sci USA 82:4526.
8. Ibrahim, J.B.T., McNamara, D.J., (1988) Biochim Biophys Acta 963:109.
9. Sorci-Thomas, M., Wilson, M.D., Johnson, F.L., Williams, D.L., Rudel, L.L., (1989) J Biol Chem 264:9030.
10. Kuo, P.C., Rudd, M.A., Nicolosi, R.J., Loscalzo, J. (1989) Arteriosclerosis 9:919.
11. Loscalzo, J., Freedman, J.M., Rudd, M.A., Vasserman, I.B., Vaughan, D.E., (1987) Arteriosclerosis 7:450.
12. Kuo, P., Weinfeld, M., Rudd, M.A., Amarante, P., Loscalzo, J., (1990)Arteriosclerosis 10:111.
13. Illingworth, D.R., Harris, W.S., Connor, W.E., (1984) Arteriosclerosis 4:270.
14. Wong, S., Nestel, P.J., (1987) Atherosclerosis 64:139.
15. Ventura, M.A., Wollett, L.A., Spady, D.K. (1989) J Clin Invest 84:528.
16. Stucchi, A.F., Vespa, D.B., Weiner, E.J., Rogers, E.J., Terpstra, A.J.M., Nicolosi, R.J., (1990) Fed Proc 4:927a.
17. Foxall, T.L., Shwaery, G.T., Stucchi, A.F., Weiner, E.J., Nicolosi, R.J., (1990) Fed Proc 4:927a.
18. Hegsted, D.M., McGandy, R.B., Myers, M.L., Stare, F.J., (1965) Am J Clin Nutr 17:281.
19. Keys, A., (1970) Circulation 41:211.
20. Mattson, F.H., Grundy, S.M., (1985) J. Lipid Res 26:194.
21. Mensink, R.P., Katan, M.B., (1989) N Engl J Med 321:436.
22. McDonald, B.E., Gerrard, J.M., Bruce, V.M., Corner, E.J., (1989) Am J Clin Nutr 50:1382.
23. Sirtori, C.R., Tremoli, E., Getti, E., et al. (1986) Am J. Clin Nutr 449:635.
24. Ginsberg, H.N., Barr, S.L., Gilbert, A., et al. (1990) N Engl J Med 322:574.
25. Grundy, S.M., (1987) Am J Clin Nutr 45:1168.
26. Holmes, J.C., Hegsted, D.M., Nicolosi, R.J., (1990) Fed Proc 4:929a

Chapter Eight

Which Saturated Fatty Acids Raise Plasma Cholesterol Levels?

Scott M. Grundy, M.D., Ph.D.

Center for Human Nutrition
University of Texas Southwestern Medical Center at Dallas
5323 Harry Hines Boulevard
Dallas, Texas 75235-9052

Multiple lines of evidence indicate that saturated fatty acids as a class raise the plasma cholesterol level. Many epidemiologic studies strongly suggest that saturated fatty acids have this action. Among these investigations, the Seven Countries Study (1) in particular showed a high correlation between intakes of saturated acids and cholesterol levels. In addition, this action has been demonstrated beyond doubt in a host of studies carried out in carefully controlled metabolic investigations (2-7). And finally, the cholesterol-raising action of saturated fatty acids has been confirmed in laboratory animals (8). In humans, and to a lesser extent in laboratory animals, the action of saturated fatty acids to increase cholesterol levels occurs independently of dietary cholesterol.

The mechanisms whereby saturated fatty acids raise serum cholesterol have yet to be determined with certainty. Their major effect however,

TABLE 8-1

Saturated Fatty Acids in the Diet

Fatty Acid	Designation[a]
Caprylic	8:0
Caproic	10:0
Lauric	12:0
Myristic	14:0
Palmitic	16:0
Stearic	18:0

[a]The first number indicates the carbon chain length, and the second, the number of double bands in the molecule.

is on low density lipoprotein (LDL) cholesterol. In most patients, they do not increase very low density lipoproteins (VLDL) or triglycerides. Although saturated acids maintain relatively high levels of high density lipoprotein (HDL), they cannot be said to have a unique HDL-raising action. In contrast, saturated fatty acids raise LDL-cholesterol levels relative to other major nutrients, i.e., unsaturated fatty acids and carbohydrates. Just how saturates increase cholesterol levels is still under investigation. One possibility is that they enhance hepatic synthesis of apolipoprotein (apo) B-containing lipoproteins. Another is that they "down regulate" the synthesis of LDL receptors. Available data favor the latter. Isotope kinetic data in humans are compatible with this mechanism (9). More direct evidence for a reduced activity of LDL receptors comes for laboratory animals. Saturated fatty acids reduce LDL receptor-mediated clearance of LDL in both hamsters (10) and primates (11,12). Just how this occurs is not known. They could potentiate the action of intracellular cholesterol to suppress LDL-receptor synthesis; or they could modify cell membrane composition so as to interfere with normal LDL-receptor function. Regardless of the precise mechanism, dietary saturated fatty acids apparently decrease the activity of LDL receptors, and by this mechanism, they delay clearance of lipoproteins having affinity for LDL receptors. These lipoproteins include LDL itself and VLDL remnants. Receptor uptake of LDL is mediated by apo B-100. Uptake of VLDL remnants in contrast is mediated largely by apo E. Since apo E has greater affinity for LDL receptors than apo B, VLDL remnants are the preferred ligand for LDL receptors. Rapid uptake of VLDL remnants decreases the fractional conversion of VLDL to LDL, i.e., the "production rate" of LDL.

There are several different forms of saturated fatty acids in the diet. These fatty acids are shown in Table 8-1. An important and practical question is whether all saturated fatty acids raise the LDL-cholesterol level. If not, then it is inappropriate to lump all saturates together when making dietary recommendations. Several lines of evidence suggest that all saturated fatty acids do not have the same effect on LDL-cholesterol concentrations. Some may not raise the levels at all, and even among those that do increase LDL levels, the degree of rise may not be identical. Thus, to examine the actions of saturated fatty acids on LDL-cholesterol concentrations, it will be necessary to consider each fatty acid separately.

Palmitic Acid

The major saturated fatty acid in the diet of most Americans is palmitic acid. It is the predominant saturated acid in beef tallow and lard, in butter fat, and even in certain vegetable fats and oils. The percentages of palmitic acid relative to all other fatty acids in various fat sources are presented in Table 8-2. There is little doubt that palmitic acid raises the serum LDL cholesterol level compared to unsaturated fatty acids. The well-known equations of Keys et al. (3) and Hegsted et al. (4) which describe the cholesterol-raising actions of saturated fatty acids, are based mainly on palmitic acid. According to Keys et al. (3), palmitic acid raises the serum total cholesterol 2.7 mg/dl for every one percent of total calories in the total diet as palmitic acid. Similarly, Hegsted et al. (4) indicate that palmitic acid increases the total cholesterol levels by 2.16 mg/dl for every one percent of dietary calories. The results of many other studies are consistent with these equations. Since palmitic acid is the major saturated fatty acid in the diet, the application of these cholesterol-raising coefficients to saturated fatty acids apply almost exclusively to palmitic acid. It must not be assumed however that all of dietary saturated fatty acids are identical in their effect compared to palmitic acid. Although precise values are not readily available, it can be estimated that approximately two-thirds to three-fourths of all saturated fatty acids consumed by Americans are palmitic acid. For most

TABLE 8-2

Palmitic Acid Contents of Common Fats and Oils

Fat or Oil	% of Total Calories
Palm Oil	45.1
Beef Tallow	26.5
Lard	24.8
Chicken	23.2
Cocoa Butter	25.8
Cottonseed Oil	24.7
Butter Fat	26.2
Coconut Oil	8.4
Palm Kernel Oil	8.0
Corn Oil	12.2
Peanut Oil	11.6
Rapeseed Oil	3.6
Soybean Oil	11.0

Americans, this would correspond to intakes of palmitic acid of approximately 8 to 10% of total calories. According to the equation of Keys et al. (3), this level of palmitate intake should cause an average rise of serum cholesterol levels above a baseline devoid of saturates of 22 to 27 mg/dl.

Myristic Acid

Another saturated fatty acid that almost certainly raises the LDL-cholesterol level is myristic acid. However, the diet normally contains much less myristic acid than palmitic acid. The percentages of myristic acid in some of its richer sources are given in Table 8-3. Most of the myristic acid in the diet comes from butter fat; coconut oil and palm kernel oil likewise have a relatively high content. According to Keys et al. (3), myristic acid raises the cholesterol level to the same extent as palmitic acid. In contrast, Hegsted et al. (4) report that myristic acid is more hypercholesterolemic than palmitic acid. If this is true, myristic acid should contribute significantly to the hypercholesterolemic influence of butter fat and tropical oils, except palm oil. There have been no recent studies to test the relative effects of myristic acid on serum cholesterol levels in humans. In addition, no studies have been designed to

TABLE 8-3

Myristic Acid Contents of Common Fats and Oils

Fat or Oil	% of Total Calories
Palm Oil	0
Beef Tallow	3.3
Lard	1.5
Chicken	1.3
Cocoa Butter	0.1
Cottonseed Oil	0.9
Butter Fat	11.7
Coconut Oil	17.6
Palm Kernel Oil	16.0
Corn Oil	0
Peanut Oil	0.1
Rapeseed Oil	0.1
Soybean Oil	0.1

directly test the influence of this fatty acid on cholesterol levels. Such studies are needed as part of a systematic evaluation of the relative effects of all the saturated fatty acids.

Lauric Acid

The influence of lauric acid on serum cholesterol concentrations in humans remains to be defined adequately. Lauric acid is on the borderline between medium-chain and long-chain fatty acids. Some workers believe that it belongs primarily with medium-chain fatty acids which seemingly have little cholesterol-raising action, whereas others assume that lauric acid is hypercholesterolemic. Keys et al. (3) equated lauric acid with palmitic acid in its cholesterol-raising action, whereas Hegsted et al. (4) postulated that it is only mildly hypercholesterolemic.

Relatively rich sources of lauric acid are indicated in Table 8-4. Two important sources of lauric acid are coconut oil and palm kernel oil. It should be pointed out that even if the lauric acid does not have a striking hypercholesterolemic action, these oils nonetheless do possess considerable quantities of myristic and palmitic acid, both of which definitely raise the LDL-cholesterol concentration (Tables 8-2 and 8-3). Therefore,

TABLE 8-4
Lauric Acid Contents of Common Fats and Oils

Fat or Oil	% of Total Calories
Palm Oil	1.1
Beef Tallow	0.1
Lard	0.1
Chicken	0.2
Cocoa Butter	0
Cottonseed Oil	0
Butter Fat	3.1
Coconut Oil	48.5
Palm Kernel Oil	49.6
Corn Oil	0
Peanut Oil	0
Rapeseed Oil	0
Soybean Oil	0

coconut oil and palm kernel oil belong in the category of cholesterol-raising oils regardless of the action of lauric acid. These oils have the potential to raise the cholesterol level at least as much as beef fat. Indeed, one study found that coconut oil is more hypercholesterolemic than beef fat (13), a finding that suggests that the high lauric acid content of coconut oil has some cholesterol-raising potential. Nonetheless, few if any studies have been designed to directly test the influence of lauric acid on LDL-cholesterol levels.

Stearic Acid

The major sources of stearic acid are shown in Table 8-5. Since stearic acid is a long-chain fatty acid it frequently is included with the cholesterol raisers. Several lines of evidence however suggest that stearic acid does not raise the serum cholesterol level. For example, early studies showed that cocoa butter is less hypercholesterolemic than butter fat itself, even though the total saturation of the two fats is similar. Cocoa butter is very rich in stearic acid, much more so than butter fat. Subsequently, largely on the basis of studies done with cocoa butter, both Keys et al. (3) and Hegsted et al. (4) postulated that stearic acid does not raise

TABLE 8-5

Stearic Acid Contents of Common Fats and Oils

Fat or Oil	% of Total Calories
Palm Oil	4.7
Beef Tallow	21.6
Lard	12.3
Chicken	6.4
Cocoa Butter	34.5
Cottonseed Oil	2.3
Butter Fat	12.5
Coconut Oil	2.5
Palm Kernel Oil	2.4
Corn Oil	2.2
Peanut Oil	3.1
Rapeseed Oil	1.9
Soybean Oil	4.0

the cholesterol level. Other studies in humans and experimental animals appeared to confirm this result. Even so, these studies were largely ignored, in dietary recommendations (14-16) and in Food and Drug Administration labeling, stearic acid has not been removed from the list of cholesterol-raising saturated fatty acids.

Because of lingering uncertainties about the effects of stearic acid, we carried out a study to more directly determine the action of stearic acid on cholesterol levels (7). A synthetic fat was produced by chemical randomization between a completely saturated soy bean oil and high-oleic safflower oil so that the stearic acid content was approximately 45%. The remainder of the fatty acids in this product were predominantly oleic acid, with about 5% palmitic acid. This synthetic fat was compared with palm oil, which has about 45% palmitic acid, and with high-oleic safflower oil, which is mainly oleic acid. The study was carried out in 11 patients under metabolic ward conditions. The results of the study showed that stearic acid did not raise the total cholesterol (or LDL cholesterol) compared to oleic acid, whereas palmitic acid markedly increased cholesterol concentrations. No other lipoprotein fraction was changed by stearic acid compared to either palmitic or oleic acids. Thus, we concluded that previous conclusions were correct; namely, stearic acid does not raise the serum cholesterol level, and more specifically, it does not increase the LDL-cholesterol concentration.

An interesting question is why stearic acid does not raise the cholesterol level. There are at least two possibilities. First, the absorption of stearic acid might be incomplete, as some workers have suggested (17). Or second, stearic acid might be rapidly converted to oleic acid in the body. We recently eliminated the first possibility by examining the fatty acid composition of chylomicron lipids following administration of a fatty meal in which stearic acid was one component (18). The percentage stearic acid in chylomicron lipids was similar to that of the dietary fat. If the absorption of stearic acid had been less than that of other dietary fatty acids, the percentage stearic acid in chylomicron lipids should have been reduced. Since this did not occur, we must assume that stearic acid is absorbed approximately as well as other fatty acids. Therefore, the lack of a cholesterol-raising action of stearic acid cannot be attributed to a lack of absorption.

The second possibility is that stearic acid is rapidly converted to oleic acid in the body. In a study in rats (19), stearic acid was found to be rapidly transformed to oleic acid, whereas palmitic acid was not. For palmitic acid to be converted to oleic acid, two steps are required—

chain elongation and desaturation. Seemingly chain elongation is a slow step, but desaturation is rapid. Thus, stearic acid is quickly converted to oleic acid, which could account for its lack of a hypercholesterolemic effect. In contrast, palmitic acid remains a saturated fatty acid for a prolonged period, and presumably this allows for it to exert an hypercholesterolemic effect. In our study (7), we found no evidence for accumulation of stearic acid in plasma lipids on the high-stearate diet even though relatively large quantities were absorbed; instead the oleic acid content of plasma lipids was increased, suggesting conversion of stearic into oleic acid. Although our results are not definitive, they nonetheless are suggestive that rapid conversion to oleic acid prevents a hypercholesterolemic action of stearic acid.

Medium-Chain Fatty Acids

These fatty acids include caprylic acid and caproic acid. They are present in moderate amounts in butter fat. Early studies suggested that they raised the serum cholesterol level, perhaps more than long-chain fatty acids. Subsequently however this concept was changed. Currently it is believed that they do not raise cholesterol levels. This belief comes from research in both animals (20) and humans (21). Seemingly, they act more like carbohydrates than saturated fatty acids, and whereas they do not raise cholesterol levels, they apparently can increase triglyceride concentrations when fed in large amounts. Nonetheless, the medium-chain fatty acids do have potential for replacement of long-chain, cholesterol-raising fatty acids in the diet. Their use for this purpose however has never been developed commercially.

Trans Unsaturated Fatty Acids

When vegetable oils undergo hydrogenation, a portion of linoleic acid is completely saturated to produce stearic acid. Another portion is converted to monounsaturated fatty acids, both of *cis* and *trans* varieties. Since the location of the single double bond can migrate during hydrogenation, several different *cis and trans* isomers are produced. The metabolic effects of *trans* fatty acids have not been fully determined. A few studies suggest that they raise the serum cholesterol level, whereas other investigations indicate that they do not. To resolve this question, further research is required. If it should turn out that *trans* monounsaturated fatty acids are cholesterol raisers, then they should be in groups with the cholesterol-increasing saturated fatty acids when dietary recommendations are made. Moreover, consideration still should be given to the possibility that these fatty acids have other effects, although to date, none have been identified.

Responsiveness to Saturated Fatty Acids

Another question of considerable interest is whether individuals vary in their responsiveness to saturated fatty acids. In other words, do some individuals develop marked increases in their cholesterol levels when moderately high intakes of saturated fatty acids are consumed, whereas others do not? If there are high responders to saturated fatty acids, what is the reason? Is hyperresponsiveness a genetic condition, or is it acquired? Before these questions can even be asked, however, the basic question of individual variation in cholesterol response to saturated fatty acids must be resolved. Some workers believe that for humans the individual variation in responsiveness is relatively small (22-24). In contrast, studies from our laboratory suggest that it may be considerable (25). This issue appears to be important, because if some hypercholesterolemic people are responsive to removal of saturated fatty acids, then dietary modification clearly will be the predominant mode of therapy. On the other hand, for nonresponders, drug therapy may be required. Further research on this interesting question therefore is definitely needed.

Role of Overnutrition

There is another way in which saturated fatty acids of all types may be cholesterol raisers. If they are consumed in excess, in conjunction with other dietary constituents, the result will be a state of overnutrition and obesity. There is increasing evidence that obesity raises the LDL cholesterol level in many people (26-31). The primary mechanism appears to be an overproduction of lipoproteins by the liver (32,33). In fact, high intakes of saturated fatty acids in obese individuals should raise the serum cholesterol in two ways. First, saturated fatty acids contribute to the overproduction of lipoproteins by obesity; and second, they specifically reduce the activity of LDL receptors, accentuating the hypercholesterolemic response.

In summary, the above considerations indicate clearly that all saturated fatty acids do not have the same effects on the metabolism of cholesterol and lipoproteins. In particular, stearic acid and medium chain fatty acids do not raise the LDL-cholesterol level. Further, lauric acid has not been proven to raise cholesterol concentrations, although it probably has at least a modest cholesterol-raising action. Two saturates—palmitic acid and myristic acid undoubtedly increase LDL-cholesterol concentrations, and when dietary recommendations are made for the purpose of lowering cholesterol levels, primary attention should be given to removing these two fatty acids from the diet. The extent to which this guideline extends to lauric acid and *trans* monounsaturated fatty acids awaits further research.

References

1. Keys, A., (1970) *Circulation.* 41: (Suppl 1).
2. Ahrens, E.H., Hirsch, J., Insull, W., Tsaltas, T.T., Blomstrand, R., and Peterson, M.L., (1957) *Lancet.* 1: 943.
3. Keys, A., Anderson, J.T., and Grande, F., (1965) *Metabolism.* 14: 776.
4. Hegsted, D.M., Mc Gandy, R.B., Myers, M.L., and Stare, F.J., (1965) *Am. J. Clin. Nutr.* 17: 281.
5. Mattson, F.H., and Grundy, S.M., (1985) *J. Lipid Res.* 26: 194.
6. Grundy, S.M., (1986) *N. Engl. J. Med.* 314: 745.
7. Bonanome, A., and Grundy, S.M., (1988) *N. Engl. J. Med.* 318: 1244.
8. Spady, D.K., and Dietschy, J.M., (1988) *J. Clin. Invest.* 81: 300.
9. Shepherd, J., Packard, C.J., Grundy, S.M., Yeshurun, D., Gotto, Jr., A.M., and Taunton, O.D., (1980) *J. Lipid Res.* 21: 91.
10. Spady, D.K., and Dietschy, J.M., (1985) *Proc. Natl. Acad. Sci. U.S.A.* 82: 4526.
11. Fox, J.C., Mc Gill, Jr., H.C., Carey, K.D., and Getz, G.S., (1987) *J. Biol. Chem.* 262: 7014.
12. Nicolosi, R.J., Stucchi, A.F., Kowala, M.C., Hennessy, L.K., Hegsted, D.M., and Schaefer, E.J., (1990) *Arteriosclerosis.* 10: 119.
13. Reiser, R., Probstfield, J.L., Silvers, A., Scott, L.W., Shorney, M.L., Wood, R.D., O'Brian, B.C., Gotto, Jr., A.M., and Insull, W., (1985) *Am. J. Clin. Nutr.* 42: 190.
14. Grundy, S.M., Bilheimer, D., Blackburn, H., Brown, W.V., Kwiterovich, P.O., Mattson, F., Schonfeld, G., and Weidman, W.H., (1982) *Circulation.* 65: 839A.
15. The Expert Panel. Report of the National Cholesterol Education Program Expert Panel on detection, evaluation, and treatment of high blood cholesterol in adults. (1988) *Arch. Intern. Med.* 148: 36.
16. Committee on Diet and Health, Food and Nutrition Board, Commission on Life Sciences, National Research Council, Washington, D.C. (1989)
17. Apgar, J.L., Shively, C.A., and Tarka, Jr., S.M., (1987) *J. Nutr.* 117: 660.
18. Bonanome, A., and Grundy, S.M., (1989) *J. Nutr.* 119: 1556.
19. Elovson, J., (1965) *Biochim. Biophys. Acta.* 106: 480.

20. Grande, F., (1962) *J Nutr.* 76: 255.
21. Hashim, S.A., Arteaga, A., and Van Itallie, T.B., (1960) *Lancet.* 1: 1105.
22. Beynen, A.C., and Katan, M.B., (1985) *Atherosclerosis.* 57: 19.
23. Katan, M.B., Beynen, A.C., De Vries, J.H., and Nobels, A., (1986) *Am. J. Epidemiol.* 123: 221.
24. Katan, M.B., and Beynen, A.C., (1987) *Am J Epidemiol.* 125: 387.
25. Grundy, S.M., and Vega, G.L., (1988) *Am. J. Clin. Nutr.* 47: 822.
26. Ashley, Jr., F.W., Jr., and Kannel, W.B., (1974) *J Chron Dis.* 27: 103.
27. Kannel, W.B., Gordon, T., and Castelli, W.P., (1979) *Am. J. Clin. Nutr.* 32: 1238.
28. Garrison, R.J., Wilson, P.W., Castelli, W.P., Feinleib, M., Kannel, W.B., and McNamara, P.M., (1980) *Metabolism.* 29: 1053.
29. Shekelle, R.B., Shryock, A.M., Paul, O., Lepper, M., Stamler, J., Liu, S., and Raynor, Jr., W.J., (1981) *N. Engl. J. Med.* 304: 65.
30. Stamler, J., in *Medical Complications of Obesity*, edited by Lewis, B., and Contaldo, F., Academic Press, London, 1979, pp. 191-216.
31. Anderson, J.T., Lawler, A., and Keys, A., (1957) *J. Clin. Invest.* 36: 81.
32. Kesaniemi, Y.A., Beltz, W.F., and Grundy, S.M., (1985) *J. Clin. Invest.* 76: 586.
33. Egusa, G., Beltz, W.F., Grundy, S.M., and Howard, B.V., (1985) *J. Clin. Invest.* 76: 596.

Chapter Nine
Effects Of Dietary Fatty Acids On Blood Pressure: Epidemiology And Biochemistry

Howard R. Knapp, M.D., Ph.D.
Department of Internal Medicine
University of Iowa
Iowa City, IA 52242

Recently, there has been a renewed interest in non-pharmacological management of mild hypertension, especially in view of the lack of demonstrable cardiac benefit in treating patients diagnosed as having this condition with anti-hypertensive medications (1,2). Considerable controversy has emerged from the trials of dietary polyunsaturated fat supplementation for the purpose of lowering blood pressure. Differences in study design, patient selection criteria, and the dose or duration of the supplementation may account for some of the discrepancies. This paper will focus mainly upon the effects of n-3 polyunsaturates with occasional comparisons made to the effects of the n-6 class.

Although most of the early studies on the vascular effects of n-3 fatty acid supplements suffered from significant design problems (3), recently there have been both carefully controlled investigations of a small number of hypertensive patients (4) as well as a population-based intervention trial (5). Both have supported the hypothesis that this class of polyunsaturates exerts favorable effects on vascular tone and blood pressure control in humans. The clinical trials of n-3 fatty acids in lowering the blood pressure of Western subjects have been reviewed recently (6). The original stimulus for investigating the vascular benefits of n-3 fatty acids in Western subjects, however, was the observation of low rates of vascular disease in Greenland Eskimos despite a diet which was as high in fat content as is Westerners (7). It would be worthwhile, therefore, to examine the epidemiologic evidence for hypotensive properties of diets high in marine oils.

Epidemiology of n-3 Fatty Acids and Blood Pressure
There are several problems in the interpretation of data correlating dietary components and blood pressure in populations. Studies be-

tween population groups often attempt to single out the consumption of specific nutrient items, but it is rare to find different groups of people whose diets are identical except for the particular nutrient in question. Most populations eating diets with a high fish content, for example, also have a high salt intake which might counteract any blood pressure-lowering effect of fish. In addition, genetic adaptation to particular dietary components may occur so that dietary items could have different metabolic effects on diverse population groups. The high intake of marine lipids over many generations by Eskimos, for example, might result in such a diet having fewer or different long-term effects on them than in Western subjects.

Since people eat foods and not isolated nutrients, it is important to keep in mind that many nutrients have a high degree of association in the diet. Frequently there is a strong correlation between a number of nutrients; people with a high dietary intake of marine lipids, for example, will also have a high intake of other nutrients associated with seafood which may have unknown effects on blood pressure. Ingestion of particular nutrients can also be indirectly related to social factors which can have an independent effect on blood pressure, such as alcohol consumption, activity level or percent of calories derived from fat. Diet-health data from population studies are also limited by the inaccuracies of measuring both the intakes of various nutrients and the health parameters in question, such as blood pressure. Because of these inherent difficulties in accumulating a data base from this type of population survey, mechanistic interpretations of epidemiologic data must be made cautiously. Such data are very useful in finding associations and generating hypotheses, but these must be tested in carefully controlled dietary intervention studies. Some of the difficulties which have confounded epidemiologic studies of the relationship between diet and blood pressure are:

- Comparisons of groups with different disease prevalences and longevity due to varied public health levels.
- Genetic differences in response to specific nutrients.
- Inaccuracy of estimates of dietary composition and intake.
- Confounding effects of social and environmental factors.
- Different methods and accuracies of blood pressure measurement.

Despite the difficulties in interpreting population surveys, some interesting observations have been made between population groups and also with changes in diet and health parameters of certain countries.

The last decade of research on possible health benefits of n-3 fatty acids was prompted by observations on Eskimos, but even when many of the initial investigations were being made in the 1940s, most members of this ethnic group had been heavily exposed to Western foods, diseases and equipment, and had begun to move away from their traditional harsh lifestyle. Although it is often mentioned in review articles that Eskimos do not get hypertension (8), this impression appears to derive from anecdotal data on patients in hospitals. The first large survey of more than 1000 Eskimos living in remote villages found in 1948 that their systolic blood pressure was slightly higher than that of a reference population living in a similarly harsh climate in Finland (9). Also, it was noted that the Eskimos' blood pressure had a similar age-related increase to that usually associated with Western societies consuming diets high in fat and salt (10).

This author (9), like other Medical Officers working in Greenland, was impressed with the premature aging of the Eskimos and their average life expectancy of 26 years. This was attributed to their primitive lifestyle, severe climate and poorly balanced diet lacking in fresh fruits and vegetables. She noted that only half of the Eskimos considered to have systolic pressures greater than 170 mm Hg had diastolic hypertension as well, and felt that this was due to early loss of arterial compliance with the Eskimos' accelerated aging process, a frequent finding among elderly Western patients. The Eskimos' lower incidence of atherosclerotic vascular disease was also largely attributed to their shorter lifespan, with only 10% living over the age of 50, compared to 36% of the population in Finland. Similar data were recorded in a 1980 survey of nearly 500 Eskimos living in remote villages, where the same distribution of blood pressure and age-related increase were found as in the Copenhagen heart study (11). Finally, a recent survey of mortality statistics in Greenland showed that there was no statistically significant difference between the mortality of male or female Greenlanders from hypertensive diseases and that of their Danish counterparts (12).

There is less data on the blood pressures of Alaskan Eskimos, but a 1958 survey of coastal inhabitants found values that were on average, higher than those expected for Caucasian Americans (13). An interesting autopsy series of native Alaskans published at about the same time suggested similar patterns of mortality from heart and vascular disease for Eskimos and Caucasian Americans, and noted evidence for hypertensive arteriolonephrosclerosis in a number of Eskimo cases (14). This finding is in contrast to the retrospective hospital chart review of Greenland Eskimos from 1950-1974 which indicated much lower rates of cardiovascular disease, but more strokes, among the Eskimos than would occur in a comparable population in Denmark (15). Another autopsy series of Alaskan natives performed between 1958 and 1968 indicated a low incidence of vascular disease; but noted more than twice as many cerebrovascular as cardiovascular deaths (16).

The issue of excess numbers of strokes in populations with a high fish consumption sounds a cautionary note in an otherwise optimistic picture of vascular benefits of n-3 fatty acid ingestion by Western people. The relationship between blood pressure, prolonged bleeding time and stroke remains uncertain, as the clinical distinction between cerebral thrombosis and hemorrhage is not clear, and diagnostic equipment was nearly non-existent in remote areas of Greenland or Alaska. The Japanese, however, have a higher consumption of seafood than is ever likely to be achieved in Western societies, and their prevalence of hypertension and incidence of stroke are among the highest in the world (17). With relatively good access to diagnostic facilities, their data on disease patterns and the marked changes in the Japanese diet in the last several decades has afforded the opportunity to make some valuable observations.

A recent report from the Honolulu Heart study provided a strong indication that the traditional Japanese diet, low in animal products and high in marine foods and salt, was correlated with the development of cerebrovascular atherosclerosis (18). Longitudinal data from Japan has found marked reductions in both bood pressure and stroke, as the consumption of animal products increased and salt declined (19). The consumption of fish, however, is not believed to have changed much in the past 20 years (20). This appears to incriminate high salt intake, with resultant hypertension, rather than high n-3 fatty acid intake as the major cause of the high stroke rate in this population. Interestingly, an epidemiologic survey in Japan found that fishermen did not have higher rates of cerebrovascular events than did farmers, who consumed only one-third as much fish but similar amounts of salt (21). Other data has indicated lower stroke rates among fishermen than farmers in Japan, but blood pressure and salt intake have been found to be higher among the latter group in other studies (22). Migration studies have shown that Okinawans moving to the United States and adopting Western dietary patterns have increased all of their cardiac risk factors except blood pressure, which declines. Yet another comparison in Oriental populations found that Taiwanese fishermen consuming largely fish had a higher intake of sodium and higher blood pressure than did farmers in

Taiwan (24). From these observations, one must at least surmise that the hypertensive effects of a high salt intake cannot be counteracted by high dietary n-3 fatty acids.

A recent survey that may be more pertinent to questions of n-3 fatty acid intake in Western populations was reported from Norway (25). In one district, the investigators compared blood pressure and cardiovascular events in subjects living on the coast with those living inland. There was no difference found in the blood pressures of the two groups, and the coastal population may have had slightly higher rates of vascular events. The blood pressure results of this survey contrast with those of a population-based intervention study in Norway on the efffects of fish oil in blood pressure (5). These workers found that subjects indicating a habitually high intake of fish had lower blood pressures at the initiation of the study, and had no further blood pressure lowering with fish oil supplements. On the other hand, subjects who had low amounts of fish in their diets, similar to those studied in the United States (4), had a significant reduction in blood pressure with the n-3 fatty acid supplements. These findings are of great interest in understanding the possible mechanisms of the antihypertensive effects of n-3 fatty acids.

Biochemical Aspects of N-3 Fatty Acid Effects

Unlike other dietary lipid components, a small portion of polyunsaturated fatty acids of both the n-6 and n-3 classes are converted in the body to extremely potent autacoids. Primarily, such bioactive compounds are produced from 20-carbon (eicosanoic) fatty acids, and as a result are often referred to as "eicosanoids". Since eicosapentaenoic acid (EPA) is identical to arachidonic acid with an additional n-3 double bond, it can be converted to an analogous series of eicosanoids the same as those from arachidonate, but with retention of the extra unsaturation. Dietary EPA appears to be metabolized by the separate eicosanoid pathways to a different extent in various organs; in some cases there is little production of EPA-derived compounds and reduced amounts of the ones produced from the competing "usual" substrate, arachidonate (26,27). In other cases, EPA forms eicosanoids easily without reducing the synthesis of those from arachidonic acid (4,28,29). In terms of biological activity, the EPA- and AA-derived analogs sometimes have similar actions and potency (i.e. PGI_2 and PGI_3), whereas other analogs have qualitatively or quantitatively different activity (i.e. TxA_2 and TxA_3). Many of the alterations in the synthesis and actions of endogenous eicosanoids, therefore, have been considered to explain physiologi-

TABLE 9-1

Possible Effects of N-3 Fatty Acid Changes in Eicosanoids

1. Direct reduction in reactivity to endogenous vasoconstrictors.
2. Decreased activity of the renin-angiotensin system.
3. Increased efficiency of excess salt and water clearance.
4. Decreased peripheral sympathetic tone.
5. Lowering of cardiac output or baroreceptor settings.

cal changes observed during polyunsaturated fatty acid supplementation. With regards to vascular function in particular, prostaglandins, thromboxanes, leukotrienes and epoxides of arachidonic acid are known to have many effects on vascular smooth muscle, renal function and renin release, and regional blood flow (Table 9-1), so it has frequently been assumed that changes in vascular parameters associated with altered dietary intake of polyunsaturates would be due to changes in the amounts or types of eicosanoids produced in the body. This hypothesis had not been tested directly, until we examined the excretion of urinary metabolites of thromboxane, prostacyclin and prostaglandin E_2 during the dietary supplementation with n-6 or n-3 polyunsaturates to white males with mild essential hypertension (4). Using ambulatory blood pressure monitors, we were able to demonstrate that high doses (50 ml/day) of menhaden oil, but not safflower oil or low-dose (10 ml/day) menhaden oil, had a significant antihypertensive effect over the four weeks of the supplementation period, and we attempted to correlate these changes with those of several urinary metabolites of vasoactive eicosanoids.

The excretion of the thromboxane metabolite by the hypertensive subjects showed a small but statistically significant reduction during supplementation with high-dose fish oil. We have found previously that the elevated thromboxane synthesis of atherosclerotic patients is markedly lowered by this fish oil regimen, in association with the amelioration of other indices of accelerated platelet turnover (28). The otherwise healthy hypertensive individuals, however, excreted normal amounts of this metabolite at baseline (4), and the reduction with fish oil ingestion was much less than that seen with low-dose aspirin (30). Aspirin has been found to exacerbate essential hypertension (31), and while selective thromboxane synthase inhibitors have been reported to attenuate hypertensive responses in some animal models (32), blood pressure lowering has not been reported in clinical trials of these agents.

On the other hand, in pregnancy-induced hypertension excess thromboxane production and platelet turnover do occur, and the blood pressure increase is markedly blunted by platelet-selective, low doses of aspirin (33). This situation is, therefore, clearly different from essential hypertension, and it would seem unlikely that the modest reduction we saw in thromboxane metabolite excretion would account for the lowering of blood pressure in our subjects.

Prostaglandin E_2 is known to be important for renal function (34) and this vasodilator is a major product of the microvascular endothelium (35). We measured the excretion of its major urinary metabolite (PGE-M,36) in our hypertensive subjects and found a non-significant trend towards lower values in those taking high-dose fish oil and slightly increased excretion in the subjects taking safflower oil, who did not have any significant change in blood pressure during the study (4). No evidence for a metabolite derived from PGE_3 was obtained. This index of systemic PGE synthesis, therefore, suggested opposite changes in PGE synthesis to those one would expect if increased PGE synthesis were involved in the lowering of blood pressure by fish oil. Other workers have also noted a similar trend to lower excretion of this metabolite in normotensive subjects taking fish oil supplements(37). This metabolite does not reflect PGE synthesis by the kidneys or other organs not readily accessible to the vasculature. Technical problems have hampered the accurate determination of urinary PGE compounds, and several small studies have reported lower excretion of urinary PGE in subjects taking fish oil (37,38), but the number of subjects was too small for statistical analysis. To understand more about the effects of fish oil on endogenous PGE synthesis, we measured the concentrations of the 1-, 2- and 3-series PGE and PGF compounds in seminal plasma of 10 subjects before and after one month of high-dose fish oil supplementation (39). The results were fairly similar to that from the systemic metabolite, with significant lowering of the n-6 fatty acid-derived 1- and 2-series compounds, and small increases in the low concentrations of 3-series ones from eicosapentaenoic acid. Thus, fish oil supplementation may act in some organs to cause cyclooxygenase inhibition. When occurring systemically as the result of cyclooxygenase-inhibiting drugs, this action is well-known to increase blood pressure and antagonize the actions of antihypertensive medications, and could not account for a lowering of blood pressure by fish oils.

The last eicosanoid metabolite assessed in our blood pressure study (4) was that of prostacyclin. Both PGI_2 (from arachidonate) and PGI_3

(from EPA) are potent vasodilators, and the synthesis of total prostacyclin metabolites increased sharply in the first week of high-dose fish oil supplementation, but did not change significantly in the other groups whose blood pressure did not change during the study. This increase was entirely due to the synthesis of PGI_3 from the EPA in the fish oil supplement. As the supplementation continued and blood pressure fell, so did the excretion of prostacyclin metabolites until, by week 4 of the fish oil period when blood pressure was at its lowest, total prostacyclin metabolites were the same as they had been during the baseline period, only now 29% of the prostacyclin being made was PGI_3 from the EPA. No rebound increase in PGI_2-M occurred when the subjects' blood pressures returned to their baseline high values after withdrawal of the fish oil, and it can be concluded that although the initial surge of prostacyclin synthesis might have altered other vasoactive hormone systems, a continued high output of this vasodilator could not be responsible for the lowering of blood pressure by fish oil.

From the above studies, it seems that changes in cyclooxygenase products are unlikely to explain the hypotensive effects of fish oil. Recently, epoxides generated by cytochrome P-450 from arachidonate have been intensively studied in regards to their renal vascular and functional effects, as well as their actions on other vascular beds (40). We have determined that similar epoxides of eicosapentaenoic acid appear in sizable quantities in the urine of volunteers ingesting n-3 fatty acid supplements (41), and it is possible that this class of compounds may provide some of the answers to a number of our questions about the vascular effects of dietary n-3 fatty acid supplements.

Fish Oils and Vascular Reactivity

Several review articles have mentioned that dietary fish oil reduces vascular reactivity in man (42,43), but only a small number of published studies deal with this question. Both human and animal studies have shown that the endogenous synthesis of prostaglandins attenuates the contractile response of blood vessels *in vivo* and *in vitro*, lending further support to the notion that changes in these local hormones mediate the vascular effects of dietary fish oil. The factors regulating *in vitro* vascular muscle responses to vasoconstrictors are complex, and the local control of prostaglandin synthesis is not limited under normal *in vivo* conditions by substrate availability. Therefore, since dietary modification of the prostaglandin precursor pool with precursor fatty acids would also change dietary fat content and other aspects of lipid metabolism, it could influence vascular reactivity in ways not directly attributable to increased or decreased release of prostaglandins. It has been found, for example, that aortae of rats fed fish oil have decreased responsiveness to vasoconstrictors (44), but similar results were obtained in another study in which the animals were fed n-6 fatty acid-rich safflower oil (45). Since dietary fish oil has been reported to decrease prostaglandin production *in vitro* (26,27) and safflower oil to increase it (46), such data are difficult to reconcile on the basis of prostaglandin synthesis alone.

A biochemical study on fish oil supplementation in male volunteers was the first to include an assessment of the effect of the n-3 fatty acids on the response to vasopressor infusions (47). Although the control values were obtained "randomly" before or after the fish oil period and the subjects were not on controlled diets, a small but statistically significant decrease was observed in the systolic pressure response to a 15 minute norepinephrine infusion. There was also a non-significant trend towards a lessened response to angiotensin II, despite an apparent increase in sodium excretion (and, presumably, intake). This is an interesting change, since in this setting (and with the observed reduction in plasma renin activity) one might expect an increase in angiotensin sensitivity. No alteration in catecholamine or prostaglandin excretion was noted, although there was a trend toward reduced excretion of the latter.

An investigation of mildly hypertensive subjects on a mackerel diet found it lowered blood pressure, but did not reduce the pressor response in a standardized psychophysiological stress test (48), indicating an unaltered responsiveness to endogenous catecholamines. Two other recent studies have confirmed this finding; neither the forearm vasoconstriction while rubbing ice over the carotid artery (49) nor the arterial pressure increase with hand immersion in ice water (50) was altered by fish oil supplementation. We have also performed a study of the effects of fish oil supplements on the response to increasing phenylephrine infusion rates in white males with mild essential hypertension (51). The subjects had a statistically significant reduction in systolic and diastolic pressures, and underwent infusion of this pure alpha adrenergic agonist at the end of their 4-week fish oil period and after 4 weeks of recovery off the supplement. Urine samples were collected before and at the end of each infusion study for measurement of prostacyclin metabolites in order to assess the role of this endogenous vasodilator in any alteration of response. The pressor response to moderate phenylephrine infusion rates (0.5 ug/kg/min) was about the same as that found in the norepinephrine infusion study mentioned earlier (47) but no difference was seen in our subjects on the two occasions. As the phenylephrine infusion rate was increased to 0.75 ug/kg/min, the subjects appeared to have a reflex bradycardia at lower arterial pressures, and so did not achieve as high a pressure during the infusion on that occasion. This sort of resetting of baroreceptors would be consistent with their actually having a chronic reduction in their blood pressures while on the fish oil (52), and this phenomenon has been noted in dogs after about 4 days of reduced pressure. Interestingly, the subjects made less prostacyclin during the infusion study done while they were on fish oil, during which lower pressures were achieved. This indicates that the lessened pressor response during fish oil ingestion cannot be related to enhanced release of this vasodepressor by the arteries. That altered prostacyclin release is not involved in this change is also consistent with animal studies finding that prostacyclin infusion can attenuate baroreflex tachycardia, but has no influence on bradycardia (53). Further studies with direct monitoring of hemodynamic parameters in subjects with known cation balance and renin status will help to elucidate the basis for these results, as well as whether dietary fish oil can directly alter alpha adrenergic responses in the human heart as it has been reported to do in rats (54).

Future Directions

There is a lack of epidemiologic support for the idea that high dietary intake of marine products leads to lower blood pressure or to less cerebrovascular disease, but any beneficial effects of n-3 polyunsaturated fatty acids could be obscured by the hypertensive influence of other dietary components, especially salt. It appears that chronic intake of more than 3.0 g n-3 fatty acids per day can reduce blood pressure in humans, and this does not clearly relate to altered systemic release of cyclooxygenase products of arachidonic or eicosapentaenoic acids, or to an altered response to catecholamines. Whether the hypotensive effect occurs via an entirely eicosanoid-independent mechanism or is related to newly discovered epoxides of n-3 polyunsaturates is the focus of much current work. A better understanding of the many effects of this fatty acid class in man will allow us to determine the eventual health benefits to be gained by their enhanced consumption in Western societies.

Acknowledgments

This work was supported in part by a grant from the National Institutes of Health, HL-35380. Dr. Knapp is an Established Investigator of the American Heart Association.

References

1. Freis, E.D., (1982) N. Eng. J. Med. 307, 306-309.
2. Medical Research Council Working Party on Mild Hypertension (1988) Br. Heart J. 59, 364-378.
3. Knapp, H.R., Whittemore, K.L., and FitzGerald, G.A., (1987) in AOCS Short Course of Polyunsaturated Fatty Acids and Eicosanoids, Lands, W.E.M., pp. 41-55, American Oil Chemists' Society, Champaign, IL.
4. Knapp, H.R., FitzGerald, G.A., (1989) N. Engl. J. Med. 320, 1037-1043.
5. Bonaa, K.H., Bjerve, K.S., Straume, B., Gram, I.T., Thelle, D., (1990) N. Engl. J. Med. 322, 795-801.
6. Knapp, H.R., (1989) Nutr. Rev. 47, 301-313.
7. Sinclair, H.M., (1953) Proc. Nutr. Soc. 12, 69-82.
8. Dahl, L.K., (1972) Am. J. Clin. Nutr. 25, 231-244.
9. Ehrström, I., (1951) Acta Med. Scand. 151,416-422.
10. Prior, I.A.M., Evans, J.G., Harvey, H.P.B., Davidson, F., Lindsey, M., (1968) N. Engl. J. Med. 279, 515-520.
11. Kromann, N., Thygesen, K., Harvald, B., (1980) Ugeskr. Laeg 142, 2278-2281.
12. Bjerregaard, P., Dyerberg, J., (1988) Int. J. Epidemiol. 17, 514-519.
13. Scott, E.M., Griffith, I.V., Hoskins, D.D., Whaley, R.D., (1958) Lancet i, 667-668.
14. Gottmann, A.W., (1960) Arch. Path. 70, 131-138.
15. Kromann, N., Green, A., (1980) Acta. Med. Scand. 208, 401-406.
16. Arthaud, J.B., (1970) Arch. Path. 90, 433-438.
17. Omae, T., Ueda, K., (1988) J. Hypertension 6, 343-349.
18. Reed, D.M., Resch, J.A., Hayashi, T., MacLean, C., Yano, K., (1988) Stroke 19, 820-825.
19. Shimamoto, T., Komachi, Y., Inada, H., Doi, M., Iso, H., Sato, S., Kitamura, A., Iida, M., Konishi, M., Nakanishi, N., Terao, A., Naito, Y., Kojima, S., (1988) Circulation 79, 503-515.
20. Nutrition Section, Ministry of Health and Welfare: National Nutrition Survey, 1969, 1975, 1983. Tokyo, Daiichi Shuppan Publishers, 1973, 1978, 1985.
21. Omoto, M., Sawamura, T., Hara, H., (1984) Japanese J. Hygiene 38, 887-898.
22. Kagawa, Y., Nishizawa, M., Suzuki, M., Miyatake, T., Hamamoto, T., Goto, K., Motonaga, E., Izumikawa, H., Hirata, H., Ebihara, A., (1982) J. Nutr. Sci.

Vitaminol. 28, 441-453.
23. Prior, I.A.M. (1984) in *Nutritional Prevention of Cardiovascular Diseases*, Lovenberg, W. and Yamori, Y., Academic Press, New York, pp. 137-153.
24. Tseng, W-P., (1967) Am. J. Epidemiol. 86, 513-525.
25. Simonsen, T., Vartun, A., Lyngmo, V., Nordoy, A., (1987) Acta. Med. Scand. 222, 237-245.
26. Croft, K.D., Beilin, L.J., Legge, F.M., Vandongen, R., (1987) Lipids 22, 647-650.
27. Hornstra, G., Crist-Hazelhof, E., Haddeman, E., ten Hoor, F., Nugteren, D.H., (1981) Prostaglandins 21, 727-738.
28. Knapp, H.R., Reilly, I.A.G., Alessandrini, P., FitzGerald, G.A., (1986) N. Engl. J. Med. 314, 937-942.
29. Fischer, S., Weber, P.C., (1984) Nature 307, 165-168.
30. Knapp, H.R., Healy, C., Lawson, J., FitzGerald, G.A., (1988) Thromb. Res. 50, 377-386.
31. Dunn, M.J., Gröne, H-J., (1985) Adv. Prost. Thromb. Leuk. Res. 13, 179-187.
32. Uderman, H.D., Jackson, E.K., Puett, D., Workman, R.J., (1984) J. Cardiovasc. Pharmacol. 6, 969-972.
33. Fitzgerald, D.J., FitzGerald, G.A., (1990) in *Hypertension: Pathophysiology, Diagnosis, and Management*, Laragh, J.H. and Brenner, B.M., pp. 1789-1807, Raven Press, New York.
34. Jackson, E.K., Branch, R.A., Margolius, H.S., Oates, J.A. (1985) in *The Kidney: Physiology and Pathophysiology*, Seldin, D.W. and Geibisch, G., pp. 613-643, Raven Press, New York.
35. Gerritsen, ME., Parks, T.P., Printz, M.P., (1980) Biochim. Biophys. Acta 619, 196-206.
36. Hamberg, M., Samuelsson, B., (1971) J. Biol. Chem. 246, 6713-6721.
37. Fischer, S., von Schacky, C., Schweer, H., (1988) Biochim. Biophys. Acta, 963, 501-508.
38. Ferretti, A., Flanagan, V.P., Reeves, V.B., (1988) Biochim. Biophys. Acta 959, 262-268.
39. Knapp, H.R., (1990) Prostaglandins 39, 407-423.
40. Hirt, D.L., Capdevila, J., Falck, J.R., Breyer, M.D., Jacobson, H.R., (1989) J. Clin. Invest. 84, 1805-1812.
41. Knapp, H.R., (1990) Clin. Res. 38, 419A.
42. Leaf, A., Weber, P.C., (1988) N. Engl. J. Med. 318, 549-557.
43. Yetiv, J.Z., (1988) JAMA 260, 665-670.
44. Lockette, W.E., Webb, R.C., Culp, B.R., Pitt, B., (1982) Prostaglandins 24, 631-639.
45. Somova, L., Hoffman, P., Förster, W., (1980) Eur. J. Pharmacol. 64, 79-83.
46. Singer, P., Berger, I., Moritz, V., Förster, D. Taube, C., (1990) Prost. Leukotr. Essent. Fatty Acids 39, 207-211.
47. Lorenz, R., Spengler, U., Fischer, S., Duhm, J., Weber, P.C., (1983) Circula-

tion 67, 504-511.
48. Singer, P., Wirth, M., Voigt, S., Richter-Heinrich, E., Gödicke, W., Berger, I., Naumann, E., Listing, J., Hartrodt, W., Taube, C., (1985) Atherosclerosis 56, 223-235.
49. Butcher, L.A., O'Dea, K., Sinclair, A.J., Parkin, J.D., Smith, I.L., Blombery, P., (1990) Prost. Leukotr. Essent. Fatty Acids 39, 221-226.
50. Hughes, G.S., Ringer, T.V., Spillers, C.R., Francom, S.F., DeLoof, M., (1989) J. Am. Coll. Nutr. 8, 435.
51. Knapp, H.R., Gregory, D., Nolan, S. (1989) in *Dietary w3 and w6 Fatty Acids*, Simopoulos, A.P. and Galli, C. pp. 283-295, Plenum Publishing Corp., New York.
52. Mancia, G., Mark, A.L., (1988) in Handbook of Physiology—The Cardiovascular System III, Chapter 20, pp. 755-793, American Physiological Society, Washington, D.C.
53. Panzenbeck, M.J., Tan, W., Hajdu, M.A. Zucker, I.H., (1988) Circ. Res. 63, 860-868.
54. Reibel, D.K., Holahan, M.A., Hock, C.E. (1988) Am. J. Physiol. 254, H494-H499.

Chapter Ten

The Effect of ω6 Dietary Fatty Acids on Blood Pressure

James M. Iacono

Western Human Nutrition Research Center
USDA-ARS
P.O. Box 29997
Presidio of San Francisco, CA 94129

Hypertension is a well established risk factor for major cardiovascular disease (CVD) and thus a great challenge to modern public health. Prospective studies show that an individual's risk increases with increasing blood pressure levels starting from levels so low that they are clinically considered normal (1). Since great numbers of people in the population have mild-to-moderately elevated blood pressure levels, the bulk of the risk attributable to hypertension in the population is in this large segment of the population (2). The pharmacological reduction of blood pressure has to be restricted to people with overt hypertension and, therefore, the need for non-pharmacological control of elevated blood pressure, applicable to the large population groups at risk, is urgent. Several possible interventions have been proposed, including weight reduction, stress management, relaxation therapy and dietary changes.

The role of nutrition in the control of blood pressure represents a challenge to scientists in the field of hypertension. For many years scientists have been concerned with the role of Na in blood pressure regulation (3-5). In spite of all that has been accomplished, the role of Na still remains controversial (6). A new and promising aspect of blood pressure regulation has come from a series of studies that have implicated the role of dietary fat (7-25).

The studies reported in this paper will summarize the data for ω6 fatty acids. Emphasis will be placed on three different experimental nutrition studies performed at Beltsville, Maryland, USA, in North Karelia, Finland (North Karelia-studies I-II) and one joint study performed in the USA, Finland and Italy (joint study). The results of these studies give strong support to the blood pressure lowering effect of dietary fat, specifically polyunsaturated fat of the ω6 type.

Experimental Procedure and Results
Beltsville study

This free-living study consisted of three periods with a switchback and cross-over design (14, 16-18). Prior to the study's commencement, a seven-day dietary history of food intake for each subject was recorded. The first 21 days was a stabilization period when all subjects consumed a 44 % energy from fat (en%) diet with a P/S ratio of 0.3. Two 30-day

TABLE 10-1

Calculated Composition of Selected Nutrients for Beltsville Study, Average Daily Intakes

Constituents	Prestudy*	Stabilization period	Experimental diets Energy as fat	
			25%	44%
Protein (% total energy)	16.7	17.3	15.7	17.2
Carbohydrates (% total energy)	42.1	39.8	59.8	39.5
Fat (% total energy)	40.9	44.2	26.4	44.2
Sat'd fatty acids	14.9	18.2	6.8	18.4
Oleic acid	16.8	15.9	10.2	15.9
Linoleic acid	5.3	5.4	6.6	5.3
P/S ratio	0.38	0.30	0.98	0.28
Cholesterol (mg)	528	770	270	845
Vitamins				
Vitamin A (IU)	7634	10615	10053	11104
Thiamin (mg)	1.46	1.76	2.11	1.92
Riboflavin (mg)	1.91	2.37	2.35	2.88
Niacin (mg)	22.3	25.4	32.9	28.4
Vitamin C (mg)	120	161	231	168
Minerals				
Calcium (mg)	767	1204	1164	1353
Phosphorus (mg)	1400	1901	1920	2134
Iron (mg)	15.5	17.4	21.6	19.0
Sodium in food (mg)	3465	2911	3315	3296
Sodium added (mg)	—	617	775	775
Total sodium (mg)	—	3530	4090	4070
Sodium chloride (g)	8.1	9.7	10.6	10.5
Potassium (mg)	2760	4070	5252	4431

Composition of nutrients calculated from data in USDA Handbook No. 8; includes updated data on cholesterol and fatty acid composition on tape (data set 8-1-1).
*Prestudy values calculated from 7-day dietary history, whereas experimental data based on values calculated from weighed food intakes.

periods followed. Ten subjects with a diastolic blood pressure greater than 88 mm Hg (hypertensive group) were fed a diet containing 25 en% (P/S ratio 1) for 30 days, while ten subjects with a diastolic blood pressure less than 88 mm Hg (normotensive group) continued on the 44

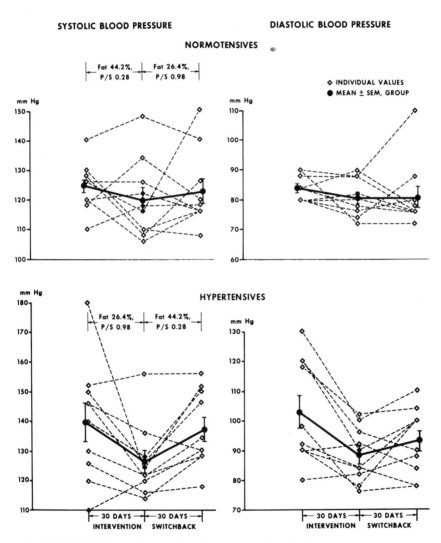

Fig. 10-1. Individual and mean blood pressure values in the normotensive and hypertensive groups at the end of each dietary period in the Beltsville study.

en% diet (P/S ratio 0.3). At the end of the 30-day period the two groups of subjects were switched from one diet to the other (switchback period).

Diet Composition. The nutrient composition of the diets is shown on Table 10-1. The dietary composition of the 25 en% and 44 en% remained constant except eggs and dairy products were added to the 25 en% diet to increase the fat content to 44 en% and to maintain a P/S ratio of 0.3. On both experimental diets, daily NaCl intake was 10.5 g. During the baseline period salt was provided in weighed shakers and used ad libitum. The subjects consumed less salt during the baseline period than during the intervention and the switchback periods.

Blood Pressure. In the hypertensive group, systolic blood pressure declined significantly during the intervention period (Fig. 10-1). When these subjects were placed on the 44 en% diet, during the switchback period, systolic blood pressure increased significantly. The diastolic blood pressure also declined significantly during the intervention period. It increased significantly to the initial level during the first half of the switchback period but declined significantly during the second half of this period. Throughout the study, neither systolic nor diastolic blood pressure changed significantly in the normotensive group.

Joint study-USA, Finland and Italy

A cross-sectional international epidemiological pilot study was carried out at Beltsville, Maryland, USA, Nurmijarvi, Finland, and Canino, Italy (15). Finland and the USA represent countries with high CHD rates and Italy a country with low CHD rates. From each area, data were collected on male farmers aged 40 to 45 years. All food was weighed or measured for seven days and the diet composition was calculated (Table 10-2). Local dietitians visited the homes of each subject and worked with the families to determine their food intake. Random daily food samples were also collected and analyzed.

Diet Composition. The average total energy content from fat in the diet was 32% in Italy, 40% in the USA and 39% in Finland. The level of dietary saturated fatty acids was highest in Finland and lowest in Italy (Table 10-2). The level of dietary linoleic acid was lowest in Italy and highest in the USA. The P/S ratio was lowest, 0.16, in Finland and was 0.25 and 0.28 in Italy and the USA, respectively. Alcohol intake differed markedly among the three areas. The Italians consumed 14% of their total energy intake as alcohol, primarily as wine. Finns and Americans reported about 1% of their total energy intake as alcohol.

TABLE 10-2
Calculated composition of diets[1] of subjects in a joint study—USA, Finland, Italy.

	Beltsville USA (n = 20)	Nurmijarvi Finland (n = 29)	Canino Italy (n = 17)
Constituents, % total energy			
Protein	15	14	13
Carbohydrate	46	47	49
Fat	40	39	32
Saturated Fatty acids	17.4	24.2	8.7
Linoleic acid	4.9	3.9	2.2
P/S ratio	0.28	0.16	0.25

[1] Calculated from data in USDA Handbook No. 8.

TABLE 10-3
Blood Pressures of the Subjects in Study 4

	Area		
Blood pressure	Beltsville (n = 20)	Nurmijarvi (n = 29)	Canino (n = 20)
Systolic (mm Hg)	123.6±1.2*[a]	136.2±2.6[b]	125.3±1.7[a]
Diastolic (mm Hg)	78.0±1.3[a]	90.4±1.4[b]	79.7±1.9[a]

Values are means ± SEM.
*Within a line, not sharing a common superscript, mean values are significantly different ($p < 0.05$).

Blood Pressure. Both systolic and diastolic blood pressure were significantly higher among the Finns than among either the Italians or Americans (Table 10-3).

North Karelia I study

This study was conducted in married couples in the community of Liperi in North Karelia, Finland (19). Prior to the six-week intervention period, a seven-day dietary history was taken for each subject, and the energy intake determined (baseline period). During the intervention period all subjects consumed a low fat diet with a high P/S ratio (Table 10-4).

TABLE 10-4
Calculated Composition of Selected Nutrients for North Karelia I Study, Average Daily Intakes

Constituents	Baseline	Intervention	Recovery
Protein (% total energy)	13.6	17.5	14.2
Carbohydrates (% total energy)	48.7	59.7	50.6
Alcohol (% total energy)	0.9	1.3	1.0
Fat (% total energy)	38.6	23.6	35.9
Sat'd fatty acids	21.9	7.6	20.1
Unsat'd fatty acids	3.1	9.1	3.1
Oleic acid	12.3	6.3	11.5
Linoleic acid	2.5	8.5	2.5
P/S ratio	0.15	1.2	0.16
Cholesterol (mg)	541	301	539
Minerals	1405	1409	1388
Calcium (mg)			
Phosphorus (mg)	2017	2150	2059
Iron (mg)	20.4	21.0	20.9
Sodium (mg)*	4128	4618	4494
Sodium chloride (g)*	10.5	11.7	11.4
Potassium (mg)	4616	5144	5437

Calculated from data in Finnish Food Table, Autoklinikan ravintotutkimuksen seuranta vuosina 1973-1975.
*By direct analysis of 30 composited duplicate diets during each period.

Thereafter, during a six-week switchback period all subjects consumed their usual diet which contained 36 en% (P/S ratio of 0.16). All participants were instructed to eat sufficient food to maintain body weight. Body weights did not change significantly during the study.

Diet Composition. The food eaten by the participants during the study was commonly available in North Karelia, Finland, and was typical for this area. During the intervention period high fat containing food items such as milk, cheese, meat, and sausages were replaced by similar items containing less fat. Margarines and oils prepared from sunflower seeds were substituted for butter and cooking oil to increase the P/S ratio of the diet. The estimated daily salt intake was 10.5 g, 11.7 g and 11.4 g for the three study periods (Table 10-4).

Blood Pressure. For men and women systolic blood pressure declined significantly when the last two readings of the intervention period were

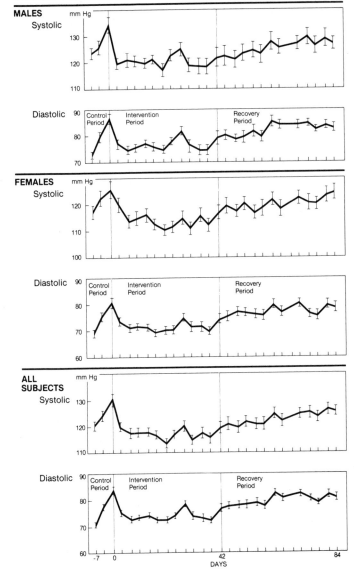

Fig. 10-2. Changes in systolic and diastolic blood pressure of the Finnish subjects in the North Karelia 1 study. Each point represents the mean of 30 values for males, 29 values for females, and 59 values for all subjects.

compared to the mean blood pressure during the baseline period ($p < 0.0004$) (Figure 10-2). There was a significant increase in systolic and diastolic blood pressure when the last two values of the recovery period were compared to the last two values of the intervention period for men and women ($p < 0.0001$). Diastolic blood pressures were also significantly different for men and women when the last two values of the baseline period were compared to the last two values of the intervention period ($p < 0.036$). The data obtained for blood pressure for this dietary intervention study were similar to those obtained in the Beltsville study.

North Karelia II study

The last study reported was conducted in two communities, Juuka and Lieksa in North Karelia, Finland (20, 21). A total of fifty-seven families were identified from the local community-based hypertension register that functions in the whole of North Karelia (22). The participants, husbands and wives, were 30-50 years old and had no major health problems and were not treated with antihypertensive drugs before they entered the study.

The families were randomly allocated into three different groups. During the intervention period Group 1 consumed a low fat diet with a high P/S ratio; Group 2 ate a diet typical for the region but low in Na; and a third group did not change their usual diet (reference group). The study consisted of three periods: baseline (two weeks), intervention (six weeks) and switchback (four weeks). During the baseline and switchback periods all the families were asked to eat their usual diets. During the intervention period the families in Groups 1 and 2 were asked to consume their respective experimental diets and the families of the reference group were asked to continue with their usual diet. Except for the alterations in the diets, the families made no other changes in their lifestyles, i.e., smoking or exercise, throughout the study.

Diet Composition. The composition of the diets consumed in this study were similar to those eaten in the North Karelia I study. In Group 1, substitutions of food items high in fat with food items low in fat were made and the energy content of the diet from fat was reduced from 39% to 23% during the intervention period and increased again during the switchback period to 37%. The respective P/S ratios were 0.27, 0.98 and 0.29. The percent of fat in the other two groups remained constant (39% with a P/S ratio of 0.29). Group 2 was asked to reduce their salt consumption during the intervention period to less than half their usual

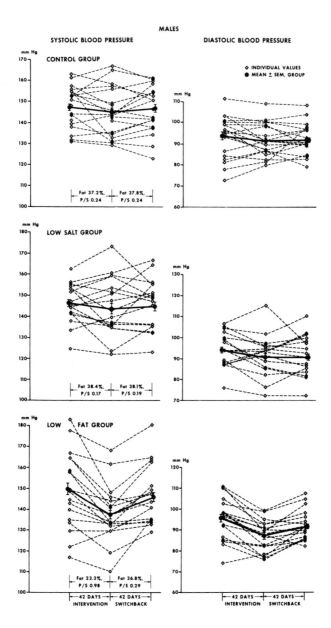

Fig. 10-3. Individual and mean blood pressure values at the end of each dietary period for men in the North Karelia II Study.

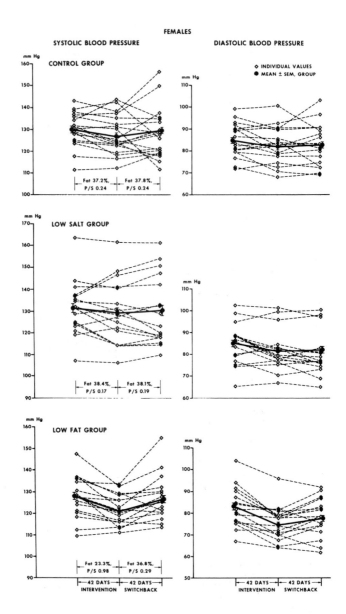

Fig. 10-4. Individual and mean blood pressure values at the end of each dietary period or women in the North Karelia II study.

intake. The families were provided with a number of low salt products. They were also directed by the dietitians to avoid salty products and were asked to prepare their food with a special low Na salt and not add salt to the foods at the table.

Blood Pressure. The mean blood pressure values for the last week of each period in the three groups are shown in Figures 10-3 and 10-4. During the intervention period the systolic blood pressure decreased 8.9 mm Hg ($p < 0.001$) and the diastolic pressure decreased 7.6 mm Hg ($p < 0.001$) in Group 1, but during the switchback period the systolic blood pressure level approached the baseline level ($p < 0.01$) and the diastolic blood pressure level also increased ($p < 0.001$). Blood pressure changes in the other two groups were small and were parallel to each other. Diastolic blood pressure decreased only slightly in both groups ($p < 0.01$) but remained at this lower level during the switchback period. The results were similar for men and women.

In the studies reported above, saturated and monounsaturated fat were decreased and PUFA were increased in the diet. This led to concern about the decrease in saturated fats or the increase of PUFA on blood pressure regulation. To resolve this dilemma, a controlled, experiment was conducted with normotensive and hypertensive male subjects (n=5) on a metabolic unit (23). They were fed diets containing 10% of energy from saturated fatty acids and 10% of energy from monounsaturated fatty acids throughout the intervention and switchback periods, with either 3% of energy as ω6 PUFA during a 40-day period or 10% of energy as ω6 PUFA during a 40-day period. Significant reductions in systolic and diastolic blood pressure were observed in the hypertensive group when 10% PUFA diet was consumed (Fig. 10-5).

The series of dietary intervention studies reported here demonstrate that blood pressure can be decreased or increased in high normotensive and hypertensive individuals by altering the fatty acid composition of the diet. The evidence implicates dietary ω6 PUFA. Significant alterations in systolic and diastolic blood pressure which occur as a consequence of change in the dietary fat take place within four to six weeks in both men and women. Mean blood pressure levels of the various groups dropped gradually during the course of the intervention periods. The full benefits and the long term implications of this type of dietary change are not known.

In view of the direct relationship between blood pressure and body weight (24, 25), participants maintained relatively constant body weights in the various studies by adjusting their calorie intakes. We can,

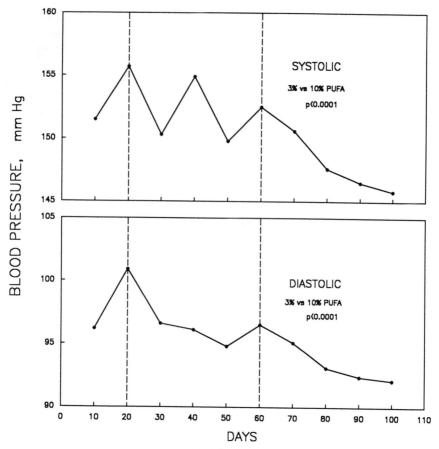

Fig. 10-5. Average blood pressure values for mild to moderate hypertensive male subjects (n=6) in a Metabolic Unit study at WHNRC; 40 days each period, intervention period I (10 en% saturated and 10 en% monounsaturated fat and 3 en% ω6 PUFA; polyunsaturated fat 40 days, intervention period II diet (10 en% saturated and 10 en% monounsaturated fat and 10 en% ω6 PUFA. Only hypertensive data shown.

therefore, rule out body weight as a factor affecting the changes observed in blood pressure in this series of experiments.

No attempt was made to alter salt intake, except in Group 2 in the North Karelia II study. An average amount of about 10-12 g per day was consumed in the Beltsville and the North Karelian studies. The values obtained for 24-hour urinary Na excretion were essentially the same as the Na intake values derived from direct chemical analysis of the diet. We conclude, therefore, that in these experiments, dietary Na was not an important factor for the blood pressure changes observed.

It was shown in the North Karelia II study that reducing dietary Na intake by about 60% in one group of hypertensive subjects, that only small changes in blood pressure were observed compared to the dramatic change observed in the group consuming the low fat, high P/S ratio diet. Salt intake and its relationship to blood pressure is controversial and requires a great deal more research.

High levels of dietary Ca have been shown to reduce blood pressure in animals while the results in man are not clear (26). The intake of Ca in North Karelia, Finland is high (1.4 g per day) because of the high consumption of dairy products. In spite of this, the blood pressure of the population of North Karelia remains relatively high suggesting that other dietary factors play a more important role in regulating blood pressure than dietary Ca. Ca intakes did not change significantly during the different periods of the two North Karelian studies.

The role of K in regulating blood pressure is also unclear. Available data suggests that a higher intake of K may reduce blood pressure, especially when the Na intake is high (27, 28). In the above discussed experiments this possibility could not completely be ruled out. For instance, in the North Karelia II study the K intake tended to increase somewhat during the intervention period (20) and it remained at the higher level when the subjects resumed their usual diets in the switchback period during which the blood pressure level increased again.

In seeking an explanation for the reduction of blood pressure in the dietary studies reported, present data implicate the action of $\omega6$ PUFA. The mechanism of action of essential fatty acids would appear to be through their conversion to prostaglandins which in turn have been repeatedly shown to have effects on blood pressure (29-35). The first epidemiological evidence linking dietary linoleic acid intake to urinary Na excretion has been reported by Oster et al. (9) and a significant positive correlation between these two factors was found.

There are still many unanswered questions to be resolved in this field. Much research needs to be done to understand the role of nutrients on blood pressure regulation before dietary recommendations can be made to the general public. However, the emerging findings concerning the association between dietary fat and blood pressure support the already existing dietary recommendations for modification of serum lipids for prevention of CHD.

References

1. The Polling Project Research Group, Relationship of blood pressure, serum cholesterol, smoking habit, relative weight and ECG abnormalities to incidence of major coronary events. Final report of the Pooling Project, American Heart Association Monograph, No. 60, Dallas, 1978.
2. Wilhelmsen, L., Salt and hypertension, in Proceedings of the 6th Scientific Meeting of International Society of Hypertension, 1979.
3. Dahl, L. K., (1972) Am. J. Clin. Nutr. 25: 231-244.
4. Freis, E. D., (1976) Circulation 53: 589-595.
5. Meneely, G. R., and Battarbee, H. D., (1976) Am. J. Cardiol. 38: 768-785.
6. Simpson, F. O., (1979) Clin. Sci. Mol. Med. 57: 463-480.
7. Iacono, J. M., Marshall, M. W., Dougherty, R. M., Wheeler, M. A., Mackin, J. F., and Canary, J. J., (1975) Prev. Med. 4: 426-443.
8. Burstyn, P. G., and Firth W. R., (1975) Cardiovascular Res. 9: 807-810.
9. Oster, P., Arab, L., Schellenberg, B., Heuck, C. C., Mordasini, R., and Schlierf, G., (1979) Res. Exp. Med. 175: 287-291.
10. Stern, B., Heyden, S., Miller, D., Latham, G., Klimas, A., and Pilkington, K., (1980) Nutr. Metab. 24: 137-147.
11. Harsha Rao, R., Brahmaji Rao, U., and Srikantia, S.G., (1981) Clin. Exp. Hypertens. 3: 27-38.
12. Hoffman, P., and Forster, W., (1981) Adv. in Lipid Res. 18: 202-227.
13. Iacono, J. M., Zellner, D. C., Paoletti, R., Ishikawa, T., Frigeni, V., and Fumagalli, R., (1973/1974) Haemostasis 4: 141-162.
14. Iacono, J. M., Marshall, M. W., Mackin, J. F., et al., in Proceedings of the 11th International Congress of Nutrition, Rio de Janeiro, Brazil, 1978, p. 101.
15. Iacono, J. M., in The Thrombotic Process in Atherogenesis, edited by A. Chandler, K. Eurenius, G. McMillan, C. Nelson, C. Schwartz and S. Wessler, Plenum Publishing, New York, 1981, pp. 309-327.
16. Iacono, J. M., Judd, J., Marshall, M. W., et al., (1981) Prog. in Lipid Res. 20: 349-364.
17. Iacono, J. M., in Atherosclerosis: Clinical Evaluation and Therapy, edited by S. Lenzi and G. C. Descovich, MTP Press Limited, London, 1982, pp. 315-332.
18. Iacono, J. M., Dougherty, R. M., and Puska, P., (1982) Hypertension 4 (suppl 2): III-34-III-42.
19. Iacono, J. M., Puska, P., Dougherty, R. M., et al., (1983) Am. J. Clin. Nutr. 38: 860-869.
20. Puska, P., Iacono, J. M. Nissinen, A., et al., (1983) Lancet i: 1-5.
21. Ehnholm, C., Huttunen, J., Pietinen, P., et al., (1982) N. Engl. J. Med. 307: 850-855.
22. Elo, J., Tuomilehto, J., Nissinen, A., and Puska, P., (1981) Med. Inf. 6: 57-72.
23. Iacono, J. M., Dougherty, R. M., Puska, P., and Pietinen, P., (1989) Ann. Med. 21: 251-254.

24. Kannel, W., Brand, N., Skinner, J., Dawber, T., and McNamara, P., (1967) Ann. Intern. Med. 67: 48-59.
25. Chiang, B. N., Perlman, L. V., and Epstein, F. H., (1969) Circulation 39: 403-421.
26. McCarron, D. A., Morris, C. D., and Cole, C., (1982) Science 217: 267-269.
27. Dahl, L. K., Leitl, H. G., and Heine, M., (1972) J. Exp. Med. 13: 318-328.
28. Skrabal, F., Auback, F. J., and Hortnagl, H., (1981) Lancet ii: 895-900.
29. Hansen, H. S., (1981) Lipids 16: 859-864.
30. Jackson, E. K., Branch, R. A., and Oates, J. A., (1980) Adv. PG LX Leuko. Res. 10: 255-302.
31. McGiff, J. C., (1981) Ann. Rev. Pharmacol. Toxicol. 21: 479-509.
32. Zollner, N., Adam, O., and Wolfram, G., (1979) Res. Exp. Med. 175: 149-153.
33. Smith-Barbaro, P., Fisher, H., Quinn, M. R., and Hegsted, D. M., (1980) Nutr. Reports Internatl. 22: 759-770.
34. Adam, O., Wolfram, G., and Zollner, N., (1982) Ann. Nutr. Metab. 26: 315-325.
35. Tobian, L., Ganguli, M., Johnson, M. A., and Iwai, J., (1962) Hypertension 4 (suppl 2): 149-153.

Chapter Eleven
Effect of Dietary Omega-3 Fatty Acids on Blood Platelet Reactivity

Bruce J. Holub

>Department of Nutritional Sciences
>University of Guelph
>Guelph, Ontario, Canada N1G 2W1

Recent statistics from the World Health Organization in Geneva, Switzerland have indicated that annual death rates per 100,000 U.S. males (aged 45-54 yr) from acute myocardial infarction, other ischemic heart diseases, and atherosclerosis are currently approximately 740% higher than that for the corresponding Japanese males. Interestingly, total blood plasma cholesterol levels in the U.S. males are only higher by 18% than the corresponding Japanese. Based on the conclusion from the U.S. consensus conference on lowering blood cholesterol to prevent heart disease, each 1% reduction of blood cholesterol level can be expected to yield approximately a 2% reduction in coronary heart disease rates (1). Based on the latter, it is apparent that the differences in blood cholesterol levels can only account for a very small portion of the marked differences in death rates from cardiovascular disease (CVD) in U.S. versus Japanese populations. In our research, we have been particularly interested in the possibility of dietary reduction of CVD and mortality via strategies which act independently of lowering blood cholesterol levels. Such approaches could complement blood cholesterol-lowering regimens and also offer protection for those with apparently normal or 'safe' blood cholesterol levels.

The work of Drs. Dyerberg and Bang suggested that the high intake of seafood (seal, whale, fish) by the Greenland Inuit population enriched in omega-3 polyunsaturated fatty acid in the form of eicosapentaenoic acid, EPA (20:5n-3) may account for the lesser mortality from myocardial infarction in this group as compared to the corresponding Danes (2). The current intake of fish and EPA in the Japanese population is approximately 7-fold that for North Americans. The reported epidemiological study from the Netherlands by Dr. D. Kromhout and colleagues suggesting an inverse relationship between fish consumption and mortality from coronary artery disease has further stimulated interest in the possible protective effects of fish/fish oils containing EPA (3). The aforementioned studies have stimulated many intervention trials evaluating the potential benefits of ingesting fish/fish oils or derived omega-3 concentrates on CVD and related risk factors. Recent review articles on the hyperlipidemic, antiatherogenic, and antithrombotic effects of oral supplements of fish oil concentrates proving EPA plus docosahexaenoic acid, DHA (22:6n-3), have appeared (4-9). Interestingly, these effects of omega-3 fatty acids have generally been observed in the absence of any lowering of total plasma cholesterol or low-density lipoprotein (LDL)-cholesterol levels.

Platelet-Vessel Wall Interactions and Platelet Reactivity

There is increasing evidence to indicate that the dietary consumption of fish or fish oils containing omega-3 fatty acids as EPA plus DHA can significantly reduce blood platelet aggregation and platelet-vessel wall interactions. A number of groups have observed that the consumption of fish or their omega-3 enriched concentrates can produce a moderate increase in bleeding times consistent with a decrease in platelet-vessel wall interactions. It is of interest to note that the bleeding times of Greenland Inuit have been reported to be considerably longer than those of their Danish counterparts. In some studies, but not others, platelet deposition in injured vessel walls appear to be significantly depressed in experimental studies where animals were given dietary fish oil. Studies using platelet-rich plasma as well as highly washed suspensions have indicated that the consumption of fish/fish oils containing EPA can significantly reduce platelet aggregation and associated events. These effects have depended upon the agonist employed to some extent, the dose level of omega-3 fatty acid supplementation, the duration of feeding, conditions used to measure platelet aggregability, and other variables. In general, the use of low level collagen as an agonist, for example, might be expected to show more consistent effects of dietary omega-3 fatty acids in this regard as compared to high levels of thrombin since, in the former case, platelet activation is markedly dependent upon the releasability of arachidonic acid, AA (20:4n-6) from membrane phospholipid and thromboxane A_2 (TxA_2) synthesis. TxA_2 is both a potentiator of platelet aggregation and a vasoconstrictor. Review articles have appeared discussing the potential of omega-3 fatty acids to influence platelet reactivity (4-9). It is noteworthy that the vast majority of these studies have employed platelet-rich plasma for conducting the aggregation studies. As recently pointed out by Packham and colleagues (10), the responses of human platelets in media with low concentrations of Ca^{++} (citrated platelet-rich plasma or artificial media to which no Ca^{++} has been added) are abnormal in at least two ways and do not correspond to the responses at physiological concentrations of Ca^{++}. In most of our experiments, we have employed the method outlined by Dr. Mustard and colleagues wherein physiological concentrations of Ca^{++} are added to washed platelet suspensions.

As well as having the potential to suppress *in vivo* platelet reactivity, omega-3 fatty acids have exhibited an influence on platelet survival in patients with pre-existing, atherothrombotic disorders. These latter studies have been of interest since platelet survival has been found to be decreased in persons with coronary atherosclerosis and to improve following coronary revascularization surgery. A prolongation of platelet survival by approximately 20% has been observed upon dietary supplementation with omega-3 fatty acids. The haemorheological effects of omega-3 fatty acids have also been investigated since viscosity and mechanical properties of the red blood cells (deformability and aggregation) are known to influence the flow properties of blood. In both healthy volunteers and patients with various forms of hyperlipoproteinemia, omega-3 fatty acids were found to produce a significant fall in overall blood viscosity including a significant decrease in blood plasma viscosity and increase in red cell deformability. Somewhat inconsistent effects of fish oil therapy have been found on overall fibrinolytic activity including variable alterations of tissue plasminogen activator or its inhibitor including factor VII and plasma fibrinogen. At high dose levels of omega-3 fatty acids (i.e., 9 gm daily), reductions in plasma levels of fibrinogen and von Willebrand factor have been observed by Schmidt et al. (11) while bleeding time, plasminogen activator antigen, and plasminogen activator inhibitor increased.

Most of the experiments on platelet aggregability and coagulation profiles that have been conducted to date with dietary marine oils have employed mixtures (naturally occurring) of EPA plus some DHA; relatively few studies have been performed using pure forms of EPA and/or DHA. A recent *in vitro* study (12) indicated that albumin-bound DHA (in free fatty acid form) at 20 μM concentration was capable of significantly inhibiting platelet activation with low level collagen as the agonist. These results are of interest since the concentration employed is attainable following fish oil supplementation of the diet.

Omega-3 Fatty Acid and Platelet Phospholipids

When dietary EPA is consumed it shows considerable accumulation in the total platelet phospholipid and has the potential to replace some of the endogenous AA present as well as other unsaturated fatty acids. While AA is widely distributed in considerable amounts across the various individual phospholipids including the choline phosphoglycerides (PC), ethanolamine phosphoglycerides (PE), serine phosphoglycerides (PS), and inositol phosphoglycerides (PI), the vast majority (approximately 95%) of the EPA accumulating in platelet phospholipid following fish oil consumption was found to reside within the total PC and PE with approximately 1.4% of the EPA mass residing in PI (5). Sphingomyelin was found to be essentially devoid of both AA and EPA in control subjects (not consuming fish oil) and in fish oil consumers. Interestingly, the ratios of EPA/AA differed considerably across the various phospholipid classes with the total phospholipid, PC, PE, PS, and PI exhibiting ratios of 0.19, 0.29, 0.22, 0.05, and 0.02, respectively, in human volunteers receiving 3.6 gm of EPA plus 2.4 g of DHA over a 3-week period. Significant enrichment of platelet phospholipid in DHA is also observed when this fatty acid is consumed in the diet although the basal level of DHA in control subjects is much higher than that for EPA at entry (only trace amounts).

When evaluating the enrichment of the various sub-classes of PC and PE with respect to EPA accumulation, we observed (13,14) that the ether-containing phospholipid form of PE (notably the 1-alkenyl 2-acyl form of PE) became particularly enriched in EPA with fish oil consumption. In contrast to the diacyl sub-class of PE, the alkenylacyl class showed significant diminution in AA levels as EPA entered phospholipid following dietary consumption.

Suppression of Thromboxane A_2 Synthesis by Dietary Fish/Fish Oils

The accumulation of EPA in the circulating platelet (membrane phospholipids) upon dietary consumption can serve to reduce the amount of AA available in the various platelet membrane phospholipids thereby reducing the availability of AA for release in stimulated platelets and diminishing eicosanoid (including TxA_2) synthesis. As well, the release of EPA in free fatty acid form upon stimulation can provide a competitive inhibitor of AA metabolism at the level of cyclooxygenase thereby further reducing TxA_2 synthesis. We have observed from both labelling

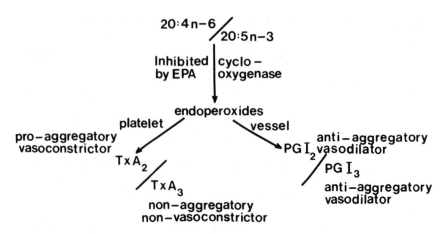

Fig. 11-1. Summary of AA (20:4n-6) and EPA (20:5n-3) metabolism as mediated via cyclo-oxygenase enzyme activity in blood platelets or vascular tissue (vessel wall).

and mass determinations that both AA and EPA are readily released from platelet membrane phospholipids upon stimulation of human platelet suspensions with thrombin as the agonist (5). As summarized in Figure 11-1, some EPA can be metabolized to thromboxane A_3 although the latter does not have the pro-aggregatory and vasoconstrictory potential of TxA_2. In vascular tissue, AA and EPA are metabolized to PGI_2 (prostacyclin) and PGI_3, respectively. These latter two compounds have similar potentials for both inhibiting platelet aggregation and enhancing vasodilation. While DHA is not readily released in free fatty acid form from platelet membrane phospholipid upon stimulation, it is known that the addition of DHA (as free fatty acid) can significantly inhibit platelet reactivity (12) as well as the cyclooxygenase-mediated generation of TxA_2 from AA.

In addition to potentially dampening platelet reactivity and vasoconstriction by reducing TxA_2 formation, the enrichment of platelet membrane phospholipids in omega-3 fatty acids may also reduce agonist-receptor interactions through a membrane (fluidity) effect which is independent of eicosanoid synthesis. Furthermore, recent research from our laboratory and that of other investigators suggest that cell signalling processes which involve the turnover of inositol-containing membrane phospholipids including second messenger generation (inositol trisphosphate and 1,2-diacylglycerol) involved with calcium mobilization and protein kinase C activation, respectively, may be significantly influenced by dietary fish oil consumption upon alteration of membrane phospholipid (fatty acid) profiles.

Vegetable Oil Consumption and EPA Enrichment of Platelet Membrane Phospholipid

Since dietary linolenic acid, LNA (18:3n-3) as found in certain vegetable oils can be converted via desaturation/elongation reactions to EPA, we have evaluated the potential for dietary canola oil in controlled feeding trials (conducted in human volunteers in collaboration with Dr. Bruce McDonald and Dr. Vivian Bruce of the University of Manitoba) to provide for EPA entry and accumulation in platelet phospholipids with particular emphasis on the alkenylacyl PE fraction. These results (15) indicated that, in contrast to the pre-experimental dietary regimen providing a dietary ratio of linoleic acid (18:2n-6, LA) to LNA of 14.8 and an EPA level of 0.6 mol% in the platelet alkenylacyl PE, those subjects given canola oil (with a corresponding ratio of 2.6) gave an EPA level of 1.4 mol% which was considerably greater than that for dietary sunflower oil (having a LA/LNA ratio of 73.7) which gave an EPA level of only 0.3 mol%. Subsequent studies comparing dietary soybean oil (LA/LNA ratio 6.8) versus canola oil-fed subjects (LA/LNA ratio 3.0) indicated a higher level of EPA accumulation in the alkenylacyl PE of platelet phospholipid (1.1 mol%) as compared to 0.6 mol% for the latter group despite the fact that both groups consumed approximately 8 gm of LNA daily. Maintaining a dietary ratio of LA/LNA at approximately 3.0 did not provide for any further enrichment of the alkenylacyl PE in EPA when the LNA intake was doubled (from 8-16 gm daily). These latter findings indicate that dietary canola oil with a relatively low ratio of LA/LNA (3.0) permits significant conversion of LNA to EPA and some accumulation of the latter in circulating human platelet phospholipid. Presumably, higher ratios of LA/LNA (n-6/n-3) reduced the convertibility of LNA to EPA (and its fatty acid products including 22:5n-3 and DHA) by competitive effects at the level of the fatty acid desaturation reactions.

References

1. The Lipid Research Clinics Coronary Primary Prevention Trial results, (1984) J. Am. Med. Assoc. 252: 351.
2. Dyerberg, J., and Bang, H.O., (1979) Lancet 2: 433.
3. Kromhout, D., Bosschieter, E.B., and Coulander, C., (1985) New Engl. J. Med. 312: 1205.

4. Herold, P.M., Kinsella, J.E., (1986) Am. J. Clin. Nutr. 43: 566.
5. Weaver, B.J. and Holub, B.J., (1988) Prog. Food Nutr. Sci. 12: 111.
6. Leaf, A. and Weber, P.C., (1988) N. Engl. J. Med. 31: 549.
7. Holub, B.J., (1989) Can. Med. Assoc. J. 131: 377.
8. Holub, B.J., (1989) Can. Med. Assoc. J. 141: 1063.
9. Hornstra, G., in: *The Role of Fats in Human Nutrition*, edited by A.J. Vergrosesen and M. Crawford, Academic Press, New York, 1989, 2nd edn., pp. 151-235.
10. Packham, M.A., N.L. Bryant, M.A. Guccione, R.L. Kinlough-Rathbone, and J.F. Mustard (1989) Thromb. Haem. 62: 968.
11. Schmidt, E., K. Varming, E. Ernst, P. Madsen, and J. Dyerberg, (1990) Thromb. Haem. 63: 1.
12. Gaudette, D.C. and Holub, B.J., (1990) Lipids. 25: 166.
13. Holub, B.J., Celi, B., and Skeaff, C.M., (1988) Thromb. Res. 50: 135.
14. Aukema, H. and Holub, B.J., (1989) J. Lipid Res. 30: 59.
15. Weaver, B.J., Corner, E.J., Bruce, V.M., McDonald, B.E., and Holub, B.J., (1990) Am. J. Clin. Nutr. 51: 594.

Chapter Twelve

Dietary Fatty Acids and Platelet Function: Mechanisms

Norberta W. Schoene

Lipid Nutrition Laboratory
Beltsville Human Nutrition Research Center
U.S. Dept. of Agriculture
Beltsville, MD 20705

The relationship between dietary fatty acids and platelet responses has received intense scrutiny in the last decade. The participation of platelets in the sequelae of myocardial infarction has prompted investigators to discover new ways to depress the aggregative propensity of this cell with drugs and with diet. Epidemiologic data on the low rate of cardiovascular disease in populations that consume long-chain n-3 fatty acids have led to renewed interest in the consumption of marine oils as a strategy for diminution of the mortality and morbidity associated with degenerative diseases of the vascular system. Mechanisms to explain the effects of n-3 fatty acids on the function of platelets have relied heavily on competitive reactions among the families of unsaturated fatty acids for enzymes that elongate and desaturate fatty acids, assemble and reassemble tissue lipids, and produce the oxygenated metabolites of arachidonic acid. In the platelet the arachidonic acid metabolite, thromboxane A_2 (TXA_2), is a major amplifier of aggregation. TXA_2 is produced when a pro-aggregative agonist binds to its receptor on the surface membrane. Amplification occurs when TXA_2 itself binds to its own receptor on the platelet membrane initiating even more aggregation.

When an agonist binds to its receptor, information from this coupling is transduced via GTP-binding proteins to the interior of the cell culminating in the production of second messengers. Under normal hemostatic conditions, pro-aggregative reactions are limited and no pathology results from their stimulation. Conditions which affect the production of TXA_2 or its ability to amplify signals will have notable effects on platelet function. The following sections assess how the methods used to examine platelet function can influence experimental results and their interpretations. In depth reviews of concepts outlined above can be found in the following references (1-4).

In Vivo Assessment Of Platelet Function
Humans
Monitoring the production of TXA_2 in humans by determining the amount of metabolites (TX-M) in the urine is a non-invasive procedure to assess platelet activation *in vivo* (5). Aspirin has been used to demonstrate that platelets are the source of 80% of TX-M found in the urine (6). Furthermore, increased excretion of TX-M compared to that seen in healthy subjects has been shown to occur in patients suffering from severe atherosclerosis (5), myocardial infarction (7), and diabetes mellitus (8). The increased excretion is consistent with *in vivo* platelet activation in these disease states. When fish oil supplements were given to patients with atherosclerosis (5), the excretion of TX-M dropped significantly. Similar reductions in the excretion of the metabolite are seen when aspirin is given (6). Both treatments, fish oil supplementation and aspirin ingestion, have been implicated in the reduction of morbidity due to cardiovascular disease (9,10). Bleeding times are also extended by these two treatments. Both Thorngren and Gustafson (11) and Harris et al. (12) have shown that a combination of a fish oil supplement with aspirin produced additive effects on bleeding time. This was regarded to be indirect evidence that n-3 fatty acids may diminish platelet responses by mechanism(s) independent of cyclooxygenase activity.

When platelets are labeled with indium-111, distribution of circulating platelets can be monitored with scintigraphy. With this technique, Isaka et al. (13) reported that deposition of platelets in the carotid artery can be observed in some patients suffering from cerebrovascular atherosclerosis. Nevertheless, platelets isolated from these patients were less responsive to ADP-induced aggregation compared to those from healthy controls and from patients who had no evidence of *in vivo* platelet deposition. These findings are an example of the conflicting results that investigators must explain when comparing *in vivo* versus *in vitro* tests of platelet function.

Animals
Arterial thrombotic tendency has been measured in animals fed diets containing various kinds of fats by determining the obstruction time of

aortic loops in rats. In general, diets high in saturated fats enhanced arterial thrombosis compared to diets containing either n-6 or n-3 polyunsaturated fatty acids (PUFA) (14). Rats fed diets lacking in both n-6 and n-3 PUFA (essential fatty acid deficient diets), had very long obstruction times which could be lowered by feeding either sunflower seed or fish oils (15), demonstrating the importance of the arachidonic acid metabolite, TXA_2, in the promotion of clot formation in the aortic loop model.

In Vitro Assessment of Platelet Function

Historically, *in vitro* platelet responses have been measured in platelet-rich plasma (PRP) in the presence of an anticoagulant, usually citrate. Studies conducted under these conditions are difficult to compare and interpret. The presence of citrate in PRP is a major obstacle in the production of physiological meaningful data on responses of platelets to various stimuli (16,17). Platelet-platelet interactions stimulated by agonists in the presence of abnormally low amounts of ionized calcium result in artifactual aggregation that has little relevance to the *in vivo* situation (16-18). When platelets are isolated, either by centrifugation or gel-filtration, other problems can arise because of the kind of buffer used, plus the presence or absence of calcium, magnesium, and albumin (3).

The manner in which the blood sample is obtained is also very important because platelets can be activated during the process of blood sampling. Prior activation of the platelets, either in circulation or during sampling, results in desensitization of membrane receptors. It is this variable desensitization of receptors which causes difficulties in producing meaningful data on the function of platelets. Critical platelet studies require the use of submaximal doses of agonists to initiate platelet aggregation since maximal stimulation can mask inefficient signal-response coupling and cause an underestimation of desensitization (19,20).

Measurement in plasma of two secreted proteins, β-thromboglobulin (β-TG) and platelet factor 4 (PF-4), can give an indication of whether platelets have been activated *in vivo* as they circulate or *in vitro* during the sampling procedure (21). This is possible because these two constituents of platelet α-granules have different lifetimes in the circulation. PF-4 decays quickly while β-TG has a much longer lifetime. Elevated values for both proteins are strong evidence that activation has occurred during sampling. If only β-TG is elevated, it is suggestive of *in vivo* activation of platelets.

Each method to assess platelet function contributes its own unique set of problems to the generation of reproducible and interpretable data. Comparison of the turbidimetric procedure to measure platelet aggregation with indices of *in vivo* platelet activation have produced discrepant results in many instances. In addition to the paradox involving scintigraphy versus optical aggregation (13), another example of contradictory results is found in smokers (22). Increased excretion of TX-M compared to non-smoking controls is evidence for in vivo activation of platelets in these subjects. However, platelets tested in PRP from these subjects revealed a refractoriness to receptor-mediated stimulation (22). With an *in vitro* procedure based on the rapid disappearance of single platelets, the quenched-flow method, Taylor et al. (23) demonstrated that platelets from hypertensive patients had a diminished sensitivity to ADP compared to those from normotensive controls. This diminution contradicted evidence for the presence of activated platelets in the circulation of hypertensive subjects as suggested by the elevation of ionized calcium concentrations above those found in platelets from normotensives (24,25).

Receptor Integrity

In 1985, Carmo et al. (26) demonstrated that human platelets pre-exposed to either arachidonic acid or to the TX mimetic, U46619, displayed decreased responsiveness to a subsequent challenge by either agonist. The decreased responsiveness could be prevented by TX receptor antagonists. These investigators concluded that arachidonic acid and U46619 desensitized platelets via the TX receptor. The desensitization by arachidonic acid was mediated by a cyclooxygenase-dependent metabolite since the desensitization process could be inhibited by reversible inhibitors of the enzyme. Furthermore, inactivation of the cyclooxygenase was not involved since TX synthesis persisted in spite of receptor desensitization. Murray and FitzGerald (27) also showed that desensitization by prior exposure to U46619 occurred very rapidly and was related to uncoupling of the receptor from a GTP-binding protein. The rapid desensitization was followed by downregulation after 24 hours of exposure to agonist, with 50% loss in receptor number. The TX receptor was also subject to heterologous desensitization since preincubation with thrombin resulted in a diminished subsequent response to U46619. These studies on the function and regulation of the TX receptor have produced data suggesting that platelet exposure to various agonists and antagonists either as they circulate in the body or as they are isolated from blood samples is a critical factor in determining the extent of response to subsequent challenges at membrane receptors.

In addition to causing a decreased excretion of TX-M, ingestion of dietary n-3 PUFA has been shown to reduce the amounts of TXB_2 in serum (5). These results are consistent with the importance of competition among the various n-3 and n-6 fatty acids for the metabolic pathways open to PUFA. However, eicosapentaenoic and docosahexaenoic acids have also been shown to be TX receptor antagonists (28,29). In addition, several lipoxygenase products of these two fatty acids inhibited platelet aggregation to varying degrees by also acting as antagonists at the TX receptor (30). Thus, the facile attribution of decreased TXA_2 formation as the mechanism by which n-3 fatty acid diminish platelet function needs further critical testing.

Recently, Hornstra's group (31) demonstrated *in vitro* that platelets from rats fed diets high in saturated fats aggregated less when stimulated by thrombin and collagen compared to platelets from rats fed diets high in PUFA, again both n-6 (sunflowerseed oil) and n-3 (fish oil) fatty acids. These results are in direct contrast to those obtained earlier by Hornstra with the aortic loop model (14,15). Furthermore, washed platelets from the animals fed the fish oil were shown to be more sensitive to stimulation by the TX mimetic and collagen than platelets from rats fed either sunflowerseed oil or hydrogenated coconut oil. The discrepancy between results from the *in vivo* animal thrombotic models and the *in vitro* platelet aggregation studies can be reconciled in part by considering the functional integrity of the TX receptor as described above. Either during circulation or during the process of sampling and cell preparation, platelets from rats fed the saturated fat or the sunflowerseed oil were most likely exposed to more TXA_2 than the platelets from rats fed the fish oil diet. This means that receptors on the platelets from rats fed either sunflowerseed oil or hydrogenated coconut oil would have been exposed to greater risks of desensitization that would result in less responsive platelets. The situation for the receptors on the platelets from the rats fed fish oil would be just the opposite. And indeed, this is what Hornstra and his colleagues found. Platelets from the rats fed fish oil were more responsive to U46619 plus collagen *in vitro*.

Our laboratory (32) has demonstrated that when gel-filtered platelets from rats fed either corn oil or fish oil diets were stimulated with fluoride, the platelets demonstrated equal responsiveness in contrast to the differences observed when the platelets were activated with collagen. Fluoride, an agent that bypasses membrane receptors, non-specifically activates GTP-binding proteins and thus can produce intracellular signaling independent of the functional sensitivity of receptor-mediated events. Our results are evidence that dietary n-3 fatty acids produce effects on receptor-mediated processes but not on processes which bypass the ligand-receptor interaction.

In summary, investigations into how dietary fatty acids and/or their metabolites affect receptor integrity will contribute to the understanding of the complexities associated with regulation of signal-response coupling in platelets. Assessments of platelet function require careful application of the latest knowledge in the rapidly evolving area of receptor research.

References

1. Sanders, T.A.B., (1983) Clin. Sci. 65:343.
2. Leaf, A. and Weber, P.C., (1988) N. Engl. J. Med. 318:549.
3. Hawiger, J. (ed.), Platelets, Receptors, Adhesion, Secretion. Part A, Volume 169, Methods in Enzymology. San Diego: Academic Press, 1989.
4. Kroll, M. and Schafer, A., (1989) Blood, 74:1181.
5. Knapp, H.R., Reilly, I.A.G., Alessandrini, P., and FitzGerald, G.A., (1986) N. Engl. J. Med. 314:937.
6. Catella, F., and FitzGerald, G.A., (1987) Thromb. Res. 47:647.
7. Henriksson, P., Wennmalm, Å., Edhag, O., Vesterqvist, O., and Green, K., (1986) Br. Heart. J. 55:543.
8. Davi, G., Catalano, I., Averna, M., Notarbartolo, A., Strano, A., Ciabattoni, G., and Patrono, C., (1990) N. Engl. J. Med. 322:1769.
9. Steering committee of the Physicians' Health Study Research Group, (1989) N. Engl. J. Med. 321:129.
10. Burr, M.L., Fehily, A.M., Gilbert, J.R., Rogers, S., Holliday, R.M., Sweetman, P.M., Elwood, P.C., and Deadman, N.M., (1989) Lancet 2:757.
11. Thorngren, M., and Gustafson, A., (1981) Lancet 2:1190.
12. Harris, W.S., Silveira, S., and Dujovne, C.A., (1990) Thromb. Res. 57:517.
13. Isaka, Y., Kimura, K., Uehara, A., Hashikawa, K., Mieno, M., Matsumoto, M., Handa, N., Nakabayashi, S., Imaizumi, M., and Kamada, T., (1989) Thromb. Res. 56:739.
14. Hornstra, G. Dietary Fats and Arterial Thrombosis, Dissertation, University of Maastrich, Limburg, 1980.
15. Hornstra, G., Haddeman, E., and Don, J., (1989) Thromb. Res. 53:45.
16. Packham, M.A., Bryant, N.L., Guccione, M.A., Kinlough-Rathbone, R.L., and Mustard, J.F., (1989) Thromb. Haemostas. 62:968.
17. Bowry, S.K. and Müller-Berghaus, G., (1986) Thromb. Haemostas. 56:172.
18. Bell, D.N., Spain, S., Goldsmith, H.L., (1990) Thromb. Res. 58:47.
19. Clark, R.B., Kunkel, M.W., Freidman, J., Gokat, T.J., and Johnson, J.A.,

(1988) Proc. Natl. Acad. Sci. USA 85:1442.
20. Lohse, M.J., Benovic, J.L., Caron, M.G., Lefkowitz, R.J., (1990) J. Biol. Chem. 265:3202.
21. Kaplan, K.L. and Owen, J., (1981) Blood, 57:199.
22. Nowak, J., Murray, J.J., Oates, J.A., FitzGerald, G.A., (1987) Circulation 76:6.
23. Taylor, M.A., Ayers, C.R., and Gear, A.R.L., (1989) Hypertension 13:558.
24. Erne, P., Bolli, P., Bürgisser, E., Bühler, F.R., (1984) N. Engl. J. Med. 310:1084.
25. Lande, K., Os, I., Kjeldsen, S.E., Westheim, A., Hjermann, I., Eide, I., and Gjesdal, K., (1987) J. Hypertension 5:401.
26. Carmo, L.G., Hatmi, M., Rotilio, D., and Vargaftig, B.B., (1985) Br. J. Pharmac. 85:849.
27. Murray, R., FitzGerald, G., (1989) Proc. Natl. Acad. Sci. USA, 86:124.
28. Hatmi, M., Lussiana, J., Junien, J., Bure, J., and Vargaftig, B., (1988) Biochem. Pharmacol. 37:481.
29. Swann, P.G., Venton, D.L., and Le Breton, G.C., (1989) FEBS Lett. 242:244.
30. Croset, M., Sala, A., Folco, G., and Lagarde, M., (1988) Biochem. Pharmacol. 37:1275.
31. Heemskerk, J., Feijge, M., Kalafusz, R., and Hornstra, G., (1989) Biochim. Biophys. Acta, 1004:252.
32. Schoene, N.W., and Church, J.P., (1991) Nutr. Res. : In press.

Chapter Thirteen
Correlations Between Fatty Acid Intake and Cancer Incidence

Maureen M. Henderson, M.D.
Head, Cancer Prevention Research Program
Fred Hutchinson Cancer Research Center
1124 Columbia St. MP-702
Seattle, WA 98104

Links between national dietary practices and patterns of cancer incidence have been hypothesized for 30-40 years (1). Much of the early focus was on naturally occurring mutagens and carcinogens in food as well as cooking products. The experimental animal research work of Carroll (2) and the analytic epidemiological work of Armstrong and Doll (3), Miller (4), Hursting (5) and Prentice (6,7), has redirected interest to the potential carcinogenic role of fatty acids usually in the context of tumor promotion.

Ecological correlations provide the most consistent and strongest human evidence in support of dietary fat as a cause of cancer. They are, however, considered a weak form of evidence by most scientists because they do not link diseased individuals directly to suspected exposures. They do, however, identify public health problems and have particular relevance if public health interventions are likely to solve those problems, i.e., they can be attacked by mass intervention rather than risk reduction in high risk individuals (8).

Analytic epidemiological studies of individual subjects within countries have failed to provide any conclusive results about the cancer risk of high fat diets. The most probable reasons for their ambiguity are the limited ranges of fat consumption resulting from more or less uniform national eating habits and the technical difficulties of making precise measurements of consumption of a wide range of nutrients—usually eaten in combination.

Meta-analyses of data from the most representative of these studies suggest that there is a definite association between the level of fat intake and both breast and colon cancer but the interpretation of the strength and significance of that relationship depends upon the perception of the amount of misclassification that results from the use of dietary instruments to document causal differences between the diets of diseased and comparison subjects (9,10,11).

USA food disappearance data suggest a steady annual increase in the average consumption of grams of fat during the last fifty years (12) (Figure 13-1). While the average amount of saturated fat used has stabilized since the 1960s, the rates of increase in the use of polyunsaturated and monounsaturated fats have accelerated fast enough to maintain an upward trend (Figure 13-2). This continued high level of fat consumption with gradually increasing proportions of polyunsaturated fat in the USA is probably representative of other western countries.

The average amounts of fat consumed are also increasing in countries that are improving their general socioeconomic conditions or adopting Westernized diets. This pattern has been well documented in Japan where dietary changes have increased the use of saturated fats relatively more than polyunsaturated fats (13). The changes from lower to higher levels of fat consumption by adding steadily increasing proportions of saturated fat is probably representative of many rapidly developing countries.

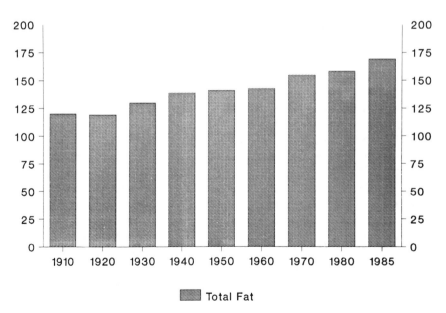

Fig. 13-1. Increase in the annual consumption of grams of fat during the past 50 years.

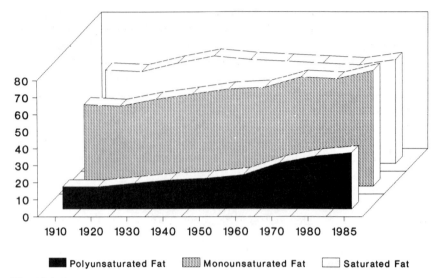

Fig. 13-2. Increases in polyunsaturated and monosaturated fats.

Analysis of secular trends in site specific cancer incidence rates in both the USA and Japan, show a steady increase in incidence rates of reproductive organ and large bowel cancers as the average use of dietary fat increases. The rate of increase within both countries is consistent with the differences in overall incidence of these cancers in countries with different levels of fat consumption (14). Systematic increases in the total amount of fat in the national diet do appear to predict systematic increases in the annual incidence of certain cancers.

The country of residence is one of the strongest risk factors for a number of cancers. The specific factors in the environment that account for the variation in rates of incidence are, however, different for cancers of different sites. Differences in rates of use of tobacco products explain international variations in lung cancer rates, and rates of stomach cancer declined as the rates of use of refrigeration for food preservation and transportation increased. Over at least twenty years analyses of available measures of national lifestyle, demographic profiles and socioeconomic conditons have pinpointed diet as the environmental factor, and fat as the nutrient, with the most influence on breast, prostate, and colon cancers (1,7,14,15,16,17). These are an interesting constellation of cancers, breast and prostate being cancers of reproductive organs likely

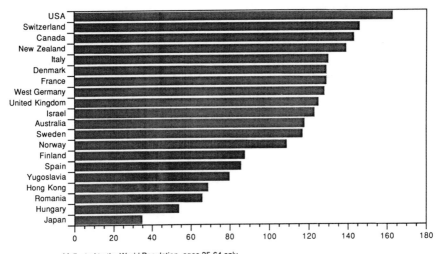

*Adjusted to the World Population, ages 35-64 only.

13-3. Breast cancer rates in various countries.

TABLE 13-1
Age Adjusted Breast Cancer Incidence Rates SEER* PROGRAM. White Females

Year of Diagnosis	Age	
	<50	≥50
1973	29.1	252.1
1975	29.9	271.0
1977	28.8	258.4
1979	27.9	265.4
1981	28.8	280.3
1983	29.3	295.4
1985	32.0	326.7
per cent change	2.8	16.9
average yearly change	0.2	1.4

NCI 1988

*Surveillance, Epidemiology and End Results

TABLE 13-2
Breast Cancer Incidence per 100,000, 1974-1986
Nine Standard SEER Registries. Females Only, All Races, by Five-Year Age Groups

Age	Year of Diagnosis												
	1974	1975	1976	1977	1978	1979	1980	1981	1982	1983	1984	1985	1986
Total	99	92	89	89	89	91	92	96	97	102	106	114	117
10-14							0						
15-19		0	0	0		0	0	0	0		0	0	
20-24	1	1	1	1	2	1	1	1	1	2	1	1	1
25-29	8	9	9	8	9	8	8	8	9	9	9	7	7
30-34	29	25	23	28	24	27	26	28	31	27	25	27	30
35-39	66	55	56	58	61	54	62	65	63	63	71	68	65
40-44	119	115	104	104	111	104	107	105	107	115	122	124	131
45-49	196	178	184	170	158	163	150	159	171	161	168	189	186
50-54	213	208	199	192	191	188	181	186	179	191	201	219	217
55-59	257	231	222	220	212	212	215	235	225	253	247	267	263
60-64	278	261	246	251	261	268	259	271	281	287	300	324	331
65-69	318	292	282	267	276	296	299	306	307	332	349	367	402
70-74	326	297	314	283	298	322	338	333	342	356	381	403	424
75-79	369	354	307	322	331	335	343	358	353	368	410	413	450
80-84	365	342	342	361	323	342	349	381	375	398	380	459	443
85+	383	357	374	401	384	386	367	408	362	385	389	414	391

to be mediated by steroidal hormones and colon a digestive organ cancer likely to arise through a more direct pathway.

Breast cancer incidence rates vary as much, if not more, than any of the other cancers related to national consumption of dietary fat (Figure 13-3). Rates in the USA are at least five times those in Japan, and four times those in Hungary and Poland. Age is the other major risk factor for breast, prostate and colon cancers. American women aged 50 years and over have ten times the breast cancer incidence of women aged 18 to 49 (Table 13-1). This country has a steady increase in rates with age and the statistical association with average fat consumption strengthens with age, a typical picture of cancer caused by cumulative environmental exposure (Table 13-2). A steady increase in year-by-year rates of breast and prostate cancer has continued for a number of decades. The annual rate of increase in breast cancer incidence is currently as high as one and half percent per year for women over 50 years of age (Table 13-1). Colon and rectal cancer rates increase steadily in earlier years, but level off in latter years. In recent years Japan has had a steady annual increase in rates of breast, prostate and colon cancers (18).

Most of the early analytic studies correlated estimates of animal or vegetable or total fat consumption with rates of death for specific

TABLE 13-3
Partial Correlation Coefficients Between Age Standardized Cancer Incidence Rates and Dietary Components

| Cancer Site | Total Fat** | | |
	Partial Correlation Coefficient	P‡	Slope*
Female			
Breast	0.72	(0.0046)	0.95
Colon	0.62	(0.0048)	0.24
Lung	0.34		0.16
Cervix	−0.17		−0.12
Male			
Prostate	0.69	(0.0011)	0.23

**Adjusted for total calories
‡P value of test of Pcc = 0, only P values below 0.10 shown
*Slope of least squares relationship
Unit = cases/100,000/g.

cancer sites taking into account only major confounding variables like Gross National Product. More recent efforts have correlated the best possible estimates of the average consumption of each fatty acid that can be derived from national food disappearance tables with reported annual rates of diagnoses of new cancers in countries with reliable and representative cancer registries (5,6). These correlation analyses have been controlled for all potentially confounding or modifying social and biological variables for which national measurements are available and partial correlations were examined. Cancers of the lung and cervix were included in some of the first of these regression analyses along with cancers of the breast, colon and prostate to test the specificity of the dietary fat associations. With cigarette smoking known to be the overwhelming risk factor for lung cancer and sexual behavior the major risk factor for cervical cancer, a finding of little or no fat-use association with these would strengthen confidence in the results.

There was no association between average fat consumption and either lung or cervical cancer rates and strong associations with rates of breast, colon and prostate cancers. The total (average) number of calories from fat were positively and significantly correlated with both mortality and incidence rates of breast, prostate, and colon cancers (Table

TABLE 13-4

Partial Correlation Coefficients (and Slopes) Between Age-Adjusted Cancer Rates and Components of Dietary Fat

	Cancer Incidence		
Fat Component†	(F) Breast	(F) Colon	Prostate
Total Fat	0.72* (0.95)	0.62* (0.024)	0.69* (0.23)
Saturated Fat	0.58* (1.80)	0.47 (0.044)	0.55* (0.43)
Monounsaturated Fat	−0.01 (−0.03)	0.004 (0.004)	0.02 (0.01)
Polyunsaturated Fat	0.51* (2.70)	−0.01 (−0.01)	0.46 (0.64)
N-6P	0.49* (2.70)	0.05 (0.09)	0.48* (0.70)
N-3P	0.16 (2.90)	−0.22 (−1.30)	−0.03 (−0.16)

*$p < .05$
P value of test of Pcc = 0
† adjusted for total calories and other fatty acids
( ) slope = slope of least squares relationship
Unit = cases/100,000/g.

13-3). The total (average) number of non-fat calories was not associated with either the incidence or mortality rates in either younger or older men (colon, prostate) or women (breast, colon). As predicted from the results of animal feeding studies monounsaturated fat had no association, saturated fat had a positive association and N_3 from fish sources tended to have negative associations with rates of all three cancers. Polyunsaturated fat was positively associated with breast and prostate cancers but had no association with colon cancer (Table 13-4). More extensive statistical analyses of international data adding ovarian and endometrial cancers as well as known confounding factors strengthened rather than weakened these associations with total fat, saturated and polyunsaturated fatty acids (7).

The links between reproductive cancers and both saturated and polyunsaturated fatty acids and between colon cancer and saturated fats fit logically with the recent patterns of cancer rates and fat and fatty acids consumption in the U.S. and Japan. The documented experience of migrants who move from countries with lower rates of breast, colon and prostate cancers to countries with higher ones back up the results of these international analyses. Some of the most recent and important studies are of changes in cancer rates during the lifetime of Australian immigrants (19). Italian women who move to Australia increase their breast cancer death rates from less than half to the same high rate as Australian born women within twenty years. Risks for colon cancer converge towards the indigenous Australian rate with 20 years of residence by immigrants from countries with higher (e.g. Scotland) and lower (e.g. Southeast Asia) colon cancer rates. National dietary survey (20) data suggest that migrants to Australia continue to cook their usual dishes but add more red meat to them. The results of linear regression of international variations in fat disappearance on site specific cancer incidence rates have been used to predict changes in cancer rates of migrants after some years of residence in the host country (7). Rates observed in migrants from Japan to the United States by an independent Japanese investigator (21) fit well with those predictions (Table 13-5).

As mentioned earlier, analytic studies of the diets of individuals with and without cancer have been constrained by the homogeneity of regional and national diets. Populations in the process of dietary change (often but not necessarily migrants) or including subgroups having very distinct dietary practices offer unique opportunities to detect links between fat and cancer. Studies in two such populations have been pub-

TABLE 13-5

Relative Cancer Incidence Risk Japanese Women Living in the U.S. and Japan

	Observed (1985)	Projected from regression analysis
Site:		
Breast	3.5	2.9
Colon	3.2	3.5
Rectum	1.5	1.5
Ovary	2.9	2.9
Endometrium	11.3	4.6

Prentice 1990

lished very recently. One took advantage of a stable but culturally diverse northern Italian population and its varying rates of breast cancer (21); the other took advantage of the Shanghai population with low indigenous levels and a similar population with rising rates of colon cancer, Chinese migrants living on the West Coast of the United States (22). The former showed an increased risk of breast cancer with diets, high in animal protein and fat and the latter an increased risk for colon cancer with the increased consumption of saturated fat. Although more results from studies in unique populations and more information about likely biological mechanisms will increase the desire to fund human intervention studies to prove or disprove the dietary fat cancer association, the need for such studies is not disputed. One of the most critical public health questions is whether the public response to heart disease prevention programs concentrated on lowering blood cholesterol will achieve this goal with substantial changes in the ratio of polyunsaturated to saturated fatty acids eaten without lowering total fat intake enough to slow down the increasing rates of reproductive organ cancer.

There are a number of feasible biological pathways by which dietary fat could influence reproductive, and large bowel cancers, and there are small amounts of epidemiologic data to support some of them. A hormonal influence is one of the most easily accepted mechanisms for the reproductive cancers and there is evidence to show that dietary fat intake can influence hormone levels in post-menopausal women who have the highest risk of breast cancer. Two groups of 180 and 600 women who followed a low fat dietary intervention in the context of a randomized trial cut their dietary fat consumption in half and maintained

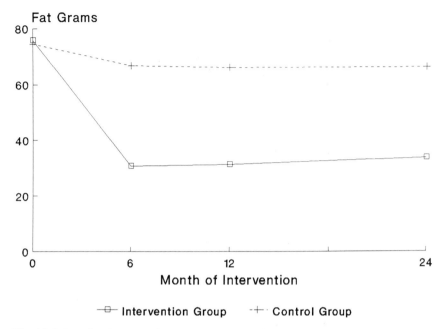

Fig. 13-4. Low fat dietary intervention program.

that new pattern of eating for one to three years (Figure 13-4) (23). They reduced their total fat and each fatty acid proportionately. Blood samples were collected during a period of four weeks when the second group of women were between 10 to 22 weeks into the intervention protocol. Hormone levels were measured in the blood samples from 73 women who were postmenopausal and had never used exogenous hormones (Table 13-6) (24). There were significant reductions from baseline levels of total and weakly bound estradiol. This reduction was accompanied by an average reduction of 12 mg/dl in total plasma cholesterol and an average 3.4 kg in body weight. A reduction of circulating hormone levels during short-term dietary fat interventions has been shown by other investigators and one of the questions raised about measurements relatively early in the process of dietary fat reduction is whether active weight loss could influence hormone levels.

A randomized 10 month feeding study in fourteen female primates (15-18 years) has just been completed. The groups of monkeys had isocaloric diets with high or low-fat composition and were in individual cages throughout. The monkeys on the low fat diet did not lose weight.

TABLE 13-6
Plasma hormone concentrations in relation to dietary fat intervention in 73 postmenopausal women not using exogenous hormones*

	Estradiol, pg/mL	Unbound estradiol, pg/mL	Weakly bound estradiol, pg/mL	Bioavailable estradiol†, pg/mL	SHBG-bound estradiol‡, pg/mL	SHBG, µg/dL
Pre-intervention	0.71 (0.26)	−0.89 (0.32)	0.44 (0.34)	0.46 (0.34)	0.28 (0.30)	0.07 (0.27)
Post-intervention	0.63 (0.26)	−0.88 (0.29)	0.36 (0.32)	0.39 (0.31)	0.18 (0.30)	0.02 (0.28)
Difference	−0.08 (0.20)	0.01 (0.26)	−0.07 (0.24)	−0.07 (0.24)	−0.09 (0.35)	−0.05 (0.30)
t value	−3.27	0.33	−2.49	−2.49	−2.18	−1.46
p value	<.001	>.70	.01	.01	.03	.14

*Values = mean and SD (in parentheses) for log (base 10) of preintervention and postintervention measurements and for their difference.
†Calculated as sum of concentrations of unbound and weakly bound (albumin-bound) estradiol.
‡Concentration of estradiol bound to sex hormone-binding globulin (SHBG) was approximated as difference between concentrations of total and bioavailable estradiol.
Source: Prentice, et al, 1990; 82:129-134.

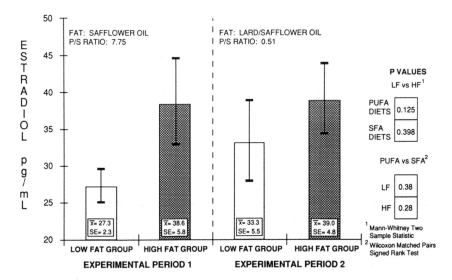

Fig. 13-5. Estradiol levels

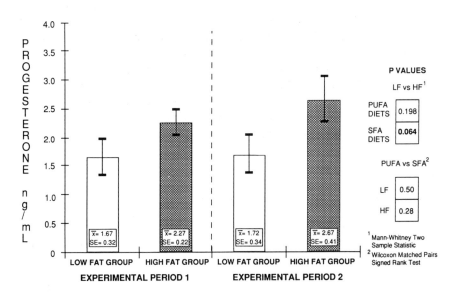

Fig. 13-6. Progesterone levels

The group of monkeys on the high fat diet had more estrus cycles and higher blood levels of both estradiol (Figure 13-5) and progesterone (Figure 13-6). This pattern was true whether the fat fed to the monkeys was mostly polyunsaturated or saturated fatty acid. The only point to be made with this illustration is that high fat diets can influence endogenous hormone levels, whether the fat is predominantly saturated or polyunsaturated fatty acid (25).

Ad libitum feeding experiments have shown that dietary fat consistently promotes spontaneous and induced mammary and colon tumors in small laboratory animals, and that both polyunsaturated and saturated fatty acids can act as promoters given the right conditions (a basic amount of essential fatty acids). On the other hand, dietary fat composition does not have the same influence on animals fed on calorie restricted (deficient) diets. Detailed meta-analysis of experimental studies on mammary (26) and colon (27) cancer tumors showed that both mammary and colon tumors were independently influenced by total energy (calories) and by fatty acid content of the diets under ad lib feeding conditions. In general, clinical investigators accept ad lib feeding conditions as most pertinent to studies of human cancers with high rates in highly developed countries and associated with migration from countries with low to countries with high dietary fat consumption.

In summary the analysis of natural human experiments and the results of animal feeding studies uniformly suggest that cancer rates rise as the fat content of the diet increases and that both saturated and polyunsaturated fatty acids can contribute to that rising rate. Explanatory analytic epidemiologic studies are fraught with logistic and technical difficulties that make their results inconclusive. Human experimental intervention studies will be needed to get conclusive answers to the questions: will low fat diets prevent cancers of the reproductive organs and colon and rectum.

References

1. Doll, R., Peto, R., (1981) JNCI 66:1191-1308.
2. Carroll, K.K., (1980) J Environ Pathol Toxicol 3:253-271.
3. Armstrong, B., Doll, R., (1975) Int J Cancer 15:617-631.
4. Miller, A.B., (1986) In: Reddy BS, Cohen LA, eds. Diet, nutrition and cancer, a critical evaluation. VI. Micronutrients and cancer. Boca Raton, FL CRC Press. 67-76.
5. Hursting, S.D., Thornquist, M., Henderson, M.M., (1990) J Prev Med 19:242-253.

6. Prentice, R.L., Kakar, F., Hursting, S., Sheppard, L., Klein, R. and Kushi, L.H., (1988) JNCI 80, 802-814.
7. Prentice, R.L. and Sheppard, L., (1990) Dietary fat and cancer: Consistency of the epidemiologic data, and disease prevention that may follow from a practical reduction in fat consumption. Cancer Causes and Control 1, 81-97.
8. Rose, G., (1985) Int J Epidemiol 14:32-38.
9. Prentice, R.L., Pepe, M., Self, S.G., (1989) Cancer Res 49:3147-3156.
10. Howe, G.R., Hirohata, T., Hislop, G., et al. (1990) JNCI 82:561-569.
11. Willett W. Nutritional Epidemiology. Oxford U Press, New York, 1990: Chapter 14.
12. United States Department of Agriculture (1988). Nutrient Content of the US Food Supply. Hyattsville, MD: Human Nutrition Service Admin Report 299-21:8-9.
13. Ministry of Health and Welfare, Bureau of Public Health (1951-1989). Kokumin-Eiyo-no Genjo (current status of national nutrition) 1949-1987. Tokyo: Dai-ichi Shuppan (in Japanese).
14. Prentice, R.L. and Sheppard, L., (1989) Prev Med 18, 167-179.
15. Grahm, S., Haughey, B., Marshall, J., et al. (1983) JNCI 70:687-692.
16. Lands, W.E.M., Hamazaki, T., Yamazaki, K., Okuyuma, H., Sakai, K., Gato, Y. and Hubbard, Y.S., (1990) Am J Clin Nutr 51:991-993.
17. Kolonel, L., (1987) Am J Clin Nutr 45:336-341.
18. Tominaga, S. and Kato, T., (1990) Changing patterns of cancer and diet in Japan. Recent Progress in Research on Nutrition and Cancer. Mettlin CJ and Aoki K, eds. New York: Wiley-Liss Inc., pp 1-10.
19. McMichael, A.J. and Giles, G.G., (1988) Cancer Res 48:751-756.
20. Cashel, K., English, R., Bennett, S., et al. National Dietary Survey of adults: 1983: 1. Foods consumed. Canberra: Commonwealth Department of Health, 1986.
21. Tominaga, S. (1985) Cancer incidence in Japanese in Japan, Hawaii and Western United States. National Cancer Inst Monograph 69:83-92.
22. Whittemore, A.S., Wu-Williams, A.H., Lee, M., Shu, R., Gallagher, R.P., Dengao, J., et al. (1990) Diet, physical activity, and colorectal cancer among Chinese in North America and China. JNCI 82:915-926.
23. Insull, W., Henderson, M.M., Prentice, R.L., et al. (1990) Arch Intern Med 150:421-427.
24. Prentice, R.L., Thompson, D.J., Clifford, C., et al. (1990) JNCI 82:129-134.
25. Henderson M. Personal Communication
26. Freidman, L.S., Clifford, C., Messina, M., (1990) Cancer Res 50:5710-5719.
27. Zhao, LP. Personal Communication

Chapter Fourteen
Fatty Acid Metabolism and Biochemical Mechanisms in Cancer

Rashida A. Karmali

>Memorial Sloan-Kettering Cancer Center
>New York, NY 10021

The relationship of dietary fat to cancer is an important area in cancer prevention and causation. High fat diets have long been associated with a higher than average risk of breast and colon cancer. Laboratory animal studies indicate that the type as well as the amount of fat in the diet influences the development of spontaneous, carcinogen-induced, and transplantable mammary tumors in mice and rats (1-3). Polyunsaturated fats (linoleic acid, C18:2n-6) promote mammary tumorigenesis more than saturated fats. However, there is no correlation between age-adjusted mortality rates for human breast cancer and total consumption of vegetable oils or percent calories of polyunsaturated fatty acids (linoleic acid) from vegetable oils (4). Even though epidemiological data do not by themselves establish a causative relationship between dietary fat or linoleic acid and cancer, the supporting evidence from animal studies has directed investigators to identify the various components of dietary fat to determine the mechanism of action. Of course, the question as to whether findings in rodent tumor models can be applied to human tumors, still remains unanswered.

Experimental Carcinogenesis

While there is evidence to suggest that saturated fat influences the initiation of mammary carcinogenesis (5) most of the evidence points to the effect of linoleic acid on the promotional stage of carcinogenesis. Linoleic acid (4% of calories) was required to elicit maximal tumor incidence in the 7,12, dimethylbenz (a) anthracene (DMBA) -induced mammary tumor model (6). In these studies the fat blends used consisted of corn oil and coconut oil. A positive trend between linoleic acid (range 0.5 to 4% of calories) and tumor incidence was observed in the experiment using the corn/coconut oil blend but not with corn/palm oil. Even though the absolute levels of linoleic acid were similar in the two fat blends, the composition of remaining fatty acids was different. The corn/coconut oil blend contained relatively large quantities of C14:0 compared with the corn/palm oil blend. The latter contained higher amounts of C16:0 and C18:1 than the corn/coconut blend. These observations suggest that linoleic acid actions are a function of overall dietary fatty acids. In this study, there was no correlation between tumor yield and prostaglandin E concentration in mammary fat pads of normal animals maintained on similar diets. The authors concluded that "linoleate may act by some other mechanism to stimulate tumorigenesis." One possible reason for the lack of correlation may be that prostaglandin mediated actions of linoleic acid have been reported to occur during the promotion phase of DMBA carcinogenesis (7). Hence, a more suitable tissue to determine whether prostaglandin E production is important in mediation of linoleic acid actions is mammary tissue taken during the promotion phase after DMBA challenge.

A positive association was found among dietary linoleic acid, tumor prostaglandin E2, and mammary tumor incidence when four different oils were studied in the N-nitrosomethylurea (NMU)-model. Cohen et al. (8,9) studied safflower (linoleic acid 82%), corn (linoleic acid 56%), olive (oleic acid 79%), and coconut oil (myristic acid 54%). Rats on safflower and corn oil diets exhibited enhanced mammary tumor yields when compared to animals fed olive or coconut oil diets. The authors suggested that the relatively neutral effects of olive oil compared to corn and safflower oils "may prove of interest epidemiologically, particularly with regard to the fact that breast cancer rates in traditional olive oil-consuming countries such as Greece and Spain lie in an intermediate position between the high risk northern European countries, the United States, and Canada, and low-risk Japan, despite the relatively high total fat consumption typical of these countries" (1,8,10,11).

Marine N-3 Fatty Acids and Tumor Inhibition

Studies of Japanese in Japan and migrants to Hawaii provide important clues on the effect of westernization of their diet and the incidence of breast and colon cancers. The traditional Japanese diet includes large quantities of fish so that total fat, currently 22-23% of total calories (12), is comprised of an appreciable portion of long chain fatty acids of the n-3 family (13).

The first studies to test the hypothesis that n-3 fatty acids may exert anti-tumor effects were based upon knowledge of the biochemical actions of eicosapentaenoic acid (C20:5n-3) and docosahexaenoic acid (C22:6n-3). These fatty acids, present in appreciable amounts in fish oil concentrates, inhibit the oxidative metabolism of arachidonic acid by the cycloxygenase pathway (14, 15). In addition, eicosapentaeonoic acid competitively inhibits the lipoxygenase pathways. Whereas arachidonic acid is the precursor of dienoic prostanoids/thromboxane and tetraene leukotrienes, eicosapentaenoic acid is the substrate for trienoic prostanoids/thromboxane and pentaene leukotrienes. All products of eicosapentaenoic acid are biologically less active than corresponding products of arachidonic acid (16,17).

We have studied the effect of feeding fish oil on four animal tumor systems—the R3230AC transplantable mammary tumor, DU-145 human prostatic transplantable tumor, DMBA-induced mammary tumor, and 13762 metastatic mammary adenocarcinoma. The sizes of the R3230AC (18) and the DU-145 (19) were significantly reduced in animals fed fish oil. Tumor dienoic prostaglandins and thromboxane were reduced in the fish-oil fed animals. Eicosapentaenoic acid and docosahexaenoic acid were incorporated into tumor phospholipids at the expense of linoleic acid and arachidonic acid. A number of studies have been reported to suggest a moderate inhibiting effect of n-3 fatty acids on DMBA-induced mammary tumor development (20,21). Metastasis of 13762 MAT: B mammary tumor cells was inhibited by dietary n-3 fatty acids (22). The balance between prostacyclin and thromboxane A2 may be disrupted in favor of platelet aggregation during tumor cell metastasis (23). Since eicosapentaenoic acid inhibits thromboxane A2 synthesis and prostacyclin (PGI3) is produced from eicosapentaenoic acid, the hypothesis we have tested is that selective inhibition of thromboxane A2 synthesis may prove a useful means of controlling the formation of hematogenous tumor metastasis. Several investigators have tested the effects of marine n-3 fatty acids in a number of different tumor models. This topic has been reviewed previously (24,25).

Plant C18:3, N-3 and N-6 Fatty Acids

An important mechanism of action by which linoleic acid exerts tumor promoting activity is synthesis of dienoic prostaglandins (7,26). When cyclooxygenase inhibitors were administered with a linoleic acid-rich diet, fewer mammary tumors developed compared to the control group. The exaggerated arachidonic metabolism in cancer tissues is also inhibited by n-3 fatty acids present in fish oil (24, 25). The working hypothesis tested in animal tumor models is that linoleic acid (n-6) acts as a tumor promoter whereas marine n-3 fatty acids do not enhance development and progression of several types of animal tumors. If the ultimate goal is to inhibit arachidonic acid metabolism, biochemical studies suggest that both dihomogamma-linolenic acid (C20:3,n-6) and eicosapentaenoic acid modulate arachidonic acid metabolism by competing for the cyclooxygenase and lipoxygense enzymes. Endogenous levels of dihomo-gamma-linolenic acid and eicosapentaenoic acid can be elevated by feeding their precursors gamma-linolenic acid (C18:3,n-6) and alpha-linoleic acid (C18:3, n-3). Blackcurrant oil was used as a source of C18:3, n-3 (16%) and C18:3, n-6 (18%). We have examined the influence of diets containing corn oil, black currant oil, fish oil plus corn oil and two mixtures of black currant oil plus fish oil. This approach was taken to compare effects of plant and marine n-3 and n-6 fatty acids to devise optimal cancer prevention interventions in the DMBA model.

Analysis of tumor incidence indicates that rats fed blackcurrant oil, fish oil plus corn oil, and 2 combinations of blackcurrant oil plus fish oil did not exhibit enhanced mammary tumor yields compared to rats fed the corn oil diet (27).

In general, fatty acid profiles of red blood cell and tumor phosphoglycerides reflected dietary fatty acid composition. Even though tumor levels of linoleic acid were similar, levels of gamma-linolenic acid, dihomo-gamma-linolenic acid and alpha-linolenic acid were higher in the blackcurrant group compared to the corn oil group. These results raise the possibility that fatty acids other than linoleic acid may alter yields of DMBA-induced mammary tumors. Incorporation of marine n-3 fatty acids in tumor phosphoglycerides was greater in the fish oil group compared to groups fed the plant type n-3 fatty acid. Since tumor yields were the lowest in the fish oil group, these results suggest that incorporation of marine n-3 fatty acids into cell membranes does not favor development of DMBA-induced mammary tumors (27).

Fatty acid composition of phosphoglycerides in nine additional tissues was measured in the groups fed corn oil or black currant oil. Results obtained indicated decreases in C18:1 n-9 and C18:2 n-6 but increases in C18:3 n-6, C-18:3n-3, C20:3 n-6, C-20:5 n-3 and C22:6 n-3 in the blackcurrant oil fed animals compared to corn oil fed animals (Tables 14-1 and 14-2).

Within the blackcurrant oil fed group, there were differences in incorporation of some fatty acids among the nine tissues. For example, heart and liver phospholipids contained both plant and marine n-3 fatty acids. However, colon, mammary gland, ovary, spleen, stomach, thymus,

TABLE 14-1
Changes in Tissue Fatty Acid Composition (%)
(Blackcurrant oil - Corn Oil)

Tissue	18:2n-6	18:3n-6	20:3n-6	20:3n-6
Colon	-4.58	+7.54	+0.77	+0.10
Mammary	-5.75	+7.90	+1.08	+0.36
Stomach	-5.45	+7.57	+0.82	-0.17
Heart	-8.91	+3.70	+3.63	+0.83
Liver	-1.96	+4.73	+3.04	+0.75
Ovary	-8.82	+7.13	+1.51	+0.63
Uterus	-7.67	+5.77	+0.46	+0.91
Thymus	-1.98	+6.67	+1.20	+0.59
Spleen	-4.13	+6.64	+1.30	+0.03

TABLE 14-2
Changes in Tissue Fatty Acid Composition (%)
(Blackcurrant oil - Corn Oil)

Tissue	18:3n-3	20:5n-3	22:5n-3	22:6n-3
Colon	+8.54	+0.25	+0.28	+0.27
Mammary	+9.12	+0.31	+0.32	+0.19
Stomach	+7.95	+0.12	+0.22	+0.12
Heart	+3.72	+2.08	+2.26	+0.11
Liver	+5.82	+2.32	+1.93	+2.05
Ovary	+7.80	+0.43	+0.63	+0.53
Uterus	+6.38	+0.27	+0.47	+0.39
Thymus	+7.58	+0.21	+0.39	+0.22
Spleen	+6.82	+0.56	+0.42	+0.28

and uterus phosphoglycerides contained plant n-3 fatty acid and only traces of marine n-3 fatty acids. The highest level of linoleic acid (51%) was found in mammary phosphoglycerides from the corn oil fed group (Table 14-3). These results demonstrate that dietary fatty acids alter the structure of several tissues besides the target for the carcinogen DMBA. Clearly the impact of varied lipid nutriture should be studied in the whole animal.

Additional biochemical studies completed demonstrate competition between 3 eicosapolyenoic acids as substrates for cyclooxygenase. Pros-

TABLE 14-3
% Linoleic Acid

Tissue	Corn oil	Blackcurrant oil
Colon	49.25	44.67
Mammary	50.95	45.20
Stomach	47.47	42.02
Heart	33.74	24.83
Liver	42.17	40.21
Ovary	48.95	40.13
Uterus	46.72	39.05
Thymus	48.60	46.62
Spleen	47.25	43.12

taglandin E2 production was reduced in the order corn oil > blackcurrant oil fish oil. Expression of H-ras in mammary tumors was in the order corn oil > blackcurrant and fish oil (28).

References

1. Carroll, K.K., and Khor, H.T., (1970) Cancer Res. 30:2260.
2. Carroll, K.K., and Khor, H.T., (1975) Prog. Biochem. Pharmacol. 10:308.
3. Rogers, A.E., and Wetsel, W.C., (1981) Cancer Res. 41:3735.
4. Carroll, K.K., Dietary Fat and Cancer (Ip, C., Birt, D.F., Rogers, A.E., and Mettlin, C., eds.) p.231. 1986. Alan R. Liss, New York
5. Rogers, A.E., Conner, R.H., Bonlanger, C.L., Lee, S.Y., Carr, F.A., and Dumouchil, W.H., in Basic and Clinical Aspects of Dietary fiber (Vahouny, G. and Kritchevski, D., eds.) 1985 Plenum Press.
6. Ip, C, Carter, C.A. and Ip, M., (1985) Cancer Res. 45:1997.
7. Carter, C.A., Milholland, R.J., Shea, W. and Ip, M.M., (1983) Cancer Res. 43:3559.
8. Cohen, L.A., Thompson, D.O., Maeura, Y., Choi, K., Blank, M.E. and Rose, D.P., (1986) J Natl Cancer Inst. 77:33.
9. Cohen, L.A., Thompson, D.O., Choi, K., Karmali, R.A., and Rose, D.P., (1986) J. Natl. Cancer Inst. 777:43.
10. Aravanis, C., and Ioannidis, P.J., in The Greek Islands heart study. Nutritional prevention of cardiovascular disease (Yamoril, Y., and Levenberg, W., eds) 125, 1984
11. Christakis, G., Fordyce, M.K., and Kurtz, C.S. in Third International Congress on the biological value of olive oil. Chania, Crete, Greece: Public Subtropical Plants and Olive Trees Institute, 85, 1980.

12. Hirayama, T.J., (1979) Natl. Cancer Inst. Monogr. 53:149.
13. Harai, A., Hamazaki, T. and Terano, T., (1980) Lancet 2:1132.
14. Needleman, P., Whitaker, M.O., Syche, A., Watters, K., Sprecher, H., and Raz, A., (1980) Prostaglandins 19:165.
15. Corey, R.J., Shih, C., and Cashman, J.R., (1983) Proc. Natl. Acad. Sci USA 80:3581.
16. Lee, T.H., Mencia-Huerta, J.M., Shih, C., Corey, E.J., Lewis, R.A., and Austen, K.F., (1984) J. Biol. Chem. 259:2383.
17. Terano, T., Salmon, J.A., and Moncada, S., (1984) Prostaglandins 27:217.
18. Karmali, R.A., Marsh, J., and Fuchs, C., (1984) J. Natl. Cancer Inst. 73:457.
19. Karmali, R.A., Reichel, P., Cohen, L.A., Trano, T., Hirari, A., Tamura, Y., and Yoshida S., (1987) Anticancer Res. 7:1173.
20. Carroll, K.K. and Braden, L.M., (1985) Nutr. Cancer 6:254.
21. Karmali, R.A., Doshi, R.U., Adams, L., and Choi, (1987) K. Adv. Prost. Thromb. Leukotr. Res. 17:886.
22. Adams, L., Trout, J.R., and Karmali, R.A., (1990) Br. J. Cancer 61:290.
23. Honn, K.V., Bockman, R.S., and Marnett, L.J., (1981) Prostaglandins 21:833.
24. Karmali, R.A., (1989) J. Int. Med. 225:Suppl., 197.
25. Karmali, R.A. in Dietary W3 and W6 Fatty Acids (Calli, G. and Simopolous, A.P., eds) 1989. Plenum Publishing Corporation.
26. Kollmorgen, G.M., King, M.M., Kosanke, S.D., and Co. (1983) Cancer Res. 43:4714.
27. Karmali, R.A., Donner, A., Gobel, S. and Shimamura, T., (1989) Anticancer Res. 9:1161.
28. Karmali, R.A., Chao, C.C., Basu, A., and Modak, M., (1989) Anticancer Res. 9:1169.

Chapter Fifteen
Omega-3 Fatty Acids as Anticancer Agents

Bandaru S. Reddy

Division of Nutritional Carcinogenesis
American Health Foundation
Valhalla, New York 10595

Cancer is the second leading cause of deaths in the United States and accounted for about 22% of all deaths in 1986 (1). Cancers of 10 sites-lung, colon-rectum, breast, prostate, pancreas, stomach, ovary, bladder, liver-biliary tract, and leukemias-account for more than 73% of all cancers in the United States (1). In searching for the causes of cancer, considerable effort has been devoted to studying both environmental and genetic factors on the incidence of cancer. In the course of this research, it has become clear that many cancers have external environmental causes, mainly dietary factors. Although the exact proportion is unknown, several researchers estimated the proportion of cancer deaths attributed to diet and other nutritional factors to be 40% in men and 60% in women (2) and about 35% overall (3).

Much of evidence on diet and cancer emerged from epidemiological and laboratory animal model studies (4). Despite some inconsistencies, both ecological and case-control studies in humans have suggested that the incidences of colon and breast cancer are mainly associated with dietary fat and that the incidence of colon cancer is correlated positively with the reduced intake of dietary fiber (4,5). A comparison of populations among the countries indicates that death rates due to cancers of breast, colon, prostate, ovaries, and endometrium are directly proportional to estimated dietary fat intakes (6-10). Animal studies also have supported a cancer-promoting role for dietary fat, and epidemiologic studies have suggested that differences in dietary fat intake may provide a meaningful key to prevention of cancer (5). Considerable uncertainties remain to be resolved about these relationship because the effects of different types of dietary fat (i.e., saturated vs. unsaturated; animal vs. plant origin; omega-3 fatty acids vs. omega-6 fatty acids vs. omega-9 fatty acids) have not been separated in most human epidemiologic studies (5). The importance of types of fat with different fatty acid composition cannot be discounted since laboratory animal model studies provided evidence that tumor promoting effect of dietary fat also depends on the type of fat. The weights of the studies thus far conducted, strongly suggest a role for dietary fat in the etiology of some types of cancer.

The purpose of this paper is to (a) evaluate the scientific evidence for the relationship between the types and amount of dietary fat with special reference to colon cancer, and (b) summarize the experiments conducted in our laboratory to test omega-3 fatty acids as anticancer agents in colon cancer model.

Dietary Fat and Colon Cancer
Evidence From Epidemiolic Studies

Dietary fat has received considerable attention as a possible risk factor in the etiology of colon and breast cancer (7). Based on Japanese data and case-control studies, Wynder et al. (8) proposed in the late 1960s that colon cancer incidence is associated with dietary fat and further suggested that dietary fat influences the composition of the colonic microflora and thus may be involved in the pathogenesis of cancer of the colon. The risk for breast cancer in women and prostate cancer in men is a correlated with total fat consumption in international comparisons (7,9). These pioneering studies led to several correlation and case-control studies on the relationship between dietary fat and cancer. The discussion on the relationship between dietary fat and cancer will be restricted to cancer of the colon.

Descriptive and correlational studies have found a strong positive association between colon cancer mortality and incidence and per capita availability in national diets of total fat, and animal fat estimated from FAO food balance sheets or food disappearance data (4). Because food availability data are known to overestimate actual food consumption in some developed countries, a recent study, in which the food availability was expressed as a percentage of total energy, showed that the availabilities of total fat and animal fat were positively associated with colon cancer mortality (11).

Several case-control studies suggest a positive association between dietary fat and colon cancer (12). Fat consumption has been associated with colon cancer risk in American blacks (13). A Canadian case-control study reported a direct association, including a dose-response, between risk of colorectal cancer and consumption of total fat, especially saturated fat (14,15). The group with the highest fat consumption was at 3.3

times the risk of colon cancer as with the groups with the least consumption. Bristol et al. (16) reported that the group consuming more than 130g fat/day (highest) had a relative risk of 7.9 as compared to the group consuming less than 83g fat/day with a relative risk of 1. Case-control study in Australia, also reported evidence of increasing risk with increased dietary fat and possibly saturated fat and colon cancer (17).

Although the above studies support a role for total dietary fat and saturated fat in the incidence of colon cancer, there were few studies which showed no association between colon cancer risk and dietary fat (18). These conflicting results could be explained on the basis that several of these studies neglected to take into consideration the other confounding factors such as dietary fiber, highly polyunsaturated fish oils, monounsaturated olive oil and other food items that have been shown to reduce the risk of or no effect on colon cancer. For example, Mediterranean countires such as Spain, Greece and Italy have colon cancer mortality rates approximately one-half that of the United States despite the fact their overall fat intake is only slightly lower than that of the United States. One possible reason for this is the high levels of dietary monounsaturated fats in these countries vis-a-vis polyunsaturated fats. In addition, populations consuming increased amount of oils derived from fish or marine animals have a reduced risk for colon cancer. Although further epidemiological studies are needed to verify the association between types of fat and colonic cancer risk and to elucidate their biologic basis, the consistency of the evidence derived from the epidemiologic and animal model studies suggests that the assocation may be casual.

Evidence from Animal Model Studies

A variety of compounds, namely 1,2-dimethylhydrazine (DMH), azoxymethane (AOM), methylazoxymethanol acetate (MAM acetate), 3,2′-dimethyl-4-amino-biphenyl (DMAB) and methylnitrosourea (NMU), that are carcinogenic in the colon have been used in a number of animal models to study the effect of dietary fat on tumorigenesis at this site (12). Several studies using animal models suggest that not only the amount but also types of fat (differing in fatty acid composition) are important factors in determining the promoting effect of various fats in colon cancer development (12). The stage of carcinogenesis at which the effect of dietary fat is exerted appears to be mostly during the promotional phase of carcinogenesis (12).

Effect of Type and Amount of Dietary Fat

Nigro et al. (19,20) studied the effect of diets containing 5 and 35% beef fat on azoxymethane (AOM)-induced intestinal tumors in Sprague-Dawley rats. Animals fed the high beef-fat diet developed more intestinal tumors and more metastases in the abdominal cavity, lungs, and liver than did rats fed the low-fat diet. Pence and Buddingh (21) reported that 1,2-dimethylhydrazine (DMH)-induced colon tumors were increased in male F344 rats fed a high-fat diet compared with those fed a low-fat diet. Studies conducted in our laboratory indicate that F344 rats fed 20% lard or 20% corn oil diets were more susceptible to DMH-induced colon tumors compared with those fed 5% lard or 5% corn oil diets (22,23). Sakaguchi et al. (24) demonstrated a significantly higher incidence of colon tumors in rats fed 5% linoleic acid than in those fed 4.7% stearic acid + 0.3 linoleic acid suggesting that unsaturated fatty acid promotes colon carcinogenesis.

The roles of type and amount of dietary fat during the promotional phase of colon carcinogenesis has been studies in several laboratories. A recent study, in which the intake of all nutrients and calories except fat calories were controlled, provided evidence for the effect of type of fat on colon carcinogenesis (25,26). AOM-induced colon tumor incidence

TABLE 15-1
Colon Tumor Incidence In Rats Fed High And Low Fat Diets

Type and amount of fat	% animals with colon tumors	Type and amount of fat	% animals with colon tumors
	Experiment[a]		
5% corn oil	17	5% olive oil	10
23.5% corn oil	46	23.5% olive oil	13
5% safflower oil	13	23.5% coconut oil	13
23.5% safflower oil	47		
	Experiment[b]		
5% corn oil	40	5% lard	53
23.5% corn oil	93	23.5% lard	90

[a]Female F344 rats were given s.c. injection of azoxymethane at a dose level of 20 mg/kg body wt.
[b]Male F344 rats were given 2 weekly s.c. injection of azoxymethane at a dose level of 14 mg/kg body wt/week.

was increased in F344 rats fed 23% corn oil, lard or safflower oil diets compared to those fed 5% corn oil, lard or safflower oil (Table 15-1). By contrast, diets high in coconut oil or olive oil had no colon tumor-promoting effect compared with diets high in corn oil or safflower oil. The fatty acid composition of olive oil and coconut oil is different from that of corn oil or safflower oil. Olive oil is rich in oleic acid (monounsaturate) and coconut oil is high in medium chain fatty acids whereas corn oil or safflower oil is high in linoleic acid, an omega-6 fatty acid. The varied effects of different types of fat on colon carcinogenesis suggest that the fatty acid composition is one of the determining factors in colon tumor promotion.

Omega-3 Fatty Acids As Tumor Inhibitors

Recently, interest in the marine oils emerged from the findings that cancer incidence rates are generally low in Eskimos in Alaska and Greenland compared to North Americans and other western population groups who consume food containing high dietary fat (27-29). Although fish oils are rarely found in western diets, food consumed by Eskimos contains large amounts of oils derived from fish and seals, and other marine animals (30,31). It is also of interest that the coronary heart disease rates are low in Greenland Eskimos (32). These studies resulted in an interest in the role of fish oils in health and disease (33). The high levels of highly polyunsaturated omega-3 fatty acids such as eicosapentaenoic acid (c20:5, n-3) and docosahexaenoic acid (c22:6, n-3) present in the marine oils make them unique dietary fats because most common animal and vegetable fats are virtually devoid of these fatty acids.

There are numerous reports from various laboratories associating the inhibitory or no promoting effect of fish oils (MAX EPA and Menhaden fish oil) in several types of cancer in animal models. The Max EPA contains about 17% eicosapentaenoic acid and 16% docosahexaenoic acid where Menhaden fish oil contains about 16% eicosapentaenoic acid and 12% docosahexaenoic acid.

In mammary carcinogenesis, Karmali (34) demonstrated that daily supplementation of the rat chow diet with 17, 33, and 67 mg eicosapentaenoic acid and 16, 32, and 64 mg docosahexaenoic acid significantly inhibited the size of the transplantable R3230 AC mammary tumor. Subsequent study using semipurified diets demonstrated a marginal reduction in size of mammary tumors only in the group receiving a diet with omega-3 to omega-6 ratio 2.0 (34). Interestingly, the animals fed the 23.5% fish oil had larger mammary tumors than those fed the 23.5% corn oil diet (34).

The effect of dietary fish oil on chemically-induced mammary carcinogensis has been studied by several investigators. Carroll and Braden (35) demonstrated that dietary Menhaden fish oil at 10 and 20% inhibited 7,12-dimethylbenz(a)anthracine (DMBA)-induced mammary carcinogenesis in female Sprague-Dawley rats. Ip et al. (36) reported that compared to a 20% corn oil diet, 20% fat diets containing either 12% Menhaden fish oil + 8% corn oil or 19% Menhaden fish oil + 1% corn oil significantly inhibited DMBA-induced mammary carcinogensis. This decrease in tumorigenesis is not due to insufficient essential fatty acid (linoleic acid) levels since the lowest tumor incidence in this study was observed in rats receiving 12% Menhaden fish oil plus 8% corn oil. There was also a much larger number of tumor regression observed in the Menhaden fish oil groups (36). Using the mammary tumor model induced by methylnitrosourea, Jurkowski and Cave (37) reported that mammary tumor development in female Buffalo rats was inversely related to the amount of Menhaden fish oil in the diet.

The effect of fish oil on the development of pancreatic cancer in rats was also examined. O'Connor et al. (38) demonstrated that a diet containing 20% Menhaden fish oil produced a significant decrease in the development of azaserine-induced pancreatic preneoplastic lesions when compared to a 20% corn oil diet in rats.

Studies on the relationship of dietary fish oil and colon cancer also revealed that fish oil protects against chemically-induced colon carcinogenesis (39,40). In the first study, the effect of diets containing 5% corn oil, 23.5% corn oil, 3% Menhaden fish oil + 1% corn oil or 22.5% Menhaden fish oil + 1% corn oil fed during post initiation phase on azoxymethane (AOM)-induced colon carcinogenesis was investigated in male F344 rats (39). The results indicated that the colon tumor incidence (% animals with tumors) and multiplicity (number of tumors/animal) were significantly inhibited in animals fed low and high Menhaden fish oil diets than in animals fed the high corn oil diet suggesting that high intake of dietary fish oil had no colon tumor promoting effect.

Although high dietary fish oil inhibited colon carcinogenesis in the above study (39), large amounts of fish oil may induce a variety of physiopathological conditions and harmful side-effects. Therefore, another study was conducted to investigate the efficacy of varying amounts of Menhaden fish oil and corn oil on colon carcinogenesis to determine the optimum dietary levels at which the combination of two

TABLE 15-2
Azoxymethane-induced Colon Tumors In Male F344 Rats Fed The Diets Containing Different Levels of Menhaden Fish Oil

Diet group[a]	Colon adenocarcinomas	
	% animals with adenocarcinomas	No. of adenocarcinomas per animal
5% CO	48[c]	0.59 ± 0.81[b,c]
23.5 CO	81	1.30 ± 0.61
1% CO + 4% MO	37[c]	0.44 ± 0.63[c]
17.6% CO + 5.9% MO	48[c]	0.78 ± 1.03
11.8% CO + 11.8% MO	56[c]	0.79 ± 1.03
5.9% CO + 17.6% MO	37[c]	0.41 ± 0.56

[a]At 7 weeks of age, groups of animals were administered s.c. injections of azoxymethane (15 mg/kg body wt/week for 2 weeks). Four days after carcinogen treatment, groups of animals were transferred to experimental diets containing corn oil (CO) and/or Menhaden fish oil (MO) and fed these diets until sacrifice at week 38.
[b]Mean ± SD.
[c]Significantly different from 23.5% CO group, $P < 0.05$.

sources of fat elicits maximum inhibition when fed during the post initiation phase of carcinogenesis (40). In this study, in addition to 5% corn oil (5% CO) and 1% corn oil + 4% Menhaden fish oil (1% CO + 4% MO) diets, high-fat diets containing 23.5% corn oil (23.5% CO), 17.6% corn oil + 5.9% Menhaden fish oil (17.6% CO + 5.9% MO), 11.8% corn oil + 11.8% Menhaden fish oil (11.8% CO + 11.8% MO) or 5.9% corn oil + 17.6% Menhaden fish oil (5.9% CO + 17.6% MO) were tested (Table 15-2). Feeding of high-fat diets containing 17.6% CO + 5.9% MO, 11.8% CO + 11.8% MO, or 5.9% CO + 17.6% MO significantly inhibited the incidence of colon adenocarcinomas as compared to 23.5% CO; but the multiplicity of adenocarcinomas was inhibited only in the group fed 5.9% CO + 17.6% MO.

Fatty acid composition of the microsomal fraction of colonic mucosa and tumors was also measured in the animals fed the experimental diets. This study demonstrated that feeding increasing levels of Menhaden fish oil altered the incorporation of fatty acids into the microsomes of colonic mucosal cells and tumors. The monounsaturated and saturated fatty acids were unaffected in colonic mucosa by feeding various levels of corn oil and Menhaden oil while the polyunsaturated fatty acids were modified by dietary corn oil and Menhaden oil. Compared to microsomes prepared from rats fed the 23.5% CO diets, microsomes from the animals fed the Menhaden oil diets were enriched with omega-3 fatty acids. The increasing levels of Menhaden oil in the diet significantly increased the omega-3 fatty acids namely eicosapentaenoic acid, docosapentaenoic acid and docosahexaenoic acid and decreased the omega-6 fatty acids such as linoleic acid and arachidonic acid. Significant differences were also observed in the polyunsaturated fatty acid composition of microsomal lipids of colonic tumors among the animals fed the various levels of corn oil and Menhaden oil. Increasing levels of Menhaden oil in the high fat diets decreased the linoleic acid, linolenic and arachidonic acid but increased the eicosapentaenoic acid, docosapentaenoic acid and docosahexaenoic acid. There was also a significant increase in monounsaturated fatty acids namely palmitoleic acid and oleic acid with increasing levels of Menhaden oil in the high fat diets.

Several mechanisms have been postulated for tumor inhibitory effect of omega-3 fatty acids. On such mechanism in colon carcinogenesis might be mediated by the active products of essential fatty acids, namely prostaglandins, since recent studies demonstrated an inhibitory effect of certain prostaglandin synthesis inhibitors such as indomethacin and piroxicam on colon carcinogenesis (41,42). In the present study, the 23.5% CO diet contained about 13.2% linoleic acid which is a precursor for prostaglandin synthesis. Eicosapentaenoic acid and docosahexaenoic acid present in Menhaden fish oil have been shown to inhibit the oxidative metabolism of arachidonic acid by the cyclooxygenase pathway that is involved in the synthesis of prostaglandins (51,52). Eicosapentaenoic is also a competitive inhibitor of lipoxygenase pathway. It is therefore possible that the lack of a colon tumor-promoting effect of Menhaden fish oil might be due to its inhibitory effect on prostaglandin synthesis.

In summary, during the last 20 years, human and/or animal model experiments indicate that dietary fat plays an important role in cancers of colon, breast, prostate and pancreas. The effect of dietary fat in carcinogenesis depends on the type of fat and its fatty acid composition. The mechanisms by which various types of fat increase carcinogenesis is not fully understood; however, in most instances, the high fat diet appears to enhance carcinogenesis through its elevation of agents that act as promoters of tumor development. In certain instances, liver and extrahepatic tissue (colon) enzymes responsible for the metabolism of a variety of carcinogens and cocarcinogens may be mediating factors in the relationship between dietary fat and colon cancer. Several studies also demonstrated that high fat diets containing high levels of fish oil induced fewer tumors in mammary gland, colon and pancreas than did the diet containing high corn oil alone. While the mechanism by which omega-3 fatty acids inhibits carcinogenesis is not clear, one underlying mechanism is that these fatty acids act through the inhibition of prostaglandin synthesis.

Acknowledgment

This research was supported in part from grants and contracts CP-33208, CA-16382, CA-17613, CA-29602, CA-36892, and CA-37663 from the National Cancer Institute. Expert editorial assistance of Ms. Donna Virgil is gratefully appreciated.

References

1. Silverberg, E., Boring, C.C., and Squires, T.S. (1990) Ca-A Cancer J. Clinicians 40, 9-26.
2. Wynder, E.L., and Gori, G.B., (1977) J. Natl. Cancer Inst. 58, 825-832.
3. Doll, R., and Peto, R., (1981) J. Natl. Cancer Inst. 66, 1191-1308.
4. Committee on Diet, Nutrition and Cancer (1982) Diet, Nutrition and Cancer, National Academy of Science, Washington, D.C.
5. Surgeon General's Report on Nutrition and Health (1988) pp.177-247, DHHS (PHS) Publication No. 88-50210, U.S. Department of Health and Human Services, Washington, D.C.
6. Kakar, F., and Henderson, M., (1985) Clinical Nutrition 4, 119-130.
7. Carroll, K.K., and Khot, H.T., (1975) Progress in Biochem Pharmacol. 10, 308-353.
8. Wynder, E.L., Kajitani, T., Ishikawa, S., Dodo, H., and Takano, A., (1969) Cancer 23, 1210-1220.
9. Rose, D.P., Boyar, A.P., and Wynder, E.L., (1985) Cancer 58, 2363-2371.
10. Mahboubi, E., Eyler, N., and Wynder, E.L., (1982) Clinical Obstert. Gynecol. 25, 5-17.
11. McKeown-Eyssen, G.E. and Bright-See, E., (1985) Nutr. Cancer 7, 251-253.
12. Reddy, B.S., (1986) Diet. Nutrition and Cancer, Boca Raton, FL., vol. 1, pp. 47-65.
13. Dale, L.G., Friedman, G.D., Ury, H.K., Grassman, S., and Williams, S.R., (1978) Am. J. Epidemiol. 109, 132-153.
14. Jain, M., Cook, G.M., Davis, F.G., Grace, M.G., Howe, G.R., and Miller, A.B., (1980) Int. J. Cancer 26, 757-768.
15. Miller, A.B., Howe, G.R., and Jain, M., (1983) Int. J. Cancer 32, 155-161.
16. Bristol, J.B., Emmett, P.M., Heaton, K.W., and Williams, R.C.N., (1985) Br. Med. J. 291, 1467-1470.
17. Potter, D.J., and McMichael, A.J., (1986) J. Natl. Cancer Inst. 76, 557-569.

18. Stemmermann, G.N., Nomura, A.M.Y., and Heilbrun, L., (1984) Cancer Res. 44, 4633-4637.
19. Nigro, N.D., Singh, D.V., Campbell, R.L., and Pak, M.S., (1975) J. Natl. Cancer Inst. 54, 439-442.
20. Bull, A.W., Soullier, B.K., Wilson, P.S., Haydon, M.T., and Nigro, N.D., (1979) Cancer Res. 39, 4956-4959.
21. Pence, B.C., and Buddingh, F., (1988) Carcinogenesis 9, 187-190.
22. Reddy, B.S., Narisawa, T., Vukusich, D., Weisburger, J.H., and Wynder, E.L., (1976) Soc. Exp. Biol. Med. 151, 237-239.
23. Reddy, B.S., and Maruyama, H., (1986) J. Natl. Cancer Inst. 77, 815-822.
24. Sakaguchi, M., Hiramatsu, Y., Takada, H., Yamamura, M., Hioki, K., Sato, K., and Yamamoto, M., (1984) Cancer Res. 44, 1472-1477.
25. Reddy, B.S., and Maeura, Y., (1984) J. Natl. Cancer Inst. 72, 745-750.
26. Reddy, B.S., and Maruyama, H., (1986) Cancer Res. 46, 3367-3370.
27. Neilson, N.H., and Hansen, J.P.H., (1980) J. Cancer Res. Clin. Oncol. 98, 287-299.
28. Blot, W.J., Lanier, A., Franmeni, B.J.F., Jr., and Bender, T.R., (1975) J. Natl. Cancer Inst. 55, 546-554, 1975.
29. Waterhouse, J., Muir, C., Correa, P., and Powell, J., (1976) International Agency for Research on Cancer Lyon, France, vol. 3.
30. Bang, H.O., Dyerberg, J., and Hjorne, N., (1976) Acta Med. Scand. 200, 69-73.
31. Murro, I., (1976) Acta Med. Scand. 200, 69-73.
32. Dyerberg, J., and Bjerregaare, P., (1987) Proceedings of the AOCS Short Course on Polyunsaturated Fatty Acids and Eicosanoids, Lands, W.E.M., American Oil Chemists' Society, Champaign, IL., pp. 2-8.
33. Simopoulos, A.P., Kifer, R.R., and Martin, R.E., (1986) Academic Press
34. Karmali, R.A., (1987) Proceedings of the AOCS Short Course on Polyunsaturated Fatty Acids on Eicosanoids, Lands, W.E.M., American Oil Chemists' Society, Champaign, IL., pp. 222-232.
35. Carroll, K.K., and Braden, L.M., (1984) Nutr. Cancer 6, 254-259.
36. Ip, C., Ip, M.M., and Sylvester, P., (1986) Progress in Clinical and Biological Research 222, 283-294.
37. Jurkowski, J.J., and Cave, W.T., (1985) J. Natl. Cancer Inst. 74, 1145-1150.
38. O'Connor, T.P., Roebuck, B.D., and Campbell, T.C., (1985) J. Natl. Cancer Inst. 75, 955-957.
39. Reddy, B.S., and Maruyama, H., (1986) Cancer Res. 46, 3367-3370.
40. Reddy, B.S., and Sugie, S., (1988) Cancer Res. 48, 6642-6647.
41. Pollard, M., and Luckert, P.H., (1980) Cancer Treat. Rep. 64, 1323-1327.
42. Reddy, B.S. Maruyama, H., and Kelloff, G., (1987) Cancer Res. 47, 5340-5346.
43. Corey, R.J., Shih, C., and Cashman, J.R., (1983) Proc. Natl. Acad. Sci. USA 80, 3581-3584.
44. Culp, B.R., Titus, B.J., and Lands, W.E., (1979) Prostaglandins Med. 3, 269-278.

Chapter Sixteen
Effect of Dietary Fats and Eicosanoids on Immune System

Simin Nikbin Meydani, DVM, PhD

Nutritional Immunology Laboratory
USDA Human Nutrition Research Center on Aging at Tufts University
711 Washington Street,
Boston, MA 02111

Interest in the role of lipids as contributing to immune function was initiated by the recognition of its modifying effect on the reticuloendothelial system (1). This interest was further stimulated by the suggestion that an association may exist between certain types of cancer and the quality and quantity of dietary lipids (2,3). Dietary fat has also been shown to affect the severity of autoimmune diseases as well as the length of allograft acceptance (4,5). Furthermore, *in vitro* addition of fatty acids (FA) to lymphocyte cultures was shown to change their mitogenic responses (6).

Cooperation between different cells of the immune system, via membrane associated events and through different protein and lipid mediators, is essential in mounting a successful immune response. Dietary lipids have the capacity to affect the immune system by influencing substrate availability in the formation of cyclooxygenase and lipoxygenase products. These products, in turn, act as lipid mediators in the control of the immune system (7,8). Furthermore, the cells of the immune system are highly dependent on cell membrane function for operations such as the secretion of lymphokines and antibodies, antigen reception, lymphocyte transformation, and contact lysis. The importance of lipids in the maintenance of membrane integrity (9) identifies them as potentially critical nutrients in the regulation of the immune function.

The immune response is divided into cell-mediated and humoral immunity. Cell-mediated immunity refers to the specific response of the system to antigens, principally directed by lymphocytes and macrophages. It is responsible for delayed-type hypersensitivity (DTH), foreign graft rejection, resistance to many pathogenic microorganisms, and tumor immunosurveillance. Cell-mediated immunity is assessed by the proliferative response of lymphocytes to antigens or T and B cell mitogens, lysis of tumor cell lines by lymphocytes and macrophages, lymphokine production, *in vitro* and by DTH *in vivo*. The humoral immune response primarily involves B cell production of antibodies and includes the complement cascade. Both the production of antigen-specific antibodies and activation of the complement cascade result in phagocytosis and neutralization of the invading antigen.

Role Of Arachidonic Acid (AA) Metabolites in Control of the Immune System

AA metabolites, prostaglandins (PG), hydroxyeicosatetraenoic acid (HETE) and leukotrienes (LT), are produced by human peripheral blood mononuclear cells (PBMC) and by mouse splenocytes in response to stimulation by mitogens or antigens and inhibit subsequent T cell proliferation. Likewise, inhibition of PG synthesis *In vitro* enhances T cell proliferation (10-15). Cellular and humoral immune responses operate under negative control by PG. *In vitro*, PGE_2 inhibits T cell prolif-

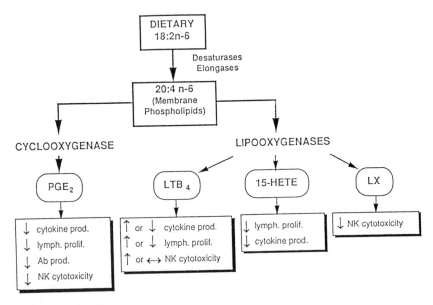

Fig. 16-1. Role of eicosanoids in regulation of immune response.

eration (10,11), lymphokine production (16), the generation of cytotoxic cells (17), and natural killer cell (NK) activity (18).

In addition to PGE_2, lipooxygenase products, i.e. LT and HETE, have been shown to inhibit lymphocyte proliferation in mouse splenocytes and human peripheral lymphocytes (19). This effect may be mediated by decreased T helper and increased T suppressor/cytotoxic cell proliferation (20,21). LTB_4, in some but not all (12) studies, has been shown to increase interleukin (IL)-1 as well as IL-2 production and lymphocyte proliferation. Lipoxins (Lx) which are products of 15-lipoxygenation of AA have been shown to inhibit human NK activity when tested against K562 target cells (22). On the other hand, LTB_4 was shown to augment human NK activity (23). The effect of AA metabolites on cell mediated immunity is summaried in Figure 16-1.

Effect of Polyunsaturated Fatty Acids (PUFA) on the Immune Response

Several investigators have evaluated the effect of dietary fat on the immune response (24,25). Review of the literature presents a confusing picture which is due mainly to the fact that the effect of PUFA on the immune response varies depending on: 1) concentration of dietary fat, 2) duration of supplementation, 3) genetic variation, 4) existence of infectious or autoimmune and inflammatory diseases, 5) age of the animal, 6) status of other nutrients such as vitamin E, the requirement of which is affected by the degree of saturation of FA, 7) presence or absence of essential fatty acid (EFA) deficiency in the control diet, 8) particular immunological test used in the experiment, and 9) species of PUFA tested, i.e. N-6 or N-3 PUFA.

We recently reviewed the effect of N-6 PUFA and the N-3 PUFA of plant origin on the immune response (26,27). The present paper will focus on the effect of N-3 PUFA contained in marine oils on cell-mediated immune responses.

Effect of the N-3 PUFA on Cell-Mediated Immunity

The lowered incidence of coronary heart disease in Greenland Eskimos (28) has been attributed to a high consumption of diets rich in N-3 FA, eicosapentaenoic acid (EPA) and docosahexaenoic acid (DHA). EPA is a precursor of the 3-series of prostanoids and the 5-series of leukotrienes (LT) which have been shown to exhibit less potent aggregatory and inflammatory properties compared to corresponding AA metabolites (29,30). These findings have renewed the interest in fish oil (FO) for potential use in the prevention and/or therapy of certain chronic cardiovascular and inflammatory diseases. Animal experiments and clinical trials have indicated a potentially beneficial effect of N-3 FA supplementation on atherosclerosis and atherothrombotic disorders (31,32), autoimmune (33,34), and inflammatory diseases (35). However, the effect of N-3 FA on the cell-mediated immunity has not been well studied. Several studies have shown that EPA and DHA decrease tissue levels of AA and therefore the formation of AA-derived eicosanoids. As mentioned above, both cyclooxygenase and lipooxygenase metabolites of AA, such as PGE_2, LTB_4, 15-HETE and Lx, are involved in the regulation of the immune response. Thus, diet enrichment with N-3 FA could potentially affect the immune response. We, therefore, studied the effect of N-3 FA supplementation on 1) NK activity and prostaglandin synthesis of young and old mice, and 2) cytokine production and lymphocyte proliferation in young and old women.

Effect of N-3 FA Supplementation on NK Activity of Young and Old Mice

NK cells have a wide range of biological activities which include immunosurveillance against neoplastic cells, viral infection, abnormal hematopoietic development, and production of lymphokines such as interferon (36). With aging, there is a distinct decline in NK activity which may partially account for the increased incidence of spontaneous tumors. Our studies (37), as well as others (38), have shown that splenocytes obtained from aged rodents have a greater capacity to produce PGE_2 compared to those from young rodents.

NK activity is under negative control by PGE_2. Roder and Klein (18) showed that PGE_2 inhibited while indomethacin enhanced murine NK activity against YAC-1 target cells. The PGE_2-mediated inhibition of NK-mediated cytotoxicity was at the level of NK and not at the level of the target cells. Macrophages obtained from tumor-bearing mice with low NK activity produced higher levels of PGE_2 compared to non-tumor-bearing mice. More recently, Lx have also been shown to inhibit human NK activity when tested against K562 target cells. On the other hand, LTB_4, a 5-lipoxygenase product of AA metabolism, was shown to augment human NK activity (39). We, therefore, compared the effect of feeding diets containing marine oil (high in N-3 FA) with that of corn oil (CO) (high in N-6 FA) (9).

Young (3 mo) and old (24 mo) C57BL/6Nia mice were fed nutritionally adequate semi-purified diets which contained CO calculated as 10% of weight or 1.2% CO plus 8.8% FO (MaxEPA) for 6 weeks. Plasma and splenocyte tocopherol levels were measured by the modified method of Bieri et al. (40) as previously described (41). PGE_2 obtained from supernatant of splencoytes stimulated with 0.5µg/ml concanavaline A (Con A) for 48 hr was measured by radioimmunoassay (RIA) (42). NK-mediated cytotoxity against (^{51}Cr)-labeled YAC-1 target cells was measured by the method of Kiessling et al. (43). To clearly establish that the observed effect of FO was, in fact, due to FO and not to an adverse effect of CO, NK activity was also measured in a group of young and old mice fed a non-purified diet (Purina Lab Chow) containing 5% vegetable oils by weight.

There was no difference in weight gain due to the diet utilized. The amount of tocopherol provided by each diet as well as serum and splenocyte tocopherol levels, are shown in Table 16-1.

No difference was observed in serum and splenocyte tocopherol concentration between young and old mice fed 30 PPM tocopherol and those fed FO and 167 PPM tocopherol.

Figure 16-2 shows NK-mediated cytotoxicity of splenic leukocytes from young and old mice fed either semi-purified diets containing CO, FO, or non purified diet (Chow). Old mice fed the nonpurified diet or CO diet had significantly lower percentage of specific lysis compared to

TABLE 16-1

Dietary, Serum and Splenocyte α-tocopherol Level in Young and Old Mice Fed CO or FO Diets (mean ± SEM)

Diet	Age	dl-α-Tocopheryl[a] acetate measured in the diet	α-Tocopherol serum[b]	α-Tocopherol splenocytes[c]
	mo	mg/kg	µg/ml	mg/1×10^7 cells
CO	3	30 ± 2	2.9 ± 0.4	—
FO	3	167 ± 3	3.5 ± 0.4	—
CO	24	30 ± 2	1.7 ± 0.3	10.9 ± 1.0
FO	24	167 ± 3	2.6 ± 0.3	11.6 ± 1.3

[a]n=3, calculated from α-tocopherol values measured in extracted samples multiplied by a correctional factor (molecular weight of α-tocopherol/molecular weight of dl-α-tocopheryl acetate)
[b]n = 8 or 9
[c]n=8

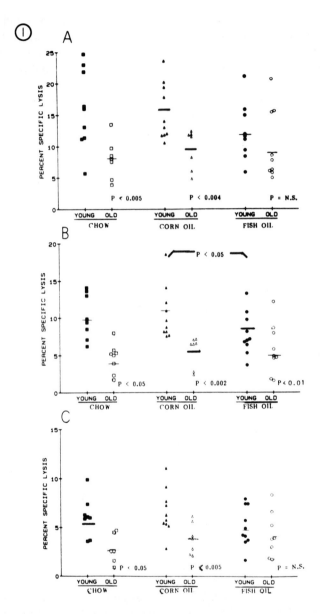

Fig. 16-2. Effect of age and dietary fat on NK-mediated cytotoxicity. A, B and C represent mean percent specific lysis value of triplicate NK assay values tested at 1:100, 1:50 and 1:25 T:E ratios, respectively.

young mice fed the same diet. This was found for all target to effector (T:E) ratios tested (P<0.05) (Fig. 16-2). However, the old mice fed FO had significantly lower NK activity than young mice fed FO only at 1:50 T:E ratio. This was due to low NK activity in young mice fed FO diet rather than high NK activity of old mice fed the FO diet. The NK activity in young and old mice fed CO diet was not different from that of mice fed the non-purified diet. Young mice fed FO diet tended to have lower percentage of specific lysis at 1:100, 1:50 and 1:25 T:E ratios compared to those fed the CO diet. However, the difference was only statistically significant at the T:E ratio of 1:50 (P<0.05). No difference was observed between old mice fed the CO or the FO diets (see Fig. 16-2).

PGE_2 synthesis by spleen cells is shown in Table 16-2. Old mice fed CO diet showed 38% higher PGE_2 production than young mice fed CO diet; however, the difference was not statistically significant. Cultures from young and old mice fed FO had significantly less PGE_2 production than those fed CO.

In agreement with other investigators (43,44), our studies demonstrate that old mice had significantly lower NK activity than young mice fed a non-purified diet or CO-based purified diet. Cultured splenic leukocytes from old mice had higher PGE_2 production than those of young mice. This agrees with our previous results (37) as well as those of others (38). PGE_2 has been shown to decrease NK activity (45) and therefore may have contributed to the lowered NK activity of old mice. However, despite a significant reduction in PGE_2 production by FO, substitution of

TABLE 16-2
PGE_2 Synthesis by Splenic Leukocytes from Young and Old Mice Fed the CO or the FO Diet (mean ± SEM)

Diet	Age	N	PGE_2[a]
	mo		ng/5×10^6 cells
CO	3	7	3.3 ± 0.6
FO	3	7	0.6 ± 0.2*
CO	24	4	4.5 ± 2.3
FO	24	6	0.1 ± 0.1

[a]5×10^6 splenic leukocytes were cultured in the presence or absence of 0.5 µg/ml Con A for 48 hr. Cell free supernant was measured for PGE_2 by radioimmunoassay. Values are ng PGE_2 produced by stimulated cells minus ng PGE_2 produced by nonstimulated cells.
*Significantly different from mice fed the CO diet at P<0.007 for young mice and P < 0.0002 for old mice.

dietary N-6 PUFA by N-3 PUFA for 6 wk in old mice did not significantly affect NK activity. The FO-fed young mice generally tended to have lower NK activity compared to CO-fed mice. The difference was statistically significant only at a T:E ratio of 1:50. Lower NK activity in FO-fed mice compared to CO-fed mice was also reported by Sandberg et al. (46). Furthermore, Yamashita et al. (47) showed that addition of 20:5 N-3 emulsion to human NK cells *in vitro* resulted in a marked depression of NK activity. More recently, Hamazaki et al. (48) demonstrated that *in vivo* injection of 20:5 N-3 or 22:6 N-3 emulsion in humans resulted in up to a 65% decrease in NK activity. In a study by Fritsche and Johnston (49), NK activity was not significantly affected by FO feeding. Cyclooxygenase (PGE_2 and lipooxygenase [LTB_4 and 5-hydroperoxyeicosatetraenoic acid (5-HPETE)] have been shown to conversely modulate NK activity, i.e., PGE_2 was shown to decrease (45) and LTB_4 and 5-HPETE were shown to augment NK activity (23,50). Therefore, it is not surprising that despite an 80-96% decrease in PGE_2 synthesis in FO-fed mice compared with CO-fed mice, NK activity was decreased rather than increased in FO-fed mice. LTB_4 and other lipooxygenase products are decreased by FO feeding (30,51). These findings imply that positive modulation of NK activity by LTB_4 and 5-HPETE may be more important than the suppression of its activity by PGE_2. The decrease in NK activity was not due to changes in tocopherol status by FO because plasma and spleen tocopherol levels in FO-fed mice were not different from those of CO-fed mice.

In summary, this study indicates that old mice have lower NK activity than young mice and this may be partially due to an increase in PGE_2 level. Substituting FO for CO at 10% dietary fat level for 6 weeks causes a moderate decrease in NK activity of young mice but does not affect NK activity in old mice.

Effect of N-3 FA Supplementation on Cytokine Production and Lymphocyte Proliferation in Young and Old Women

Billar et al. (52) demonstrated that IL-1 production from Kuppfer cells, obtained from rats fed FO (15 en %) for 6 weeks, was significantly lower compared to rats fed 15 en % CO. Short-term supplementation with 4.6 g/day of N-3 FA has been shown to decrease the inducible production of IL-1 and tumor necrosis factor (TNF) (53). The effect of lower levels of supplementation with N-3 FA for longer periods of time on IL-1, TNF, other cytokines, and lymphocyte proliferation of healthy subjects has not been studied. Furthermore, the question of age difference in N-3 induced changes has not been addressed. The latter point is especially important in light of the age-associated changes of cell-mediated immune function.

Aging is associated with an altered regulation of the immune system (54). Age-related functional changes have been well characterized in both humoral and cell-mediated immune responses. However, the major alterations in immune function occur in the T cell-mediated response. *In vitro*, the proliferative response of human and rodent lymphocytes to phytohemagglutin (PHA) and Con A becomes depressed with age (55). Several groups have shown that antigen and mitogen-stimulated IL-2 production declines with age and contributes to T cell-mediated defects observed with aging (56,57-59) while changes in B cell response and IL-1 production are equivocal (58,60-62). We, therefore, investigated the effect of supplementation with 2.4 g/day of N-3 FA for up to 3 mo on cytokine production and lymphocyte proliferation of young and older females (63).

Six healthy young (23-33 yr) and six healthy older (51-68 yr) women were recruited from the Boston area. Subjects with unusual dietary habits, high alcohol consumption, users of oral contraceptives, corticosteroids, nonsteroidal antiflammatory drugs, smokers and those over 110 percent, or under 90 percent, of their ideal body weights were excluded. All older women were post-menopausal.

Each subject's usual diet was then supplemented with N-3 FA contained in six capsules of Pro-Mega (Parke Davis, Warner Lambert Co., Morris Plains, NJ) daily for 12 wk. The capsules provided each subject with 1680 mg of EPA, 720 mg of DHA, 600 mg of other FA and 6 IU of vitamin E per day. The total amount of fat contributed by the FO capsules was 3 g or approximately 1.5% of their caloric intake.

Compliance was monitored by measurement of total plasma FA. Blood was collected on two consecutive days from young women during the follicular phase of their menstrual cycle (days 4-7) and on two consecutive days from older women. The means of these two determinations were used for further analysis. Samples were collected at baseline and at the end of 1, 2 and 3 mo of supplementation with FO. Heparinized blood (40 ml) was collected for *in vitro* immunological tests and 6 ml of blood was collected in EDTA for WBC differential, FA and vitamin E analysis. Subjects were weighed weekly. PBMC were separated from heparinized blood according to the procedure of Boyum et al. (64).

Mitogenic response of lymphocytes to T cell mitogens Con A and PHA was measured as decribed before (65). Con A stimulated IL-2 production was measured as described by Gillis et al. (66). Con A stimulated IL-6 production was measured by RIA as previously described (67). Endotoxin and staphylococcus epidermis (staph.)-stimulated IL-1β and TNF production were measured by RIA (68,69). PHA-stimulated PGE_2 production was measured by RIA (42).

Compliance was confirmed by a significant increase in plasma EPA and DHA and a significant decrease in AA/EPA ratio. These changes were more dramatic in older women than young women so that the AA/EPA ratio decreased 12 fold in older women but only 4 fold in young women. (Table 16-3). Similarly the decrease in PGE_2 production was more dramatic in older women than young women (71% decrease in older women and 31% decrease in young women, Table 16-3). The total number of WBC and the percentage of mononuclear and polymorphonuclear cells in peripheral blood did not change as a result of FO consumption and was not affected by the age of subjects. Plasma tocopherol level did not change by N-3 FA supplementation.

IL-1β, TNF, and IL-6 production was not significantly different between young and older women prior to FO supplementation. FO supplementation significantly decreased production of these cytokines in both young and older women. The decrease was more dramatic in older wom-

TABLE 16-3
Percentage Change[a] in Plasma EPA, DHA, AA/EPA Level and PBMC PGE_2 Production in Young and Older Women Following N-3 FA Supplementation[b]

Age	EPA	Plasma FA		PGE_2[c]
		DHA	AA/EPA	
Young	+462	+63	− 324	−31
Older	+900	+144	−1109	−71

[a]Values calculated with the following formula:
$$\frac{\text{Post-Supplementation Value - Pre-Supplementation Value}}{\text{Pre-Supplementation Value}} \times 100.$$
[b]Women supplemented their typical American diet with 2.4 g/day of EPA and DHA for 3 mo.
[c]1×10^6 PBMC/ml were cultured in RPMI 1640 + 10% autologous plasma in presence or absence of 10 μg/ml PHA for 48 hours. Cell-free supernatant were analyzed by RIA.

TABLE 16-4

Effect of N-3 FA Supplementation on PBMC Cytokine Production and Lymphocyte Proliferation of Young and Older Women[a]

Parameter	Young baseline[b]	% change[c]	Older baseline[b]	% change[c]
IL-1β (ng/ml)[d]	3.67±0.63	-48	5.97±1.2	-90
IL-6 (ng/ml)[e]	0.57±0.05	-30	0.49±0.04	-60
TNF (ng/ml)[d]	1.62±0.23	-58	1.55±0.30	-70
IL-2 (u/ml)[e]	88.2±27.8	-57	60.4±29.5	-63
Mitogenic response to PHA (CCPm)[f]	84400±15706	-7	53867±5972	-36

[a] Young (23-33 yr) and older (51-68 yr) women supplemented their typical American diet with 2.4 g of N-3 FA for a period of 3 mo.
[b] Mean ± SEM in n=6
[c] Represent percent change after 3 mo of supplementation with N-3 FA compared to baseline value.
[d] 5×10^6 PBMC/ml were stimulate with 1 ng/ml LPS for 24 hr. Total i.e. cell-associated plus secreted IL1-β and TNF was determined by RIA
[e] 1×10^6 PBMC/ml were cultured in presence of 10μg/ml Con A or PHA in presence of autologous plasma for 48 hr. Cell free supernatant were measured by bioassay using CTLL cells for IL-2 and by RIA for IL-6.
[f] 1×10^6 PBMC/ml were cultured in presence or absence of 5 μg/ml PHA for 72 hr in presence of autologous plasma. Lymphocyte proliferation was measured by incorporation of 3H thymidine into DNA after a 4 hr pulse. Data represent corrected counts per minute (CCPM) which is the CPM of stimulated cultures minus CPM of unstimulated cultures.

en than young women so that older women had significantly lower production of IL-1β, TNF and IL-6 than young women after 3 mo of FO supplementation (Table 16-4). Older women had significantly lower production of IL-2 and mitogenic response to PHA and Con A than young women (P < 0.01 for IL-2 and p < 0.04 for mitogenic response) (Table 16-4). FO supplementation resulted in a significant reduction in IL-2 production and mitogenic response of lymphocytes to PHA in older women only. A statistically non-significant reduction was also observed in young women.

Endres et al. (53) demonstrated that N-3 FA supplementation (4.69 g/day in healthy males for 6 wk reduces IL-1β and TNF total synthesis. The amount of IL-1β and TNF produced after 6 wk of supplementation was 60 and 80% of baseline values respectively. In the present study, by using less N-3 FA (2.4 mg/d) the synthesis of IL-1β and TNF produced after 8 wk of supplementation was less than 50% of baseline values. Further reductions were observed after 12 wk of supplementation. This demonstrates that substantial reduction in cytokine production can be achieved without the consumption of large quantities of N-3 FA. Although the pre-supplementation production of IL-1β and TNF was not different between young and older women, the N-3 supplementation induced a greater reduction in older women compared to younger women. This was associated with a larger increase in plasma EPA and DHA and a greater decrease in AA/EPA ratio seen in older women compared to young women following N-3 supplementation (Table 16-3). The reason for higher incorporation of EPA and DHA into plasma lipids of older women is not clear. The analysis of a food frequency questionnaire indicates that the diet of young and older women contained a similar amount of total fat, saturated fat, monounsaturated fat, polyunsaturated fat and P:S ratio. Furthermore, plasma FA profiles prior to FO consumption were similar in young and older group. One possible reason for a higher incorporation of EPA and DHA into plasma lipids of older women is a more efficient absorption of N-3 FA by older women compared to young women. Hollander et al. (70) reported a more efficient absorption of linoleic acid by intestinal segments of old rats compared to young rats. The differences observed may also be due to hormonal differences between the young and old women because all older women were post-menopausal. This, however, unlikely since Suzuki et al. (71) also reported a larger increase in plasma EPA of older male rats than in that of young rats following FO consumption.

The reduction by N-3 supplementation in IL-2 production and PHA mitogenesis in older women is of great interest since T cell functions decrease with aging. The decline in T cell-mediated function has been implicated as a contributory factor in the increased incidence of infectious diseases and tumors in the elderly.

Payan et al. (72) found an increase in PHA induced T cell proliferation in asthma patients after 8 wk of supplementation with 4 g of EPA and Catchart et al. (73) observed an increase in Con A-induced mitogenic response in mice following 4 wk of a FO diet. On the other hand, Santoli and Zurier (74) recently showed that *in vitro* addition of EPA to human PBMC inhibited IL-2 production in some but not all donors. Alexander and Smythe (75) showed reduced ConA-induced mitogenesis in BALB/c mice fed FO compared to those fed lard or CO. It is interesting to note that in the same experiment autoimmune prone NZB/NZW mice fed 2% FO had similar mitogenic response to those fed lard or CO. This may explain the different results observed in our experiment and those of Payan et al. (72). Furthermore, the subjects in the study by Payan et al. (72) were young. In our study significant reduction in PHA-stimulated mitogenesis was observed only in older adults. This decrease in cytokine production and lymphocyte proliferation may compromise cell-mediated immunity and is supported by the study of Yoshino and Ellis (76) who showed that Sprague-Dawley rats fed FO concentrate had lower delayed type hypersensitivity response than those fed water, oleic acid or safflower oil.

The decrease in cytokine production and lymphocyte proliferation can not be readily explained by a decrease in PGE_2 production. PGE_2 has been shown to suppress IL-1, IL-2 and lymphocyte proliferation (9,15,77). We have previously shown that decrease in PGE_2 production by tocopherol supplementation enhances IL-2 production and lymphocyte proliferation in old mice (37) and elderly human subjects (65). The effect of N-3 FA supplementation, therefore, appears to be independent of PGE_2 changes. On the other had, a reduction in LTB_4 by N-3 FA can suppress IL-1, IL-2 production and the subsequent lymphocyte proliferation since LTB_4 in some but not all (11) studies has been shown to increase IL-1 as well as Il-2 production and lymphocyte proliferation (78). Santoli and Zurier (74) showed that polyunsaturated FA can reduce IL-2 production directly and independently of changes in cyclooxygenase products. Furthermore, it is not clear whether the decrease in IL-2 production and lymphocyte proliferation is due to a direct effect of N-3 FA on IL-2 production or whether it is mediated by the decrease in IL-1 and IL-6.

The clinical implications of our findings need to be determined. IL-1, TNF, and IL-6 have been implicated in the pathogenesis of inflammatory diseases and a reduction in the synthesis of these cytokines by N-3 FA of FO may contribute to their reported beneficial effect in rheumatoid arthritis (35,79) and amyloidosis (73). Furthermore, IL-1 is implicated in the pathogenesis of osteoporosis (80). The incidence of both arthritis and osteoporosis increases in older women, therefore, N-3 FA supplementation may prove to be beneficial in retarding the development of these disease states. On the other hand, the reduction in older women of IL-2 and IL-6 production may compromise B and T cell functions. Further clinical trials are needed to define the level of N-3 supplementation which provides an anti-inflammatory effect and minimizes the reduction of cell-mediated immunity.

References

1. DiLuzio, N.R., (1972) in Advances in Lipid Research, Paoletti, R., and Kritchevsky, D., Academic Press, New York: Academic Press, pp. 43-88.
2. Carroll, R.K. and Khor, H.T., (1975) Prog. Biochem. Pharmacol. 10:308-353.
3. Tannenbaum, A. and Silverstone, H., (1953) in Advances in Cancer Research, Academic Press, New York, pp. 451-501.
4. Mertin, J. and Hunt, R., (1976) Proc. Nat. Acad. Sci. USA 73:928-931.
5. Ring, J., Seifert, J., Mertin, J., and Brendel., (1974) Lancet 2:1331.
6. Mertin, J. and Hughs, D., (1975 Int. Arch. Allergy Appl. Immunol. 48:203-210.
7. Goodwin, J.S. and Webb, D.R., (1980) Clin. Immunol. Immunolopath. 15:106-122.
8. Rola-Pleszczynski, M., (1985) Immunol. Today 6:302-307.
9. Stubb, C.D. and Smith, A.D., (1984) Biochem. Biophys. Acta. 779:89-137.
10. Goodwin, J.S., Messner, R.P. and Peake, G.T., (1974) J. Clin. Invest. 54:368-378.
11. Webb, D.R., Rogers, T.J. and Nowowiejski, I., (1980) Proc. NY Acad. Sci. 332:260-270.
12. Rola-Plaszczynski, M. and Lemaire, I., (1985) J. Immunol. 135:3958-3961.
13. Metzger, Z., Hoffeld, J.T., and Oppenheim, J.J., (1980) J. Immunol. 124:983-988.
14. Fisher, R.I. and Bostic-Bruton, F., (1982) J. Immunol 129:1770-1774.
15. Muscoplat, C.C., Rakich, P.M., Thoen, C.O. et al., (1978) Infec. Immunol. 20:627-631.
16. Gordon, D., Bray, M. and Morely, J., (1976) Nature 262:401-402.
17. Plaut, M., (1979) J. Immunol. 123:692-701.
18. Roder, J.C. and Klein, M., (1979) J. Immunol 123:2785-2790.
19. Goodman, M.G. and Weigle, W.O., (1980) J. Immunol. 125:593-600.
20. Payan, D.G., (1984) Proc. Nat. Acad. Sci. 81:3501-3505.
21. Gualde, N., Mexmain, S., Aldigier, J.C., Goodwin, J.S., and Rigaud, M., (1984) in Icosanoids and Cancer, Thaler-Dao Asrastes de Paulet, H., Paoleti, R., Raven Press, NY, pp. 155-168.
22. Ramstedt, U., Ng, J., Wigzell, H., Sermhan, C.N., and Samuelsson, B., (1985) J. Immunol. 135:3434-3438.
23. Rola-Pleszcynski, M., Gagnon, L., and Sirois, P., (1983) Biochem. Biophys. Res. Commun. 113:531-537.
24. Johnston, P.V., Marshall, L.A., (1984) Prog. Food Nutr. Sci. 8:3-25.
25. Erickson, K.L., (1986) Int. J. Immunopharmac. 8:529-543.
26. Dupont, J., White, P.J., Carpenter, M.P., Schaefer, E.J., Meydani, S.N., Elson, C.E., Woods, M., and Gorbach, S.L., J. Am. Coll. Nutr., in press.
27. Meydani, S.N., Lichenstein, A., White, P.J., Goodnight, S.M., Elson, C.E., Woods, M., Gorbach, S.L., and Schaefer, E.J., J. Am. Coll. Nutr., in press.
28. Bang, H.O., Dryerberg, J. and Sinclair, H.M., (1980) Am. J. Clin. Nutr.

33:2657-2661.
29. Dryerberg, J., Bang, H.O., Slofferson, E., Moncada, S., and Vane, J.R., (1978) Lancet 2:117-119.
30. Lee, T.H., Hoover, R., Williams, J.D., Sperling, R.I., Raralese, J. III, Spur, B.W., Robinson, D.R., Corey, E.J., Lewis, R.A., and Austen, K.F., (1985) N. Engl. J. Med. 312:1217-1224.
31. Kromhout, D., Bosschieter, E.B., de Lezenne, and Coulander, C., (1985) N. Engl. J. Med. 312:1205-1209.
32. Weiner, B.H., Ockene, I.S., Levine, P.H., Cuenoud, H.F., Fisher, M., Johnson, B.F., Natale, A., Vaudrevil, C., and Hoogasian, J.J., (1986) N. Eng. J. Med. 315:841-846.
33. Prickett, J.D., Robinson, D.R. and & Steinberg, A.D., (1981) J. Clin. Invest. 68:556-559.
34. Kelley, V.E., Ferretti, A., Izui, A., and Storm, T.B., (1985) J. Immunol. 134:1914-1919.
35. Kremer, J.M., Jubiz, W., Michalek, A., et al., (1987) Ann. Intern. Med. 106:497-502.
36. Herberman, R.B., Natural Killer Cell Mediated Immunity Against Tumors, Academic, New York, 1980.
37. Meydani, S.N., Meydani, M., Verdon, C.P., Blumberg, J.B., and Hayes, K.C., (1986) Mech. Aging Devel. 34:191-201.
38. Rosenstein, M.M. and Strauser, R., (1980) J. Reticuloendothel. Soc. 27:15-166.
39. Meydani, S.N., Yogeeswaran, G., Liu, S., Baskar, S., and Meydani, M., (1988) J. Nutr. 118:1245-1252.
40. Bieri, J.G., Tolliner, T.J. and Catigani, G.L., (1979) Am. J. Clin. Nutr. 32:2143-2149.
41. Meydani, S.N., Shapiro, A.C., Meydani, M., MaCauley, J.B., and Blumberg, J.B., (1987) Lipids 22:345-350.
42. McCosh, E.J., Meyer, D.L. and Dupont, J., (1976) Prostagl. 12:472-486.
43. Kiessling, R., Klein, E. and Wigzel, H., (1975) Eur. J. Immunul. 5:112-117.
44. Herberman, R.B., Nunn, M.E. and Lavrin, D.H., (1975) Int. J. Cancer 16:216-223.
45. Brunda, M.J., Heberman, R.B. and Holden, H.T., (1980) J. Immunol. 124(6):2682-2687.
46. Sandberg, L., Troyer, D., Talal, N., and Fernandes, G., (1987) Fed. Proc. 46:1173 (abs.4988).
47. Yamashita, N., Yokoyama, A., Hamazaki, T., and Yano, S., (1986) Biochem. Biophys. Res. Commun. 138:1058-1067.
48. Hamazaki, T., Yamashita, N., Yokoyama, A., Sugiryama, E., Urakaze, M., and Yano, S., (1987) Proc. Am. Oil Chem. Soc., 127-132.
49. Fritsche, K.L. and Johnston, P.V., (1987) Fed Proc. 46:1172.
50. Bray, R.A. and Brahmi, Z., (1986) J. Immunol. 136:1783-1790.
51. Meydani, S.N., Stocking, L.M., Shapiro, A.C., Meydani, M., and Blumberg,

J.B., (1988) Ann. N.Y. Acad. Sci. 524:495-497.
52. Billiar, T.R., Bankey, P.E., Svingen, B.A. et al., (1988) Surg. 104:343-349.
53. Endres, S., Ghorbani, R., Kelley, V.E., Georgilis, K., Lonnemann, G., Van der Meer, J.W.M., Cannon, J.G., Rogers, T.S., Klempner, M.S., Weber, P.C., Schaefer, E.J., Wolff, S.M., and Dinarello, C.A., (1989) N. Engl. J. Med. 320:265-271.
54. Siskind, G.W., (1980) in Biological Mechanism in Aging, Schimke, R.T., USDA NIH, pp. 455-467.
55. Kay, M.M.B., (1978) Mech. Age. Dev. 9:39-59.
56. Thoman, M.L. and Weigle, W.O., (1981) J. Immunol. 127:2101-2106.
57. Miller, R.A. and Stutman, O., (1981) Eur. J. Immunol. 11:751-756.
58. Chang, M.P., Makinodan, T., Peterson, W.J., and Strehler, B.L., (1982) J. Immunol. 129:2426-2430.
59. Gillis, S., Kozak, R., Durante, M., and Menkler, M.K., (1982) J. Clin. Invest. 67:937-942.
60. Inamiza, T., Chang, M.P., & Makinodan, T., (1985) Immunol. 55:447-455.
61. Becker, M.J., Farkas, R., Schneider, M., Drucker, A., and Klajman, A., (1979) Immunol. Immunopathol. 14:204-210.
62. Cobleigh, M.A., Braun, D.P., & Harris, J.E., (1980) Clin. Immunol. Immunopathol. 15:162-173.
63. Meydani, S.N., Endres, S., Woods, M.N., Goldin, R.D., Soo, C., Morrill-Labrode, A., Dinarello, C.A., and Gorback, S.L., (1990) FASEB J. 4:A795.
64. Boyum, A.I., (1968) Scand. J. Clin. Lab Invest. 97(suppl 21):77-89.
65. Meydani, S.N., Barklund, M.P., Liu, S., Meydani, M., Miller, R.A., Cannon, J.G., Morrow, F.D., Rocklin, R., Blumberg, J.B., (1990) Am. J. Clin. Nutr., in press.
66. Gillis, S., Fern, M.M., Ou, W., and Smith, K.A., (1978) J. Immunol. 120:2027-2032.
67. Schindler, R., Mancilla, J., Endres, S., Ghorbani, R., Clark, S.C., and Dinarello, C.A., (1990) Blood, in press.
68. Endres, S., Ghorbani, R., Lonnemann, G., van der Meer, J.W.M., and Dinarello, C.A., (1988) Clin. Immunol. Immunopath. 49:424-438.
69. Van der Meer, J.W.M., Endres, S., Lonnemann, G., et al., (1988) J. Leukocyte Biol. 43:216-223.
70. Hollander, D., Dadufabza, V.D. and Sletten, E.G., (1984) J.L.R. 25:129-134.
71. Suzuki, H., Hayakawa, S., Tamura, S., Wada, S., and Wada, O., (1985) Biochem. Biophy. Acta. 836:390-393.
72. Payan, D.G., Wong, M.Y.S., Chernov-Rogan, T., et al., (1986) J. Clin. Immunol. 6:402-410.
73. Cathcart, E.S., Leslie, C.A., Meydani, S.N., and Hayes, K.C., (1987) J. Immunol. 139:1850-1854.
74. Santoli, D. and Zurier, R.B., (1989) J. Immunol. 143:1303-1309.
75. Alexander, N.J. and Smythe, N.L., (1988) Am. Nutr. Metab. 32:192-199.
76. Yoshino, S. and Ellis, E.F., (1987) Int. Arch. Allergy Appl. Immunol. 84:233-240.

77. Knudsen, P.J., Dinarello, C.A. and Storm, T.B., (1986) J. Immunol. 31:89-94.
78. Goodwin, J.S., Atluru, D., Sierakowski, S., and Lianos, E.A., (1986) J. Clin. Invest. 1244-1250.
79. Leslie, C.A., Gonnermann, W.A., Ullman, M.D., Hayes, K.C., Franz-Blau, C., and Cathcart, E.S., (1985) J. Exp. Med. 162:1336-
80. Gowen, M. and Mundy, G.R., (1986) J. Immunol. 136:2478-2482.

Chapter Seventeen

Effect of Dietary Fatty Acids on Cell Mediated Immune System

Darshan S. Kelley

Western Human Nutrition Research Center
Agricultural Research Service, USDA
P.O. Box 29997
Presidio of San Francisco, CA 94129

Cell Mediated immunity (CMI) refers to the protection provided by sensitized lymphocytes and activated macrophages. *In vivo* examples of CMI include delayed hypersensitivity (DHS) and granulomatous reactions. Clinical conditions involving CMI include skin reactions, graft rejections, graft vs. host reactions, viral infections, and autoallergic diseases. The mechanisms of cell mediated toxicity may involve direct killing of target cells by sensitized killer T cells (TK), or indirect killing by the lymphokines released from the sensitized effector T lymphocytes (T_D), or natural killing by the non-sensitized lymphocytes (NK), antibody dependent cell mediated cytoxicity (ADCC) involving non-sensitized lymphocytes (Null cells), polymorphonuclear cells and macrophages, or phagocytosis and digestion by activated macrophages. Commonly used techniques to evaluate CMI in humans include determining the number of T lymphocytes and their sub-sets in the peripheral blood, *in vitro* proliferation in response to antigens and T cell mitogens (Phytohemagglutinin = PHA, and Concanavalin A = ConA), *in vitro* production of lymphokines in response to mitogens, cytolysis or killing of target cells by sensitized (T_K) or non-sensitized (NK) lymphocytes, chemotaxis, phagocytosis, *in vivo* DHS skin response to recall antigens, graft rejection, and intervention with some of the autoimmune diseases. There are limitations to each of these methods, however, a reasonable estimate of CMI can be obtained by using multiple of these methods.

Fatty acids in the diet may be saturated or unsaturated. Saturated fatty acids contain only single carbon-carbon bonds, while the unsaturated fatty acids contain double carbon-carbon bonds. Unsaturated fatty acids are called monounsaturated when they contain one carbon-carbon double bond and polyunsaturated when they contain two or more carbon-carbon double bonds. In the Genevan or the older system of nomenclature, the carboxyl carbon is numbered carbon number 1 and the position of the double bond is stated by counting from the carboxyl end the number of the first carbon with the double bonds. In the Omega system of nomenclature, the methyl carbon which is farthest from the carboxyl end is designated as W and the position of the first double bond is specified in relation to the W carbon. The terms W and n are interchangeably used. Thus, the Genevan designations for the oleic (OA), linoleic (LA) and the α-linolenic acid (ALA) are 18:1; 9, 18:2; 9, 12 and 18:3; 9, 12, 15, respectively. The Omega designation for these fatty acids are W9, C18:1, W6, C18:2, and W_3, C18:3 respectively. Other polyunsaturated fatty acids with significant metabolic role include arachidonic acid (AA, W6, C20:4), eicosapentaenoic acid (EPA, W3, C20:5) and docosahexaenoic acid (DHA, W_3, C22:6). The LA and ALA are considered essential fatty acids (EFA) for man because of the body's inability to synthesize them. The body is presumable capable of elongating and desaturating these EFA.

The information regarding the effects of dietary fats on CMI has been gathered from experiments with cultured cells, animal models and human experiments. Results obtained with cells in culture and with animal models have been discussed in several recent reviews (1-9) and will be only summarized here. Human experiments investigating the effects of dietary fats on CMI are still very limited and will be discussed in detail. The use of these three models in studying the effects of dietary fatty acids on CMI is reviewed as follows:

Fatty Acids and Growth of Cells in Culture

A role for the EFA in the regulation of CMI was first suggested by Mertin et al. (10) who observed that addition of AA or LA to the cultures of human peripheral blood lymphocytes (PBL) suppressed their proliferation in response to PHA. Since then a number of reports have shown that the addition of fatty acids of both saturated and unsaturated type to the PBL in culture suppressed their growth. Particularly noteworthy are the findings of Kelly and Parker (11) who found AA at concentrations less than 1 µg/ml stimulated PBL proliferation in response to PHA. At concentrations above 20 µg/ml, the suppression of PBL growth by the added fatty acids was dependent on the fatty acid concentration (12). Recently it has been reported that the n-3 fatty acids were as effective as the n-6 fatty acids in suppressing the growth of a leukemic cell line (13). All these experiments suggest that lower concentrations of the fatty acids are required for cell growth and the higher concentrations are inhibitory of cell growth. Saturated as well as polyunsaturated fatty acids of both n-3 and n-6 type can inhibit the growth of immune cells. The physiological significance of such *in vitro* findings is not clear because of the detergent-like properties of the fatty acids and the effects of the fatty acid carriers or solvents on cell growth.

Dietary Fat and CMI in Animal Models

Table 17-1 includes a summary of the findings regarding the effects of dietary fats on the indices of CMI in animal models and in humans. It is clear from this table that both the concentration and the type of the dietary fats influence a number of indices of CMI, including proliferation of PBL and splenocytes (SPC) in response to mitogens, DHS response, NK activity, graft rejections and tumor immunity. Most of these reports with animal models support the following generalizations regarding the effects of dietary fats on CMI: 1. EFA are required to maintain a healthy CMI system and their deficiency suppresses some of the indices of CMI. 2. Diets containing high concentration of fats, suppress some of the indices of CMI, the suppression seems to be dependent on the concentration of fat in the diet. 3. Excess of both saturated and polyunsaturated fatty acids (PUFA) inhibit CMI; at a given concentration PUFA seems to be more potent inhibitor of CMI than the saturated fats. 4. The n-3 fatty acids have been reported to both suppress and enhance CMI in different animal models.

There are many exceptions to the above generalizations, which may result from a number of factors including the concentration (how much) of the dietary fat, the fatty acid composition of the diets including P:S and n3:n6 ratios, carbon chain length of the fatty acids, physical form and route of administration of the fatty acids, the length of feeding, species, strain and age of the animals used, type of the control diet, tests used to evaluate CMI. In tissue-culture experiments, additional interference comes from the fatty acid content of the serum added to the culture medium, which may sometimes mask the effects of dietary fats.

Dietary Fatty Acids and CMI in Humans

The indications that dietary fatty acids may have a role in the modulation of human CMI first came from epidemiological and clinical studies. Millar et al. (43), reported that when the diets of multiple sclerosis (autoimmune disease of CNS) patients were supplemented with sun-

TABLE 17-1
Effect of Dietary Fats on Cell Mediated Immunity

Dietary Fat	Animal Species and Strain	Immunological Test and Results	Reference
1 or 9 Wt % corn oil or 9 Wt % lard	(NZBXNZW) F_1 Mice	SPC proliferation in response to ConA was suppressed in both groups fed 9% fat compared to 1% fat. NK activity in the lard group was higher than the other two groups at 4M but it was lower than the 1% group at 7 M. DHS to DNFB was not affected by the diet.	Morrow et al. (14)
10 Wt % hydrogenated coconut oil, or linseed oil, or corn oil.	Male and female Sprague Dawley Rats	SPC proliferation in response to ConA & PHA was twice as much in the coconut oil group than in the other two groups.	Marshall and Johnston, (15)
5 Wt % fish oil, or corn oil, or coconut oil	C57BL/6J Mice	SPC proliferation in response to ConA & PHA was higher in the fish oil than in the corn oil group.	Meydani et al. (16)
Linoleic, linolenic, or arachidonic acid injected SC 3.6 mg/day for 10 d	Male C57BL/6J Mice	SPC proliferation in response to ConA & PHA was reduced by 70%, and mixed lymphocyte responses by 90% with all 3 fatty acids.	Ellis et al. (17)
5 or 20 Wt % soybean oil	Female 3 CH/OUJ Mice	SPC proliferation in response to ConA & PHA, and cell mediated cytotoxicity were lower in the 20% than in the 5% oil fed mice.	Olson et al. (18)

TABLE 17-1 — continued
Effect of Dietary Fats on Cell Mediated Immunity

Dietary Fat	Animal Species and Strain	Immunological Test and Results	Reference
20 Wt % lard, or corn oil, or fish oil	NZBXNZW mice	SI for the SPC proliferation in response to ConA in the fish oil group was higher than the other 2 groups at 9M but not at 5M.	Alexander & Smythe (19)
Same as above	BALB/C mice	SI for SPC proliferation was lower in the fish oil group than in the lard group.	Same as above
High fat (HF) 20 Wt % corn or saturated coconut oil low fat (LF) 2 Wt % linoleic acid	Female Sprague-Dawley rats.	SPC proliferation in response to ConA was suppressed in the corn oil group compared to the low fat group. Suppressive effect seemed to be serum mediated.	Kollmorgen et al. (20).
2, 8, 16, or 24 Wt % coconut or safflower oil	Female C57BL/6J mice	SPC proliferation in response to ConA decreased by an increase in the concentration of safflower oil but not with coconut oil.	Erickson et al. (21).
8, 14, or 20 Wt % corn oil or tallow	Female C57BL/6J mice	SPC proliferation in response to ConA at 8 and 14% was lower in corn oil than in tallow group. No difference at 20%.	Ossmann et al. (22).
0, 1.4, 20, or 40 en% safflower or coconut oil	Female C57BL/6J mice	SPC proliferation in response to all alloantigens (SPC from BALB/C) mice was suppressed in mice fed 0, 20 or 40% safflower or coconut oil compared to those fed 1.4% safflower oil.	Erickson et al. (23).

TABLE 17-1 — continued
Effect of Dietary Fats on Cell Mediated Immunity

Dietary Fat	Animal Species and Strain	Immunological Test and Results	Reference
5 Wt % mixed fat 24 Wt % saturated or polyunsaturated or mixed	Male Sprague-Dawley rats.	SPC proliferation in response to ConA, PHA was suppressed in the group fed PUFA diet compared to the other 3 groups.	Locniskar et al. (24).
31 en % corn or coconut oil	Cebus and squirrel monkeys	When cultured in autologus sera PBL proliferation in response to PHA and ConA was suppressed for both strains fed corn oil compared to coconut oil fed monkeys. Results were mixed with FCS.	Meydani et al. (25).
35 en % palm oil, or sunflower seed oil	Adult male Dutch rabbits	Proliferation of APC and PBL in response to ConA & PHA was not different statistically although it was less than one-half in the palm oil group than the sunflower group at 6M.	De Deckere et al. (26).
10 or 35 en % palm oil, or sunflower oil	Male Wistar Rats	SPC proliferation in response to ConA and PHA was not different among the 4 fats, however the serum from high fat groups suppresses SPC proliferation.	Same as above

TABLE 17-1 — continued
Effect of Dietary Fats on Cell Mediated Immunity

Dietary Fat	Animal Species and Strain	Immunological Test and Results	Reference
23 en % hydrogenated soybean oil, or safflower oil, linseed oil, or menhaden oil	New Zealand White male rabbits	Proliferation of SPC and PBL in response to ConA & PHA was higher in the linseed oil fed rabbits than in the other three groups.	Kelley et al. (27).
20 Wt % tallow or corn oil	Albino Guinea Pigs	DTH to PPD and KLH was suppressed in the corn oil group.	Friend et al. (28).
EFA free, or 13 or 50 en % corn oil	Male A/J Mice	DHS to DNFB reduced by EFA deficiency compared to 13 or 50% corn oil, which were not different from each other	Dewille et al. (29).
EFA free, or 0.5 en % EFA, or 8 and 20% coconut oil or safflower oil.	Female BALB/cAuN Mice	DTH to allogenic melanoma cell line was suppressed in 20% fat fed and EFA deficient groups compared to 0.5% group. Rejection of allogenic SPC into irradiated mice was suppressed by the 20% safflower oil.	Thomas & Erickson (30).
10 Wt % corn oil, or 1.2 Wt % corn oil + 8.8 Wt % fish oil	Male C57BL/6NNia Mice	In the younger but not in the older mice, fish oil group had a moderately lower NK activity than the corn oil group.	Meyandi et al. (31).
5 or 20 Wt % palm oil or safflower oil.	Female C57BL/6N and C3H/HeN Mice	NK activity not affected by the level or type of the dietary fat.	Erickson et al. (32).

TABLE 17-1 — continued

Effect of Dietary Fats on Cell Mediated Immunity

Dietary Fat	Animal Species and Strain	Immunological Test and Results	Reference
Adipose tissue fatty acid composition used as an index of dietary fatty acid intake.	Men, average 47 yrs	PBL proliferation in response to PHA, ConA, PWM, and mixed lymphocytes, and NK Activity did not show correlation with any of the fatty acids in the adipose tissue.	Berry et al. (33).
30 en % or less mixed dietary fat for 3M	Men	NK activity was significantly increased by reducing the fat intake to 30 en % or below compared to the base line values.	Barone et al. (34).
22 en % fat followed by 22 en % fat + 15 g coconut or safflower oil/day	Young men, mean age 31 yr	NK activity was significantly suppressed by the addition of extra fat from either oil. There was a 0.79% increase for each 1% decrease in fat calories. Type of dietary fat did not affect the NK activity.	Hebert et al. (35).
Stabilization diet with 30 en % fat and 6 en % PUFA. Intervention diets with 25% en % fat with 3.5 or 12.9 en % PUFA	Young men, mean age 35 yr	Numbers of T cells in the peripheral blood and their proliferation in response to PHA and ConA was significantly enhanced by the reduction of fat intake compared to the base line values; there was no difference in these indices between the two PUFA groups.	Kelley et al. (36)

TABLE 17-1 — continued
Effect of Dietary Fats on Cell Mediated Immunity

Dietary Fat	Animal Species and Strain	Immunological Test and Results	Reference
23 en % hydrogenated soybean oil, or safflower oil, linseed oil, or menhaden oil	New Zealand White male rabbits	Proliferation of SPC and PBL in response to ConA & PHA was higher in the linseed oil fed rabbits than in the other three groups.	Kelley et al. (27).
20 Wt % tallow or corn oil	Albino Guinea Pigs	DTH to PPD and KLH was suppressed in the corn oil group.	Friend et al. (28).
EFA free, or 13 or 50 en % corn oil	Male A/J Mice	DHS to DNFB reduced by EFA deficiency compared to 13 or 50% corn oil, which were not different from each other	Dewille et al. (29).
EFA free, or 0.5 en % EFA, or 8 and 20% coconut oil or safflower oil.	Female BALB/cAuN Mice	DTH to allogenic melanoma cell line was suppressed in 20% fat fed and EFA deficient groups compared to 0.5% group. Rejection of allogenic SPC into irradiated mice was suppressed by the 20% safflower oil.	Thomas & Erickson (30).
10 Wt % corn oil, or 1.2 Wt % corn oil + 8.8 Wt % fish oil	Male C57BL/6NNia Mice	In the younger but not in the older mice, fish oil group had a moderately lower NK activity than the corn oil group.	Meyandi et al. (31).
5 or 20 Wt % palm oil or safflower oil.	Female C57BL/6N and C3H/HeN Mice	NK activity not affected by the level or type of the dietary fat.	Erickson et al. (32).

TABLE 17-1 — continued
Effect of Dietary Fats on Cell Mediated Immunity

Dietary Fat	Animal Species and Strain	Immunological Test and Results	Reference
Fish oil 4.0 g/d for 6 wks	Human	Feeding fish oil suppressed neutrophil phagocytic activity compared to the values prior to feeding fish oil.	Virella et al. (41).
Fish oil 18 g/day for 6 wks	Men, mean age 28 yr	Feeding fish oil significantly suppressed the production of $Il_{1\alpha}$, $Il_{1\beta}$ and TNF by the PBMNC cultured with endotoxin compared to values prior to the feeding of fish oil. It also suppressed the chemotactic activity of the neutrophils.	Endres et al. (42)

Abbreviations used: Wt % = weight %, en % = energy %, SPC = splenocytes, PBL = peripheral blood lymphocytes, ConA = Concanavalin A, PHA = phytohemagglutinin, PWM = pokeweed mitogen, NK = Natural killer cells, SI = stimulation index, Il = interleukin, TNF = tumor necrosis factor, PUFA = polyunsaturated fatty acids, EFA = essential fatty acids, ALA = α-linolenic acid, EPA = eicosapentaenoic acid.

flower oil which is rich in LA, the relapses tended to be less severe and of shorter duration than if the diet was supplemented with olive oil which is rich in OA. Dil'man et al. (44), found that PBL proliferation in response to PHA was suppressed in patients with cardio-vascular disease who had elevated levels of serum fatty acids; PBL proliferation was restored when the serum fatty acids concentration was brought to normal levels by treatment with phenformin. McHugh et al. (45), reported that the survival of the transplanted kidneys in humans was improved if the immunosuppressive drug therapy was accompanied by EFA supplementation. Despite these early reports regarding the possible effects of EFA on CMI, until recently EFA supplementation has found only limited use in treating disorders of human immune system. This is perhaps because of the more dramatic effects produced by the drugs on CMI compared to the small effects produced by the fatty acids.

During the last few years, several human studies regarding the effects of the concentration and type of dietary fats on CMI have been conducted. Berry et al. (33), examined the fatty acid composition of the buttock adipose tissue in 94 men, and used it as an index of the dietary fatty acid intake. They also examined the proliferation of the PBL in response to ConA, PHA, pokeweed, and in mixed lymphocyte cultures, and also the NK activity. The effects of the concentrations of individual fatty acids in the adipose tissue were analyzed on the various indices of immune status. The concentration of none of the fatty acids was associated with the indices of immune status examined. We (36) conducted a study with 8 healthy young men, who were maintained at the metabolic suite of the Western Human Nutrition Research Center for 95 days. Prior to entering the study these men were consuming the typical American diet which contains about 40 energy % (en %) fat. During the course of the study, the nutrient intake and the physical activity of the subjects were strictly controlled. For the first 14 days, all 8 subjects were fed a stabilization diet containing 30 en% fat (6 en% PUFA). From day 16 to 95 (intervention period) the fat content of the diet was reduced to 25 en% for all the subjects and they were divided into 2 groups of 4 each depending upon the PUFA content of their diet. The two levels of PUFA were 12.9 and 3.5 en%. The saturated fat content of the two diets was maintained constant, while the PUFA levels were changed by adjusting the level of the monounsaturated fat. Several indices of CMI were examined twice during the stabilization period and several times during the intervention period. The moderate differences in the level of PUFA between the two intervention diets did not affect any of the indices of CMI. Such differences in the level of PUFA are adequate to provide some of their desirable effects to lower the risk from cardio-vascular diseases. Several indices of CMI were significantly enhanced upon feeding the low fat, nutritionally balanced diet when compared to the base line values. As an example of these results, proliferation of PBL in response to PHA is shown in Fig. 17-1. Similar results were obtained with ConA. There was a significant increase in the number of circulating lymphocytes with time and a concomitant decrease in the number of circulating neutrophils. The increase in lymphocyte count was reflected in T as well as B lymphocytes. Both the helper and suppressor sub-sets of T cells were increased; helper/suppressor remained unchanged. One possible explanation for the increase in the indices of CMI was the nutritionally balanced low fat diet that was fed during the intervention period. Other factors, such as confinement, stress, or a latent viral infection might

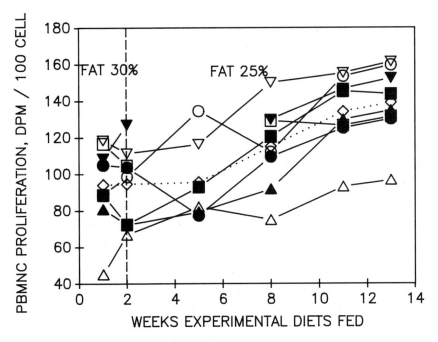

Fig. 17-1. Effect of concentration of dietary fat on the proliferation of PBMNC in response to PHA. Data taken from Kelley et al. (36). Solid lines joining different symbols represent each individual subject, while the dotted line represents the mean of the 8 subjects.

result in some of the changes observed in this study. We do not believe such factors caused the observed changes in CMI because the health status of these men were monitored daily. Studies including appropriate simultaneous controls need to be conducted to affirm the stimulation of CMI by the low fat diets.

Barone et al. (34) examined the effects of concentration of dietary fat intake on NK activity. Seventeen young men were advised to select foods low in fat during the base line period of 1.5 to 2 months, so as to lower their fat intake to less than 30 en%. The fat contents of the diets were calculated from the 4-day food diaries of the subjects. The NK activity was examined prior to the start of consuming low fat diets and then 3 months after all the subjects had been consuming the low fat diets. There was a significant increase in the NK activity at the end of the low fat diet compared to the base line values prior to the start of low fat diet. There was a 0.53% increase in NK activity for every 1% drop in fat cals. At the end of 3 months, the low fat diet of the 8 subjects was supplemented with safflower oil (15 g/day) for 2 months; while the diet of the remainder of the subjects was supplemented with the same amount of coconut oil (35). This 2 month period was called the first intervention phase and it was followed by a wash out period of 1 month, when all subjects again consumed a low fat diet. The wash out period was followed by the second intervention phase of 2 months when the diets of the two groups were again supplemented with safflower or coconut oil, however, the oil supplements during the second intervention phase were crossed-over to those of the first intervention phase. The NK activities were examined at the ends of first and second intervention phases and these data were analyzed with a general linear model to evaluate the effects of dietary fat on NK activity. There was significant decrease in the NK activity with the increase in fat intake. The P:S ratio of the diets had no significant effect on the NK activity, although during the first intervention phase the safflower oil diet seemed to be suppressive while the coconut oil did not suppress the NK activity. During the second intervention phase both oils seemed equally suppressive. These results are very interesting and seem reasonably convincing because the effects of the fat content of the diet on NK activity was reversible. However, additional studies with groups of subjects fed control and experimental diets simultaneously under controlled conditions are necessary to confirm these findings.

A number of recent reports have examined the effects of the dietary n-3 fatty acids on the indices of CMI. Most of these reports indicate suppression of various indices of CMI by the dietary n-3 fatty acids.

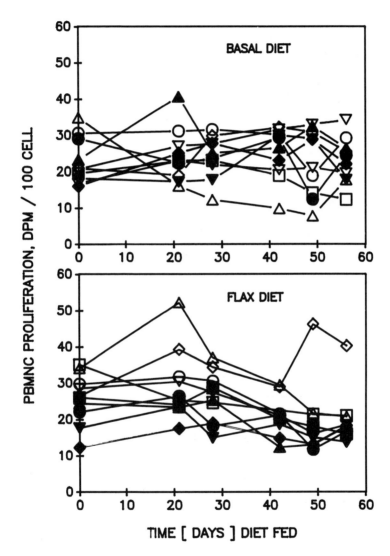

Fig. 17-2. Effect of basal and flax diets on proliferation of PBMNC cultured with PHA. Data are taken from Kelley et al. (39), and are shown individually for each of the ten subjects.

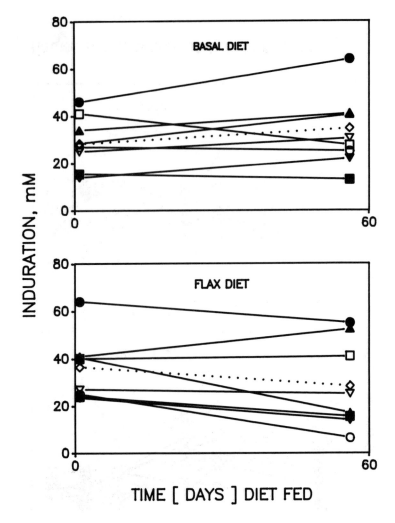

Fig. 17-3. Effect of basal and flax diets on the sum of induration diameters produced in response to 7 recall antigens. Data are taken from Kelley et al. (39). Solid lines represent each of the 8 subjects separately and the dotted lines represent the group means.

Bjerve et al. (38) found the PBL proliferation in response to PHA, ConA and pokeweed were suppressed when ALA and EPA were supplemented in the diets of 3 ALA deficient patients for 6 weeks. Similarly, supplementing the diet of healthy men with fish oils for 6 weeks was reported to suppress neutrophil adherence and chemotaxis (40) and phagocytosis (41) and the *in vitro* production of 11-1β, 11-1α and tumor necrosis factor by the peripheral blood mononuclear cells (PBMNC, 42). We (39) recently examined the effect of flax seed oil (which is about 55% ALA by weight) supplemented diets on several indices of CMI. Ten men were fed a stabilization diet that contained 25 en % fat and 0.3 en % ALA for 2 weeks and then divided into 2 groups of 5 each. From day 15 to 70 (intervention period 1), 5 subjects continued to consume the basal diet, while for the other 5 flax seed oil proved 10% calories (replacing 6% carbohydrate and 4% fat calories of the basal diet). The fat and the ALA content of the flax diet were 30 and 6 en % respectively. From day 71 to 126 (intervention period 2) the diets between the two groups were crossed over. Several indices of CMI were examined twice at the end of stabilization period and several times during the two intervention periods. The data from the two intervention periods from each diet were pooled and analyzed with ANOVA using general linear models. Flax diet suppressed PBL proliferation in response to PHA (p = 0.041, Fig. 17-2) and ConA (p = 0.054). Only 8 subjects participated in the DHS skin response; the induration (Fig. 17-3) as well as number of positive responses was suppressed in 5, unchanged in 2 and enhanced in 1 subject upon the feeding of flax diet. Because of the small number of subjects and the variation in the DHS assay, suppression of DHS by the flax diet did not attain statistical significance. Since the effect of flax diet on PHA and ConA stimulation of PBL and on the DHS response were in the same general direction, it may be safe to conclude that flax diet suppressed CMI. Other indices of CMI, including the numbers of T cells in peripheral circulation and their sub-sets, and the *in vitro* production of 11-2 and 11-2R by the PBMNC were not affected by the flax diet. In contrast to the several reports regarding the suppression of the indices of CMI by the n-3 fatty acids in the healthy men, fish oil intake was found to enhance PBL proliferation in response to PHA and also the helper/suppressor ratio in asthmatic patients (37). This conflicting result may be due to the health status or the continued intake of prescription drugs by the asthmatic patients, while taking fish oil supplements.

In general the results from human experiments support those obtained with animal models. Some indices of CMI seem to be suppressed by an increase in the concentration of dietary fat and the converse also seems to be true by the reduction in fat intake. Moderate changes in the intake of n-6 PUFA did not affect several indices of CMI, while supplements of n-3 PUFA suppressed several indices of CMI. Further experiments regarding the effects of dietary fatty acids on indices of CMI are necessary. If the additional experiments support the preliminary findings that low fat diets enhance CMI and that n-3 PUFA suppress CMI, then such dietary manipulations may find clinical use in the management of some disorders of the immune system.

In summary, there is a reasonable agreement in the results obtained from the experiments conducted with cells in culture, animal models and human subjects regarding the effects of dietary fatty acids on CMI. Taken together, These results suggest EFA are required to maintain a healthy immune system, while excess of the dietary fats suppress some indices of CMI. The amounts of the different fatty acids required to maintain optimal *in vivo* activity of the various indices of CMI are not well defined yet. Furthermore, the concentration that may be optimal for one particular index, may be sub-optimal or suppressive for the other indices. We need to understand the effects of dietary fatty acids on the indices of CMI individually and what do these changes mean in the overall expression of CMI. Also we need to view the effect of dietary fats on CMI within the frame work of a nutritionally balanced diet. Standardization of the techniques used to evaluate different indices of CMI and that of the dietary manipulations are very important to resolve some of the controversies regarding the effects of dietary fatty acids on CMI. It seems likely that the modulation of CMI by dietary fatty acids will find clinical use someday.

References

1. Meade, C.J., and Mertin, J., (1978) Adv. Lipid. Res. 16:127-165.
2. Gross, R.L., and Newberne, P.M., (1980) Physiol. Revs. 60:188-288.
3. Vitale, J.J., and Broiteman, S.A., (1981) Cancer Res. 41:3706-3710.
4. Beisel, W.R., (1982) Am. J. Clin. Nutr. Feb Supplement, 35:417-468.
5. Gur, M.I., (1983) Prog. Lipid Res. 22:257-287.
6. Johnston, D.V., and Marshall, L.A., (1984) Prog. Food and Nutr. Science 8:3-25.
7. Simopoulos, A.P., (1988) Nutrition Today 23:12-18.
8. Hwang, D. FASEB J 3:2052-2061. (1989)
9. Kinsela, J.E., Lokesh, B., Broughton, S., and Whelan, J., (1990) Nutrition 6:24-44.
10. Mertin, J., Shenton, B.K., and Field, E.J., (1973) Br. Med. J. 2:777-778.
11. Kelly, J.P., and Parker, C.W., (1979) J. Immunol. 122:1556-1562.
12. Mertin, J. and Hughes, D., (1975) Int. Archs Allergy Appl. Immunol. 48:203-210.

13. Chow, S.C., Sisfontes, L., Bjorkhem, I. and Jondal, M., (1989) Lipids, 24:700-704.
14. Morrow, W.j.W., Ohashi, Y., Hall, J., Pribnow, J., Hirose, S., Shirai, T. and Levy, J.J., (1985) Immunol. 135:3857-3863.
15. Marshall, L.A., and Johnston, P.V., (1985) J. Nutr. 115:1572-2580.
16. Meydani, S.N., Shapiro, A., Meydani, M., Macanley, J.B., and Blumberg, J.B., (1985) Fed. Proc. 44:929.
17. Ellis, N.K., Young, M.R., Nikcevich, D.A., Newby, M., Plioplys, R., and Wpsic, H.T., (1986) Cell. Immunol. 102:251-260.
18. Olson, L.M., Clinton, S.K., Everitt, J.I., Johnston, P.V., and Visek, W.J., (1987) J. Nutr. 117:955-963.
19. Alexander, N., and Smythe, N.L., (1988) Ann. Nutr. Metab. 32:192-199.
20. Kollmorgen, G.M., Sansing, W.A., Lehman, a.A., Fischer, G., Longley, R.E., Alexander, Jr. S.S., King, M.M., and McCay, P.B., (1979) Cancer Res. 39:3458-3462.
21. Erickson, K.L., McNeill, C.J., Gershwin, M.E., and Ossmann, J.B., (1980) J. Nutr. 110:1552-1572.
22. Ossmann, J.B., Erickson, K.J., and Canolty, N.L., (1980) Nutr. Reports International 22:279-284.
23. Erickson, K.L., Adams, D.A., McNeill, C.J., (1983) Lipids 18:468-474.
24. Lockniskar, M., Nauss, K.M., and Newberne, P.M., (1983) J. Nutr. 113:951-961.
25. Meydani, S.N., Nicolosi, R.J., and Hayes, K.C., (1985) Nutr. Res. 5:993-1002.
26. DeDeckere, E.A., Verplanke, C.J., Blok, C.J., and Van Nielen, W.G.L., (1988) J. Nutr. 118:11-18.
27. Kelley, D.S., Nelson, G.J., Serrato, C.M., Schmidt, P.C., and Branch, L.B., (1988) J. Nutr. 118:1376-1384.
28. Friend, J.V., Lock, S.O., Gur, M.I., and Parish, W.E., (1980) Int. Archs Allergy Appl. Immunol. 62:292-301.
29. Dewille, J.W., Fraker, P.J., and Romsos, D.R., (1981) J. Nutr. 111:2039-2043.
30. Thomas, I.K., and Erickson, K.L., (1985) J. Nutr. 115:1528-1534.
31. Meydani, S.N., Yogeeswaran, G., Liu, S., Baskar, S., and Meydani, M., (1988) J. Nutr. 118:1245-1252.
32. Erickson, K.L., and Schumacker, L.A., (1989) J. Nutr. 119:1311-1317.
33. Berry, E.M., Hirsch, J., Most, J., McNamara, D.J., Cunningham-Rundles, S., (1987) Nutr. Cancer 9:129-142.
34. Barone, J., Hebert, J.R., Reddy, M.M., (1989) Am. J. Clin. Nutr. 50:861-867.
35. Hebert, J.R., Barone, J., Reddy, M.M., and Backlund, J.C., (1990) Clin. Immunol. and Immunopath. 54:103-116.
36. Kelley, D.S., Branch, L.B., and Iacono, J.M., (1989) Nutr. Res. 9:965-975.
37. Payan, D.G., Wong, M.Y.S., Chernov-Rogan, T., Valone, F.H., Pickett, W.C., Blake, V.A., Gold, W.M., and Goetzl, L.J., (1986) J. Clin. Immunol. 6:402-410.
38. Bjerve, K.S., Fischer, S., Wammer, F., Egeland, T., (1989) Amer. J. Clin. Nutr. 49:290-300.

39. Kelley, D.S., Branch, L.B., Love, J.J., Taylor, P.C., Rivera, Y.M., and Iacono, J.M., (1991) Am. J. Clin. Nutr., 53:42-46.
40. Lee, T.H., Hoover, R.L., Williams, J.D., Sperling, R.I., Ravalese, J., Spur, B.W., Robinson, D.R., Corey, E.J., Lewis, R.A., and Austen, K.F., (1985) N. Eng. J. Med. 312:1217-1224.
41. Virella, G., Kilpatrick, J.M., Rugeles, M.T., Hyman, B. and Russell, R., (1989) Clin. Immunol. and Immunopath. 52:257-270.
42. Endres, S., Ghorbani, R., Kelley, V.E., Georgilis, K., Lonnemann, G., Meer, J.W.M.V., Cannon, J.G., Rogers, T.S., Klempner, M.S., Weber, P.C., Schaefer, E.J., Wolfe, S.M., and Dinarello, C.A., (1989) N. Eng. J. Med. 320:265-271.
43. Millar, J.H.D., Zilkha, K.J., Langman, M.J.S., Payling-Wright, H., Smith, A.D., Belin, J., and Thompson, R.H.S., (1973) Br. Med. J. 1:765-768.
44. Dil'man, V.M., Henirovsky, V.S., Ostroumova, M.N., L'Vovich, E.G., Blagorklonnayer, Y.V., Uskova, A.L., Marenko, A.I., Kondrat'ev, V.B., Semiglazov, V.F., Bershtein, L.M., Bobrov, Jr. F., Vasil'eva, I.A., Isveibah, A.S., and Gelfond, M.Z., (1976) Vopr. Onkol. 12:13-17.
45. Mchugh, M.I., Wilkinson, R., Elliott, R.W., Field, E.J., Dewar, P., Hall, R.R., Taylor, R.M.R., and Uldall, P.R., (1977) Transplantation 24:263-267.

Chapter Eighteen

Suppression of Autoimmune Disease by Purified N-3 Fatty Acids

Dwight R. Robinson, M.D.[1], Li-Lian Xu, M.D.[1], Walter Olesiak[2], Sumio Tateno, M.D.[3], Christopher T. Knoell[1], Robert B. Colvin, M.D.[4]

[1]Arthritis Unit of the Department of Medicine
Massachusetts General Hospital and Harvard Medical School
Boston, Massachusetts 02114

[2]c/o Sono Aibe, 904 Koizumi Building
3-29-11 Nishiwaseda
Shinjuku-Ku, Tokyo 169, Japan

[3]Sakura National Hospital
National Kidney Transplantation Center of Japan
2-36-2 Ebaradai Sakura
Chiba, Japan Code No. 285

[4]Department of Pathology
Massachusetts General Hospital and Harvard Medical School
Boston, Massachusetts 02114

Previous studies have demonstrated that diets containing alternative polyunsaturated fatty acids (PUFA) may modify inflammatory and immune reactions, and thus diets varying in their PUFA content may be considered as potential therapeutic approaches for inflammatory diseases. Autoimmune disease often leads to tissue injury through immune-induced inflammatory reactions. These diseases comprise a large number of important human diseases, such as rheumatoid arthritis and systemic lupus erythematosus which are poorly understood and therapy is either insufficient or accompanied by serious side-effects. A large number of studies (many reviewed elsewhere in this symposium) have clearly documented that dietary n-3 PUFA ameliorate tissue injury in several disease states, but the mechanisms of these potentially beneficial interventions are poorly understood. Anti-inflammatory effects of n-3 fatty acids may at least, in part, be related to the induction of synthesis of pro-inflammatory prostaglandins and laukotrienes, but other possible contributing mechanisms include the inhibition of cytokine release and alterations in signal transduction. The purpose of the studies reported here was to contribute to the understanding of the mechanisms of the beneficial effects of marine lipids on autoimmune diseases.

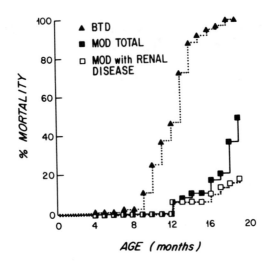

Fig. 18-1. Dietary marine lipid reduces the severity of glomerulonephritis in (NZB x NZW)F$_1$ mice. BTD = beef tallow diet. MOD = menhaden oil diet. Mortality due to renal disease was estimated from those animals with severe glomerulonephritis histologically. The experimental diets each contained 25 wt% of lipid. Mice were fed these diets beginning at age 5-6 weeks throughout the lifespan of the mice. (Reproduced from ref. [2]).

Protection From Autoimmune Glomerulonephritis by Dietary Fish Oil

Early studies by our laboratories (1-3) as well as of Kelley et al. (4) have documented that experimental diets containing marine lipids reduced the severity of autoimmune glomerulonephritis. Some representative early results are shown in Figure 18-1. In this study, female (NZBxNZW)F$_1$ mice were fed diets with either fish oil (MO) or beef tallow (BT) as lipid sources. Additional studies demonstrated that ordinary lab chow was similar to BT diets. These fish oil diets in these studies suppressed the frequency of severe glomerular disease to ca 16% of mice over the 19 month duration of the experiments whereas 100% of the BT controls all developed severe disease. Mortality was also reduced significantly although not as dramatically as the reduction in renal disease.

Fish oil diets also reduced the development of glomerulonephritis in other autoimmune mice, including the MRL/lpr and BXSB strains (3,4).

In addition, the intervention of a menhaden oil diet after the development of early glomerulonephritis was still capable of reducing the progress of renal disease compared to BT-fed controls (4). We have also documented that the protective effect of menhaden oil diets increased with increasing dose from 2.5 to 11 MO % with 25 MO % being similar to the 11 MO % diet (% by weight) (5).

Protection Of Autoimmune Diets by Purified n-3 Fatty Acids

Although we presumed that the protective effect of marine lipid diets on autoimmune disease was related to the n-3 fatty acid content of these oils, our more recent experiments have documented the effects of specific n-3 fatty acids by utilizing purified eicosapentaenoic and docosahexanoic acids as their ethyl esters. A quantitative histologic grading scale was used to measure the severity of glomerulonephritis after a defined period of experimental diets. Because of limited quantities of pure fatty acid ethyl esters, we assigned groups of NZBxNZWF$_1$ mice to experimental diets at the age of 16 weeks and continued these diets for 13 additional weeks, when all remaining mice were sacrificed. The controls (BT), at this time, had moderately severe pathological changes which could be compared with other groups. In these experiments the BT diet, consisting primarily of saturated and monoenoic fatty acids served as the control since it lacked signficant quantities of n-3 fatty acids. This control was compared to a purified fish oil triglyceride (Nissui 28) at two dose and the fish oil and BT diet preparations were compared to diets containing the n-3 ethyl esters. Each diet contained an additional 2% lipid as safflower oil to avoid any question of essential fatty acid deficiency. Diets containing less than 10% of n-3 fatty acid ethyl esters or fish oil had added beef tallow to bring the total lipid content up to 12% in each group. At the time of sacrifice, kidneys were removed for histologic analysis, and spleens were snap-frozen in liquid N$_2$ for fatty acid analyses. Some of the results of histologic studies are summarized in Table 18-1. Values for mean + SEM glomerular capillary wall thickening are given for each group of mice, along with the numbers (%) of the glomeruli present in each renal section which were essentially normal. The histologic scale ranged from zero (normal) to 4.0 (most severe). These results confirmed previous studies, described above, that the renal disease was significantly less severe in FO-fed mice compared to BT-fed, and the protection by FO was dose-dependent, and was only seen with the 10% FO diet. Both the EPA-E and DHA-E diets at the highest doses used were as effective in suppressing renal pathology as the 10% oil diet. However, several conclusions may be drawn from a comparison of these different diets. First, it is clear that DHA-E is more effective in preventing renal disease than EPA-E by both these criteria of capillary wall thickening and the ability to maintain normal glomeruli. The 6% DHA-E diet is at least as effective as the 10% FO, whereas 6% EPA-E is similar to the BT diet. When sufficiently large quantities of EPA-E are given (10%), reduction of the renal disease is seen. Second, it is clear that the renal effect of the 10% FO diet cannot be accounted for by its content of EPA alone, since EPA comprises 28% of the fatty acid composition of the FO preparation, and therefore the 10% FO diet contains almost the same content of EPA as does the 3% EPA-E diet. Even the 6% EPA-E diet is ineffective although it contains a slightly greater quantity of n-3 fatty acids than the 10% FO diet (5.5% n-3). These observations suggest that other components of the fish oil diet may make a major contribution to the protective effect of FO autoimmune disease. Other explanations may also account for these results, including the possiblity that the EPA-E was less efficiently absorbed than the FO diets. This seems unlikely since the ability of n-3 fatty acid ethyl esters to become incorporated into n-3 fatty acids into phospholipids was similar to the FO diets when comparing diets with similar n-3 fatty acid contents, based on analyses of spleen phospholipids from animals in these experiments (data not shown). This observation also indicates that n-3 fatty acid esters could be incorporated into phospholipids with an efficiency similar to these fatty acids in triglycerides. A further experiment has provided evidence for a synergistic effect of EPA and DHA in suppressing autoimmune renal disease. In this experiments, a diet consisting of 3.3% EPA-E and

TABLE 18-1

Suppression of Autoimmune Glomerulonephritis By Purified N-3 Fatty Acids.

Lipid	BT	FO		EPA-E			DHA-E		
wt%	10%	5%	10%	3%	6%	10%	3%	6%	10%
mean±SD	1.8±1.3	1.5±1.1	0.5±0.9	2.0±1.1	1.4±0.9	0.3±0.6	1.1±1.2	0.1±0.5	0.1±0.3
% normal, glomeruli	17	23	64	7.7	8.3	60	36	93	92

a = significant (p<0.05) vs 10% BT, b = significant vs 10% FO, c = glomerular capillary wall thickening, on a scale of 0 = normal, to 4 = most severe.

1.3% DHA-E provided approximately the same quantity of these fatty acids as present in the 10% FO diet. Although neither of these n-3 fatty acid ethyl esters would be expected to offer protection from renal disease based on the results shown in Table 18-1, there was highly significant protection, to an extent at least as great as the 10% FO diet (data not shown). Thus, these two n-3 fatty acids, EPA and DHA appear to act synergistically in their ability to prevent the development of autoimmune renal disease. These studies suggest that isolated n-3 fatty acid preparation such as EPA alone may not be as effective as anti-inflammatory agents as preparations containing n-3 fatty acid mixtures.

Effects Of n-3 Fatty Acid Ethyl Ester Diets On Phospholipid Fatty Acid Composition

We have carried fatty acid analyses of phospholipids in spleen, a lymphoid organ which is likely to be important in autoimmune disease, which lead to the following general conclusions. (1) The n-3 fatty acids from all of the n-3 fatty acid-containing diets are extensively incorporated into all major phospholipid classes including PE, PC, PS, PI, PE plasmalogens and alkyl ether PC. (2) The total PUFA remain relatively constant but incorporation of n-3 fatty acids is accompanied by marked reductions in 20- and 22-carbon n-6 fatty acids. (3) Extensive incorporation of EPA elongation of EPA to 22:5, n-3 is seen, but there is little or no delta-4 desaturation to DHA, when the mice are fed EPA-E. (4) There is incorporation of DHA and retroconversion of DHA to 22:5, n-3 and EPA, when the mice are fed DHA-E. (5) The DHA-E diets are at least as effective as the EPA-E diets in suppressing levels of arachidonic acid and 22-carbon, n-6 fatty acids.

In summary, the glomerulonephritis associated with spontaneous marine autoimmune disease is markedly suppressed by marine lipid diets containing fish oil. The same degree of protection can be achieved with either purified eicosapentaenoic acid or docosahexaenoic acid given as their ethyl esters. These two n-3 fatty acids appear to act synergistically in the therapy of autoimmune disease. Extensive incorporation of both fatty acids occurs into all major phospholipid classes including phosphatidylethanolamine plasmalogens and phosphatidylcholine alkyl ether. Elongation of EPA occurs but no significant desaturation to DHA is seen with these high polyunsaturated fat diets. A large degree of retroconversion of DHA is observed.

References

1. Prickett, J.D., Robinson, D.R., and Steinberg, A.D., (1981) J. Clin. Invest. 68, 556-559.
2. Prickett, J.D., Robinson, D.R., and Steinberg, A.D., (1983) Arth. & Rheum. 26, 133-139.
3. Robinson, D.R., Prickett, J.D., Makoul, G.T., Steinberg, A.D., and Colvin, R.B., (1986) Arth. & Rheum. 29, 539-545.
4. Kelley, V.E., Feretti, A., Izui, S., and Strom, T.B., (1985) J. Immunol. 134, 1914-1919.
5. Robinson, D.R., Prickett, J.D., Polisson, R., Steinberg, A.D., and Levine, L., (1985) Prostaglandins 30, 51-75.

Chapter Nineteen
Relationship Between Diet Fat, Plasma Membrane Composition and Insulin Stimulated Functions in Adipocytes

M.T. Clandinin, C.J. Field, M. Toyomizu, A.B.R. Thomson and M.L. Garg

Nutrition and Metabolism, Research Group
Departments of Foods & Nutrition and Medicine
University of Alberta
Edmonton, Alberta, Canada T6G 2C2

Physiological change in the composition of diet fat consumed alters cell membrane composition (1) by mechanisms that involve fatty acid desaturation (2) and biosynthesis of membrane phosphatidylcholine de novo (3,4). These diet-induced alterations in membrane phospholipid composition influence membrane proteins by changing the lipid environment in which these proteins function.

Normal variation in dietary fatty acid intake can alter the fatty acid composition of adipose tissue triacylglycerols and phospholipids (5,6). However, little is known about the role of the adipocyte plasma membrane phospholipid and the influences of fat intake or disease state on the composition and function of this membrane.

The insulin receptor is embedded in the plasma membrane bilayer (7). The insulin receptor (8,9) and insulin-stimulated functions (10) appear sensitive to the surrounding lipid environment. Altered microsomal rates of fatty acid Δ^6 and Δ^9-desaturation also occur in experimental models of diabetes mellitus (11,12). Insulin therapy corrects this defect in desaturase activity, and partially normalizes the altered fatty acid composition of microsomal fractions (11).

Diet fat and adipocyte membrane

On the premise that composition of the adipocyte plasma membrane is an integral determinant of insulin-stimulated functions in the adipocyte, the following experiments were designed to examine the effect of alterations in dietary fat composition on the fatty acid composition of adipocyte membrane phospholipids, on insulin binding to its receptor in the plasma membrane, and on insulin-stimulated transport and utilization of glucose. Diets representing the physiological range of dietary fatty acid composition consumed by humans were used. Control and diabetic rats were compared to assess whether increasing consumption of polyunsaturated fatty acids would normalize the decreased amounts of desaturase products expected in the diabetic state and alter insulin binding and insulin responsiveness.

Experimental Procedure

Weanling male Sprague-Dawley rats (59 ± 2 g) were fed semi-purified high fat diets containing 27% (w/w) high protein casein, 38% (w/w) carbohydrate as corn starch and 20% (w/w) fat. The composition of this basal diet has been reported in detail (4). Diets differed only in the proportion of safflower oil and hydrogenated beef tallow to provide polyunsaturated/saturated fatty acid ratios (P/S) of from 0.20 (low P/S) up to 2.0 (high P/S) (13). Linseed oil was added to obtain a total ω-3 fatty acid content of 1% (w/w) of the diet fat. Diets were cholesterol-free by analysis. After the diets had been fed for 21 days, diabetes was induced in animals in each diet group by intravenous injection of streptozotocin (45 mg/kg body weight). Animals with non-fasting blood glucose greater than 200 mg/dl after 21 days of streptozotocin injection were considered diabetic. Animals were continued on their respective diet treatment for an additional 14 days. Adipocyte plasma membrane was isolated, membrane phospholipids separated and fatty acid composition analyzed as described earlier (13). Insulin binding (13), glucose transport (14) and glucose utiliztion (15) were assessed.

Results

Effect of diet fat on adipocyte plasma membrane fatty acyl composition.

Dietary fat treatments significantly altered the fatty acid composition of the major adipocyte plasma membrane phospholipids in both control and diabetic animals (Table 19-1). Feeding a high polyunsaturated fat diet (P/S=1.0) as compared with a low polyunsaturated fat diet (P/S=0.25) increased the total polyunsaturated fatty acid content and P/S ratio in all five membrane phospholipids analyzed from control animals. For example, consumption of the high P/S diet by control animals increased the content of $C20:4(5,8,11,14)$ in phosphatidylethanolamine, phosphatidylinositol, phosphatidylserine and sphingomyelin, the con-

TABLE 19-1
Effect of Dietary Fat and the Diabetic State on the Contents of Major Fatty Acids in Adipocyte Plasma Membrane Phospholipids.

Phospholipid Group	Diet P/S Ratio	C18:2(9,12)	sats	ω-6	U.I.
Phosphatidylcholine					
Control	1.0	25.3±1.7[a]	53.5±1.3	37.2±1.3[a]	108.6±4[a]
	0.25	19.1±1.6[b]	56.3±1.5	30.4±2.2[b]	100.0±6[ab]
Diabetic	1.0	22.9±2.0[ab]	56.1±1.7	29.8±2.0[b]	91.9±3[b]
	0.25	20.7±1.4[ab]	56.7±1.3	27.6±1.7[b]	90.8±4[b]
Phosphatidylethanolamine					
Control	1.0	17.2±1.6[a]	44.6±1.8[a]	39.7±1.3[a]	145.5±4[a]
	0.25	11.9±1.4[b]	55.4±2.7[b]	25.6±2.1[b]	99.8±6[b]
Diabetic	1.0	16.0±1.8[ab]	48.7±2.0[ab]	32.4±3.3[c]	121.6±9[c]
	0.25	15.4±1.5[ab]	54.5±0.7[b]	28.1±1.8[bc]	104.6±4[b]
Phosphatidylinositol					
Control	1.0	7.5±0.8	58.8±1.6[a]	23.1±1.4[a]	101.7±5[a]
	0.25	6.7±1.1	63.7±2.8[ab]	13.2±1.4[b]	68.6±6[bc]
Diabetic	1.0	7.2±0.9	63.6±3.0[ab]	17.4±2.5[b]	78.0±10[b]
	0.25	8.3±0.8	68.5±1.4[b]	12.9±1.0[b]	54.6±3[c]
Phosphatidylserine					
Control	1.0	15.2±1.1[a]	52.3±1.6[a]	32.7±2.0[a]	121.5±7[a]
	0.25	11.7±1.3[b]	59.8±2.4[b]	22.5±1.9[b]	94.2±8[b]
Diabetic	1.0	18.6±0.7[a]	56.4±2.2[ab]	29.9±2.5[a]	102±10[ab]
	0.25	10.9±1.4[b]	56.3±3.0[ab]	23.0±1.5[b]	96.0±7[b]
Sphingomyelin					
Control	1.0	7.0±0.8[ab]	67.5±2.0	13.1±1.2[a]	64.4±5[ab]
	0.25	4.6±0.5[b]	72.7±2.1	8.0±0.8[b]	47.6±5[b]
Diabetic	1.0	8.1±1.1[a]	71.9±2.2	13.7±1.1[a]	69.2±9[a]
	0.25	6.9±1.1[ab]	70.4±2.1	11.1±1.2[ab]	60.8±5[ab]

Values are means ± S.E.M. (n=10) for control and diabetic animals given the dietary treatments: P/S, polyunsaturated/saturated fatty acid ratio of 1.0 or 0.25. Only major fatty acids are reported. Abbreviation used: U.I., unsaturation index (total number of unsaturated bonds). Values without a common superscript are significantly different (<0.05).

tent of C18:2(9,12) in phosphatidylcholine and phosphatidylethanolamine. The total number of double bonds expressed as unsaturation index increased in fatty acids found in phosphatidylethanolamine, phosphatidylinositol and phosphatidylserine of adipocyte plasma membranes in rats fed high P/S diet (Table 19-1).

The tendency towards higher phospholipid content of polyunsaturated fatty acids in diabetic animals fed the high P/S diet was also evident. Feeding the high P/S diet compared with the low P/S diet to diabetic animals increased the polyunsaturated fatty acid content in phosphatidylserine and phosphatidylinositol, the P/S ratio in phosphatidylethanolamine and phosphatidylinositol, and the unsaturation index of phosphatidylinositol and phosphatidylethanolamine (Table 19-1). A higher content of C18:2(9,12) in phosphatidylserine (Table 19-1) and C20:4(5,8,11,14) in sphingomyelin was oberved in plasma membranes obtained from diabetic animals fed the high P/S diet compared with the low P/S diet.

Effect of diet on insulin binding in normal and diabetic animals

For all insulin concentrations used to test insulin binding, adipocytes from control animals fed the high P/S diet (P/S=1.0) bound significantly more insulin than cells from control animals fed the low P/S diet (P/S=0.25). From Scatchard analysis of binding in control animals, increased insulin binding is associated with an increased number of available high affinity low capacity insulin-binding sites (13). An effect of diet on insulin binding was not observed when comparing adipocytes obtained from diabetic animals (13). At lower insulin concentration (0.1-10 ng/ml), adipocytes from diabetic animals bound significantly more insulin than did adipocytes obtained from control animals fed the low P/S diet (13). At higher insulin concentration (50 or 100 ng/ml), cells from diabetic animals bound significantly less insulin than control cells from animals fed the high P/S diet, but the amount of insulin bound at these concentrations did not differ from that in cells from control animals fed the low P/S diet.

To test that a direct relationship exists between the P/S ratio of dietary fat consumed, the composition of the major adipocyte plasma membrane phospholipids and insulin binding, animals were fed one of ten diets varying in P/S ratio between 0.14 and 1.8. The response surfaces for total specific bound insulin over the entire range (Fig. 19-1A) and what might be considered a physiological range (Fig. 19-1B) of insulin was calculated using data for all five insulin concentrations measured and using only the data for the three lower insulin concentrations (0.4, 1.2, 10 ng/ml). A significant positive relationship was found between the P/S ratio of the diet and the amount of insulin bound at every insulin

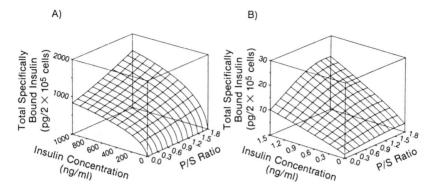

Fig. 19-1. *Relationship between diet P/S and insulin binding to adipocytes.* The response surfaces of the total specific bound insulin for animals fed the ten experimental diets was calculated over the entire range (0-1000 ng/ml) (Fig. 19-1A) and what is likely a more physiological range (0-10 ng/ml) (Fig. 19-1B) of insulin concentration. Equations to describe the response surfaces for the insulin bound (I) as functions of dietary P/S ratio (PS) and insulin concentration (C) were as follows:

A) $\text{LOG}(I) = 1.042 + 0.149 \times \text{PS} + 0.910 \times \text{LOG}(C)$
$\quad -0.094 \times \text{LOG}(C) \times \text{LOG}(C)$ $\quad (R^2 = 0.99)$

and

B) $\text{LOG}(I) = 0.879 + 0.403 \times \text{PS} - 0.122 \times \text{PS}$
$\quad \times \text{PS} + 0.687 \times \text{LOG}(C) + 0.172 \times \text{LOG}(C)$
$\quad \times \text{LOG}(C)$ $\quad (R^2 = 0.98)$

concentration (Fig. 19-1A). However, when the lower insulin levels within a smaller range of insulin values were examined, the amount of insulin bound increased to attain a plateau with increasing diet P/S (Fig. 19-1B).

Relationship between diet, membrane composition and insulin binding

The diet P/S ratio influenced the content (% w/w) of the major membrane fatty acids in adipocyte membrane phospholipids. The content of several fatty acid constituents in phosphatidylcholine and most major fatty acids in phosphatidylethanolamine were found to relate significantly to both change in the diet P/S ratio and the amount of insulin bound at insulin concentrations of 0.4, 1.2, 10 and 100 ng/ml. By mathematical modeling using a perspective program (16), a three dimensional relationship model was obtained to illustrate the relationship between change in dietary P/S ratio, levels of fatty acid constituents in plasma membrane phospholipids, and insulin binding at a concentration of 1.2 ng/ml insulin (Fig. 19-2). The amount of insulin bound increased as the content of polyunsaturated fatty acids in phosphatidylethanolamine and the content of C18:0 in phosphatidylcholine increased. Insulin binding decreased with increasing content of saturated and monounsaturated fatty acids in phosphatidylethanolamine and C16:0 in phosphatidylcholine. Although not illustrated, insulin binding was also found to be positively related to the C18:2(6) and P/S ratio of phosphatidylethanolamine, and negatively related to C16:1 levels in phosphatidylcholine, C16:0 and C18:1 levels in phosphatidylethanol-

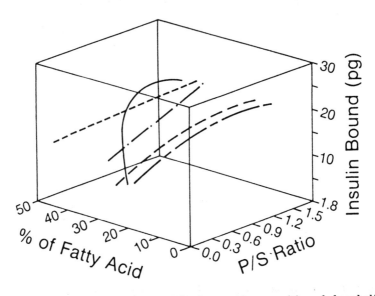

Fig. 19-2. *Relationship between diet P/A, fatty acid composition of phospholipids and insulin binding.* A three dimensional model was developed to illustrate the relationship between dietary P/S ratio, membrane phospholipid fatty acid composition and insulin binding to adipocytes at an in vitro insulin concentration of 1.2 ng/ml. In developing the figure, two equations were joined, one predicting the relationship between membrane composition and diet, and the second predicting the relationship between membrane composition and insulin binding. Abbreviations as defined in Table 19-1. The lines are: ------- for PE_{sats}, ––– for $PE_{monounsats}$, ––– for $PE_{polyunsats}$, —●— for $PC_{C18:0}$, – – – for $PC_{C16:0}$.

amine. Figure 19-2 suggests that an increase in the dietary P/S ratio between the level normally consumed by the North American population (P/S=0.35) and that recommended (P/S=1.0), results in a remarkable increase in the membrane polyunsaturated fatty acid content (primarily ω-6 fatty acids) of phosphatidylethanolamine and that this increase in polyunsaturated fatty acids is associated with increased binding of insulin to adipocytes. Although the polyunsaturated fatty acid content of phosphatidylcholine, phosphatidylinositol and phosphatidylserine were higher in animals fed the high P/S (1.8) as compared to the low P/S (0.14) diet, a significant relationship with insulin binding was not found.

Relationship between diet, insulin binding and glucose transport and metabolism

Diabetic cells transported less glucose ($P<0.001$) than cells from either control group (Fig. 19-3). At all insulin concentrations tested, adipocytes from control animals fed the high P/S diet (P/S=2.0) transported significantly more glucose than control animals fed the low P/S diet ($p<0.02$). At insulin concentration less than 25 ng/ml insulin, diet did not affect glucose transport in diabetic animals. However, at the two higher insulin concentrations (100, 1000 ng/ml), glucose transport was improved in cells from animals fed the high P/S diet ($p<0.05$). The tendency for cells from diabetic animals fed the high P/S diet to transport more glucose at 1000 ng/ml insulin (glucose concentration 0.5 mM) was observed. Change in insulin stimulated glucose transport expressed as a percent of the amount of glucose transported at insulin concentration of 25 ng/ml for each group is illustrated (Fig. 19-3). This figure clearly shows that, for both control and diabetic animals fed the high P/S diet, the relative increase in glucose transport at the higher insulin concentrations measured is greater than for animals fed the low P/S diet.

The mean amount of glucose transported per insulin bound is reduced in diabetic animals (Fig. 19-4). Diet influenced this relationship. For both control and diabetic animals fed the low P/S diet (P/S=0.2), mean glucose transport reached a maximum at approximately 350-500 pg insulin bound/2.0×10^5 cells. In animals fed the high P/S diet (P/S=2.0), glucose transport continued to increase as more insulin was bound.

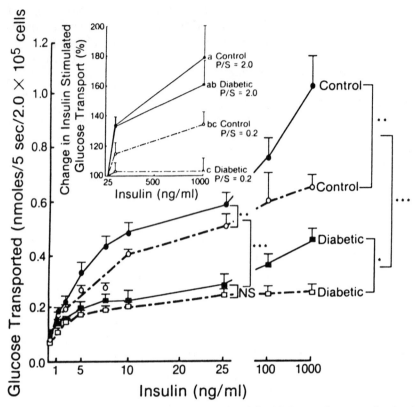

Fig. 19-3. The amount of glucose transported at 0.5 mM glucose for control animals fed the high P/S diet (●—●); control animals fed the low P/S diet (○--○); diabetic animals fed the high P/S diet (■—■); diabetic animals fed the low P/S diet (□--□). Values are group means ± S.E. (n=5/group). The level of significance is indicated (* $p<0.05$), (** $p<0.01$), (*** $p<0.001$). Statistics were conducted across the lower insulin concentration (0-25 ng/ml) and the higher insulin concentrations (100, 1000 ng/ml). Using the data illustrated in Fig. 19-3, the change in insulin-stimulated glucose transport is expressed as a percent of the amount of glucose transported at 25 ng/m. (100%) for each treatment. Values without a common superscript are significantly different ($p<0.05$).

Adipocytes from control animals oxidized significantly more glucose than diabetic adipocytes (Fig. 19-5). However, feeding diabetic animals the high P/S diet (P/S=1.0) as compared with the low P/S diet (P/S=0.25) significantly increased the amount of glucose oxidized for the seven insulin concentrations tested. Diet did not significantly alter the

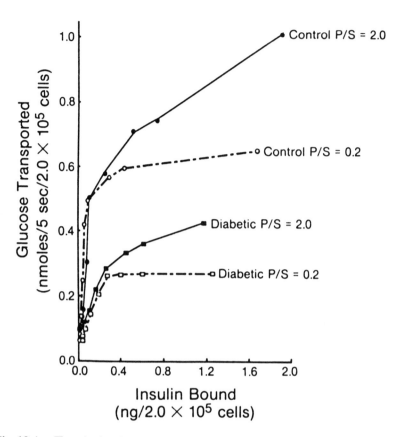

Fig. 19-4. *The relationship between insulin bound and glucose transported.* Values illustrated are group means calculated from the data illustrated in Fig. 19-1 (amount of insulin bound at each insulin concentration) for control animals fed the high P/S diet (●—●); control animals fed the low P/S diet (○--○); diabetic animals fed the high P/S diet (■—■); diabetic animals fed the low P/S diet (□--□).

amount of glucose oxidation in control adipocytes at the insulin concentrations measured. A significantly lower basal oxidation rate (at 0 ng/ml insulin) was found for diabetic animals fed the low P/S diet as compared with diet-matched control animals (10.4 ± 3.0 nmoles and 16.0 ± 3.6 nmoles, respectively). The basal oxidation rate for cells from high P/S-fed diabetic animals did not differ significantly from either control group. At sub-maximal oxidation rates (at 0-1.0 ng/ml insulin) the amount of glucose oxidized by diabetic animals fed the high P/S diet was

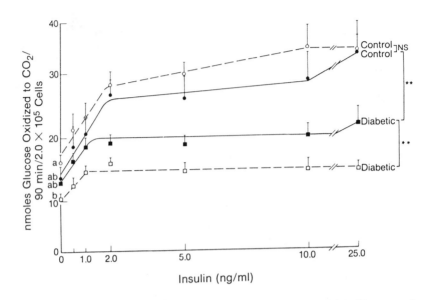

Fig. 19-5. *Relationship between glucose oxidation to CO_2 and insulin concentration.* Values reported are group means ± S.E. (n=10 animals/group): (●—●) control P/S= 1.0; (○--○) control P/S=0.25; (■—■) diabetic P/S=1.0; (□--□) diabetic P/S=0.25. Groups were compared to analysis of variance calculated over 7 insulin concentrations tested (** $p<0.01$). Basal oxidation rates were compared by analysis of variance. Values without a common superscript are significantly different ($p<0.05$).

not differ significantly from cells of either control group. At greater than observed for diabetic animals fed the low P/S diet and did these insulin levels diabetic adipocytes from animals fed the low P/S diet oxidized significantly less glucose than cells from the other groups.

Glucose incorporation into lipids

Feeding a high P/S diet (P/S=1.0) compared with a low P/S diet (P/S=0.25) significantly improved glucose incorporation into lipids by adipocytes from control and diabetic animals (Fig. 19-6). Adipocytes from diabetic animals fed the high or low P/S diet synthesized less lipid from glucose than cells from diet-matched control animals. Glucose incorporation into lipids by adipocytes from diabetic animals fed the high P/S

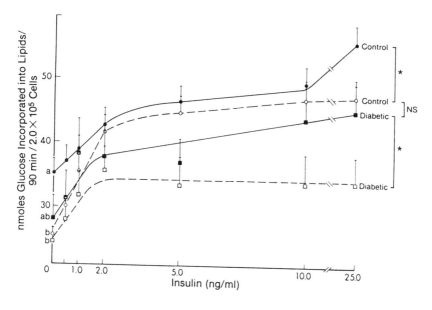

Fig. 19-6. *Relationship between glucose incorporation into lipid and insulin concentrations.* Values reported are group means ± S.E. (n=10 animals/group): (●—●) control P/S=1.0; (○--○) control P/S=0.25; (■—■) diabetic P/S=1.0; (□--□) diabetic P/S=0.25. Groups were compared by analysis of variance calculated over 7 insulin concentrations tested (* $p<0.05$; ** $p<0.01$). Basal lipogenesis rates were compared by analysis of variance. Values without a common superscript are significantly different ($p<0.05$).

diet did not differ significantly from the amount of glucose incorporated by control animals fed the low P/S diet. Basal lipid synthesis (at 0 ng/ml insulin) was significantly higher in adipocytes from control animals fed the high P/S diet than adipocytes from either diabetic group.

Discussion

The present study demonstrates that feeding animals diets providing a fat content and fatty acid composition analogous to that consumed by segments of the North American population (6), significantly alters the fatty acyl composition of the major phopholipids of the adipocyte plasma membrane in both control and diabetic animals. Individual phospholipid classes respond to dietary fatty acid manipulation to different degrees. Although the molecular control mechanism through which dietary fat composition influences the fatty acyl composition is unknown, differences in rates of synthesis of phospholipids de novo (3), redistribution of fatty acyl chains via phospholipase (17) or acyltransferase (4) and direct desaturation of membrane phospholipid-linked fatty acids (2) have been demonstrated to be altered by dietary fat composition. The availability of fatty acids at specific sites of synthesis may be influenced by dietary fat, as adipose tissue represents a large pool of available fatty acids, the composition of which to a large extent reflects the dietary fatty acid composition (4).

Specific diet-induced transitions in membrane phospholipid fatty acid composition were parallelled by changes in insulin binding at what are considered both physiological and supraphysiological insulin concentrations. The degree of change occurring in membrane polyunsaturated fatty acid content of phosphatidylethanolamine appears to be greater than that observed for other essential fatty acids, especially when related to concomitant changes occurring in insulin binding. Further, attaining a plateau for membrane polyunsaturated fatty acid content and the leveling off of monounsaturated fatty acid content of phosphatidylethanolamine for animals fed the higher P/S diets follows a similar trend to insulin binding at the lower and likely more physiological insulin levels (Fig. 19-1).

Feeding the high P/S diet tended to increase the amount of glucose transported per insulin bound in adipocytes in both the normal and diabetic states. This suggests that diet may influence the coupling between the insulin receptor and the glucose transporter. Although diabetic animals transported less glucose at a given amount of insulin bound, feeding the high P/S diet to diabetic animals tended to normalize this function. The molecular events subsequent to the hormone receptor interction causing the metabolic action of insulin on glucose transport are unknown. However, due to contact with membrane lipids, several membrane-mediated events might be influenced by diet-induced alterations in the lipid bilayer. In this regard, insulin-stimulated phosphorylation of the tyrosine residues on the β-subunit of the receptor and the activation of endogenous insulin receptor kinase are postulated to be critical steps in insulin action. Our current research indicates that this activity may be altered by transitions in membrane composition, thus resulting in altered glucose utilization.

In summary, the present study demonstrates that normal variations in dietary fat intake: 1) alter the composition of structural lipids found in the adipose organ, and 2) in the short-term diabetic state alter the membrane response to a high polyunsaturated fatty acid diet. These diet-induced alterations in membrane composition appear to influence insulin binding to adipocyte membranes. It is therefore logical to hypothesize that localized changes in adipocyte plasma membrane microenvironment may play some role in modulating insulin action within cells and may be of particular importance in dietary management of diabetes.

Acknowledgments

This work was supported by grants from the Canadian Diabetes Association and the Natural Sciences and Engineering Research Council of Canada. C.J. Field was a recipient of a Medical Research Council of Canada Studentship and an Alberta Heritage Foundation for Medical Research Independent Research Allowance. M.T. Clandinin is a Scholar of the Alberta Heritage Foundation for Medical Research.

References

1. Clandinin, M.T., Field, C.J., Hargreaves, K., Morson, L., and Zsigmond, E., (1985) Can. J. Physiol. Pharmacol. 63, 546-556.
2. Garg, M.L., Sebokova, E., Thomson, A.B.R., and Clandinin, M.T., (1988) Biochem. J. 249, 351-356.
3. Hargreaves, K.M. and Clandinin, M.T., (1987) Biochem. Biophys. Res. Commun. 145, 309-315.
4. Hargreaves, K.M. and Clandinin, M.T., (1987) Biochim. Biophys. Acta 918, 97-105.
5. Field, C.J. and Clandinin, M.T., (1984) Nutr. Res. 4, 743-755.
6. Field, C.J., Angel, A. and Clandinin, M.T., (1985) Am. J. Clin. Nutr. 42, 1206-1220.
7. Schlessinger, J., Schlechter, Y., Willingham, M.C., and Pastan, I., (1978) Proc. Natl. Acad. Sci. U.S.A. 75, 2659-2663.
8. Ginsberg, B.H., Brown, T.J., Ido, S., and Spector, A.A., (1981) Diabetes 30, 773-780.
9. Gould, R.J., Ginsberg, B.H., and Spector, A.A., (1982) J. Biol. Chem. 257, 477-484.
10. Sandra, A., Fyler, D.J., and Marshall, S.J., (1984) Biochim. Biophys. Acta 778, 511-515.
11. Faas, F.H. and Carter, W..J., (1980) Lipids 15, 953-961.
12. Worcester, N.A., Bruckdorfer, K.R., Hallinan, T., Wilkins, A.J., Mann, J.A., and Yudkin, J., (1979) Br. J. Nutr. 41, 239-252.
13. Field, C.J., Ryan, E.A., Thomson, A.B.R., and Clandinin, M.T., (1988) Bio-

chem. J. 253, 417-424.
14. Whitesell, R.R. and Abumrad, N.A., (1985) J. Biol. Chem. 260, 2894-2899.
15. Rodbell, M., (1964) J. Biol. Chem. 239, 375-380.
16. DISSPLA. User's manual: display integrated software system and plotting language. Computer Associates, U.S.A.
17. Van den Bosch, H., (1980) Biochim. Biophys. Acta 604, 191-246.

Chapter Twenty

Studies Of Dietary Supplementation With Omega-3 Fatty Acids In Patients With Rheumatoid Arthritis

Joel M. Kremer, M.D.

Department of Medicine
Division of Rheumatology
Albany Medical College
Albany, New York 12208

Studies on the use of omega-3 dietary supplementation in patients with rheumatoid arthritis first appeared in the scientific literature in the mid-1980s. Interest concerning these supplements in patients with autoimmune-induced inflammatory disease was derived from earlier investigations of their use in animal models in which dietary modifications employing omega-3 fatty acids significantly improved disease manifestations and survival. The purpose of this review will be to summarize our investigations employing omega-3 supplements in clinical investigations in patients with rheumatoid arthritis. Data on the effects of omega-3 supplements on inflammatory and immune parameters will also be discussed. Lastly, we will speculate on directions of future research efforts.

Studies in Patients with Rheumatoid Arthritis

The possible influence of dietary alterations on the disease process in rheumatoid arthritis has generated interest for some time. A Chinese physician who developed the disease claimed that he was cured when he reverted to a diet of rice, vegetables, and fish that he consumed as a youth in his native China. He published a popular book advocating his diet as treatment for arthritis. A study published in 1983 examined the effects of this diet on patients with active rheumatoid arthritis and found no discernible differences when compared to a control diet [1]. The authors did, however, note that several patients on the rice-fish diet did improve significantly from baseline, although the improvement in the entire study cohort did not achieve statistical significance.

In a pilot study published in 1985 [2], 17 patients with rheumatoid arthritis consumed an experimental diet high in polyunsaturated fat and low in saturated fat, with a daily supplement of 1.8 grams of EPA and 0.9 grams of DHA provided by 10 Max-EPA (Scherer) capsules. A control group consumed a diet with a polyunsaturated/saturated ratio of 1/4 and also took a capsule containing indigestible paraffin wax (Efamol Research). Compliance was measured by patient diaries, pill counts and gas chromatographic analysis of plasma lipids in order to document a rise in EPA in patients consuming fish-oil. The study design was double-blind, controlled, randomized and of 12 weeks duration with a follow-up evaluation 1-2 months after the diets and supplements were discontinued. Standard clinical measures of arthritis activity were performed at baseline and after 4, 8 and 12 weeks and then at the time of the follow-up. The results showed a significant difference in morning stiffness between the 2 groups at the time of the 12 week evaluation, which represented a worsening in the control group while the fish-oil/low fat group remained unchanged. There were improvements in the mean number of tender joints at 12 weeks in the experimental group when compared with baseline ($p=0.001$), which did not achieve significance vs. the control group at that time ($p=0.16$). At the follow-up visit,

TABLE 20-1
Overall Assessment, Pain Assessment, and ARA Class

	Baseline	4 wk	8wk	12wk	Follow-up
ARA class (1-4)					
C	2.2	2.3	2.3	2.3	2.3
E	2.0	1.9	1.9	2.1	2.0
Patient Pain*					
C	2.6	2.6	2.7	2.8	2.8
E	2.8	2.5	2.6	2.5	3.6+
Patient Overall*					
C	3.0	2.9	3.0	2.9	2.9
E	2.8	2.6	2.9	2.7	3.6+
Physician Pain*					
C	3.0	2.6	3.0	3.0	2.8
E	2.9	2.6	2.7	2.6	3.1+
Physician Overall*					
C	3.1	2.8	3.0	3.0	2.9
E	2.9	2.7	3.0	2.6	3.1+

*1 = none, 5 = very severe. C = control, E = experimental
+$p<0.05$ for difference between follow-up and 12 week evaluations.
Reprinted with permission from *Lancet* 1:184-187, 1985

a significant worsening was observed in the experimental group in patients' rating of pain and overall condition (p=0.02), phyiscians' pain rating (p=0.03), and physicians' overall evaluation (p=0.04) (Table 20-1).

A change in hemoglobin concentration between the experimental and control groups was significant at 12 weeks (p=0.03), but it represented an exaggeration of a baseline difference, and the change from baseline was not significant. There was, however, a significant prolongation of the IVY bleeding time in the experimental group from 5.15 minutes at baseline to 6.97 minutes at 12 weeks. The 12 week bleeding time is still within the normal range and would not result in clinically significant bleeding. It should be noted that all patients were taking aspirin or a non-steroidal anti-inflammatory drug throughout the study.

In a subsequent clinical investigation, the effect of fish-oil dietary supplementation alone was investigated in a 14 week double-blind crossover investigation with a 4 week washout period between study arms [3]. Patients with acute rheumatoid arthritis received 2.79 grams of EPA and 1.8 grams of DHA in the form of 15 MAX-EPA capsules (Scherer) or olive oil. The crossover design allowed investigators to compare the effects of fish oil vs. olive oil supplementation in the same individuals while they maintained their own background diets and medications without any alterations. Thirty-three patients completed the study with satisfactory compliance documented by pill counts and gas chromatographic analysis of plasma fatty acids.

After 14 weeks on either fish oil or olive oil, patients had significantly fewer tender joints (p=0.007) compared to when they ingested olive oil. The time interval to the first experience of fatigue also improved in patients consuming fish oil (p=0.05). No other statistically significant clinical improvements were observed in the experimental group vs. olive oil, although all of the 10 other clinical parameters measured favored fish oil. After 14 weeks significant improvements were also observed from baseline in the group consuming fish oil in American Rheumatism Association functional class, physicians global assessment of disease activity, the number of tender joints and the number of swollen joints (Table 20-2).

Ionophore-stimulated neutrophil leukotriene B_4 (LTB_4) production also decreased by 57.8% (p=0.001) when patients received the fish-oil fatty acid supplement compared with when they ingested olive oil. This is of potential significance as LTB_4 is a potent pro-inflammatory substance. A significant Pearson correlation (r=0.393, p=0.036) was seen between decreases in neutrophil leukotriene B_4 production observed in

TABLE 20-2
Mean Values and 95% Confidence Intervals for the Fish Oil and Placebo Effects on Rheumatoid Arthritis at 7 and 14 Weeks in Thirty-Three Patients

Variable	Fish Oil 7 weeks	Fish Oil 14 weeks	Placebo 7 weeks	Placebo 14 weeks
Morning Stiffness, min	−2.7 (−20.9 to 5.5)	−5.9 (−22.6 to 10.8)	22.4 (−7.7 to 52.5)	49.4 (−12.8 to 111.4)
Time to Fatigue, min	94.0 (8.3 to 179.7)	176.8 (83.0 to 270.6)*	11.8 (−86.3 to 109.9)	8.4 (−98.9 to 115.7)
Grip strength, mm Hg	−3.4 (−11.6 to 4.8)	9.7 (−0.1 to 19.5)	−2.0 (10.0 to 6.0)	2.9 (−7.1 to 12.9)
ARA Class (I to IV)	−0.13 (−0.25 to −0.01)*	−0.18 (−0.3 to −0.06)*	−0.06 (−0.2 to −0.08)	−0.03 (−0.19 to 0.13)
Physician Assessment of Pain	−0.06 (−0.36 to 0.24)	−0.06 (0.36 to 0.24)	0.14 (−0.11 to 0.39)	0.06 (−0.14 to 0.26)
Patient Assessment of Pain	−0.15 (−0.38 to 0.10)	−0.21 (−0.52 to 0.10)	−0.06 (−0.36 to 0.24)	0.0 (−0.18 to 0.18)
Physician Global Assessment	−0.17 (−0.39 to 0.05)	−0.27 (−0.52 to −0.3)	−0.0 (−0.14 to 0.14)	−0.9 (−0.27 to 0.09)
Patient Global Assessment	−0.06 (−0.36 to 0.24)	−0.11 (−0.35 to 0.13)	−0.9 (−0.27 to 0.09)	0.0 (−0.16 to 0.16)
50-ft (15 m) walking time, s	−0.01 (−0.34 to 0.32)	−0.22 (−0.69 to 0.25)	0.39 (−0.36 to 1.14)	0.39 (−0.45 to 1.53)
Tender Joints, n	−2.0 (−3.4 to −0.6)*	−3.5 (−5.2 to 1.8)*	−0.8 (−2.8 to 1.2)	0.01 (−1.19 to 1.21)
Swollen Joints, n	−0.4 (−4.7 to 3.9)	−2.8 (−4.3 to 1.3)*	−0.3 (−1.7 to 1.1)	−1.0 (−2.5 to 0.5)
Erythrocyte sedimentation Rate, mm/h	−2.3 (−6.4 to 1.8)	−0.8 (−6.8 to 5.2)	−1.11 (−4.8 to 2.58)	−2.07 (−6.89 to 2.75)

*The univariate confidence intervals not containing 0 correspond to statistical significance at $p<0.05$. All values for patients at 14 weeks on fish oil would remain significant if the Bonferroni correction were used, except the number of swollen joints. It should be observed that all the variables except sedimentation rate changed in a direction favorable to the fish-oil supplementation. ARA = American Rheumatism Association.

Physician and patient assessments are graded on a scale of 0 to 4.

Reprinted with permission of *Annals of Internal Medicine* 106:497-503, 1987.

individual patients with decreases in the number of tender joints. A Spearman rank correlation on the same data showed a higher degree of association (r=0.55, p=0.01) between the variables in individual patients. Interestingly, the neutrophil LTB_4 values in the group ingesting fish oil prior to olive oil remained below the baseline value for as long as 18 weeks after these supplements were discontinued. The fact that patients were not ingesting fish-oil during the follow-up period was confirmed by gas chromatographic analysis of plasma. Subjects were noted to do better clinically during the olive oil phase which occurred after (rather than before) fish oil and it was felt that the prolonged suppression of neutrophil LTB_4 production might account for the continued clinical benefits observed after the period of discontinuation of fish oil. Prolonged effects on the immune system were subsequently reported in normal volunteers ingesting fish oil and will be discussed in a subsequent section. Because of these observations, it appears that a crossover format is not appropriate to study the clinical or immune effects of fish oil in patients with inflammatory disease.

Before reviewing the next clinical investigation of the effects of fish oil dietary supplementation in patients with rheumatoid arthritis, it is of some interest to reflect on the previously summarized investigations in order to define certian commonly observed phenomena. Clinical benefits derived from fish oil improve from baseline vs. a control group but may not achieve statistical significance. When significant improvements are observed, they often do not occur until at least 12 weeks of dietary supplementation. This is of some interest in that Sperling et al. demonstrated that significant alterations of leukotriene metabolism occur in neutrophils and monocytes after 6 weeks in RA patients consuming fish oil [4]. Moreover, Cleland et al. observed that neutrophils LTB_4 and 5-HETE production increased towards baseline as soon as 4 weeks after discontinuing fish oil dietary supplements in patients with RA [5]. This is of note in view of the seemingly paradoxical observation that clinical benefits are maintained for up to 18 weeks following the discontinuation of fish oil [3].

There is thus a discrepancy in timing between the ex-vivo changes in leukotriene metabolism and the clinical improvements induced by fish oil. Why are clinical improvements delayed until 12 weeks and why are they sustained for so long when discontinuing fish oil? A study by Endres et al. may help to explain these observations [6]. Nine healthy volunteers consumed 2.75 grams of EPA and 1.8 grams of DHA daily for 6 weeks. Interleukin-1B and α (IL-IB-IL-1α) and tumor necrosis factor

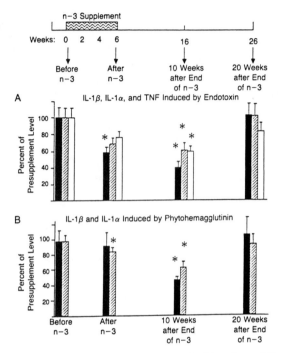

Fig. 20-1. Synthesis of IL-1 (solid bars), IL-1 (hatched bars), and Tumor Necrosis Factor (TNF; open bars) by Mononuclear Cells Stimulated with 1 ng of Endotoxin per Milliliter (Panel A) or 3 μg of Phytohemagglutinin per Milliliter (Panel B).

The concentration of total cytokine (i.e. cell-associated plus secreted) was determined by radioimmunoassay. Concentrations are presented as percentages of presupplementation levels. With endotoxin stimulation, the concentrations were 7.4 ng of IL-1β per milliliter and 14.0 ng of IL-1α per milliliter. Each bar represents the mean of 27 determinations (nine donors assayed on three days each). The error bars denote the SEM for the nine donors. An asterisk denotes a significant difference from the level before dietary n-3 supplementation (at p<0.05). Reprinted with permission of *The New England Journal of Medicine* 320:265-271, 1989.

(TNF) was measured at baseline, after 6 weeks and then 10 and 20 weeks after discontinuing the supplement. IL-1B production decreased by 43% after 6 weeks of fish-oil supplementation (p=0.048, but a further decrease was observed 10 weeks after discontinuing the supplement when production had decreased by 61% from baseline (p=0.005) (Figure 20-1). The production of IL-1B returned to pre-supplement values 20 weeks after discontinuing the fish oil.

IL-1 has significant potential impact on the RA disease process through a variety of mechanisms [7]. It is thus of relevance that fish oil dietary supplementation inhibits the production of this cytokine and that the chronology of these inhibitory effects differ from those observed with leukotriene production. It is therefore possible that fish oil induced suppression of IL-1 contributes to the amelioration of clinical signs and symptoms of disease activity in patients with RA to a greater extent than does inhibition of leukotriene metabolism. That is, the clinical benefits observed in the studies reviewed above may be "delayed" relative to leukotriene inhibition becuase of the later inhibition of the production of IL-1.

An investigation which would examine the effects of fish-oil dietary supplementation on the clinical, inflammatory and immune parameters of RA over periods of greater than 12-14 weeks was needed. In addition, it was unclear whether dose dependent effects of fish oil occur. The above investigations employed the same dose of fish oil dietary supplementation in all patients regardless of body weight. A comparison of different doses of fish oil in patients with active disease over extended periods would become a logical extension of the previous work.

In a recently completed study, 49 patients with active rheumatoid arthritis consumed either "high" or "low" dose fish or olive oil over a period of 6 months (24 weeks) [8]. The study designed was randomized, prospective parallel and doubleblind. The "low dose" fish oil group ingested 27 mg/kg/day EPA and 18 mg/kg/day DHA and the "high dose" group ingested twice this amount. Fish oil was supplied as an ethyl-ester (Pharmacaps®) containing 33 mg EPA and 240 mg DHA per capsule. The olive oil group consumed 9 capsules/day. Patients maintained their background medications for arthritis without change during the study. No special dietary instructions were provided to study subjects. Clinical investigations occurred at baseline and every 6 weeks while immune parameters including ionophore-stimulated neutrophil LTB_4 and LTB_5, macrophage Il-1 and IL-2 production, T and B cell response to mitogen proliferation and immunoglobulin production was measured at baseline and after 24 weeks.

Results showed that multiple clinical parameters improved from baseline in the groups consuming fish oil. The improvements were noted more commonly in the high dose fish-oil group in which 21/45 clinical measures evaluated at weeks 6 through 24 improved significantly from baseline, compared with 8/45 in the low dose subjects and 5/45 in the olive oil consuming patients. Moreover, significant changes from baseline increased with increasing duration of fish oil ingestion beyond 12 weeks. Only 5 clinical outcomes during weeks 6 and 12 of the study showed significant improvement in patients consuming fish oil, while 24 outcomes achieved significance at the time of the 18, 24, or 30 week evaluation.

It should be noted that only the grip strength clinical outcome improved significantly when compared with the olive oil consuming patients. Reasons for this could include common non-significant improvements observed in the olive oil group from baseline and the elimination of 11 patients during the study from this group for medication adjustment required by increased symptoms. (The need for increased medication during the period of investigation of dietary supplementation was considered a protocol violation). Olive oil also has potential to favorably affect the immune response in inflammatory disease [9-12].

Laboratory analysis showed that IL-1 production and release from macrophages decreased by 40.6% from baseline in the low dose fish-oil group (p=0.059) and by 54.7% in the high dose group (p=0.0005). IL-1 also decreased by 38% in the olive oil group, but the change was not statistically significant (Table 20-3). Tritiated thymidine incorporation after mitogen stimulation increased significantly in all 3 groups after 24 weeks compared to baseline measurements. Increased thymidine incorporation was also noted after PHA stimulation but was only significant in the high dose fish-oil group. Thymidine incorporation after PWM stim-

TABLE 20-3
Fish Oil (FO) Effects on LPS-Induced Production of IL-1 by PBMC *In Vitro*

Treatment	N	Change from Baseline Week 0-24
Olive Oil	11	-243.1 (-540.4 to 54.2)
Low Dose FO	18	-239.9 (-490.4 to 10.6)+
High Dose FO	17	-416.2 (-623.0 to 209.4)

*=Values are expressed as units/ml and are mean 95% confidence interval; 1 unit is the 50% maximal proliferative point in the C3H/HeJ co-stimulation assay (see Methods).
+p = 0.59 from baseline.
p = .0005
LPS = lipopolysacharide
PBMC = peripheral blood mononuclear cell
Reproduced with permission of *Arthritis and Rheumatism*, 1990; 33:810-820 copyright, 1990.
Used buy permission of the American College of Rheumatology.

TABLE 20-4
Significant Improvement (p<0.5) in RA Patients Ingesting Dietary Olive and Fish Oil*

Clinical Variable	Olive Oil	Fish Oil	
		Low Dose	High Dose
Number of tender joints	No	Yes	Yes
Number of swollen joints	No	Yes	Yes
Grip strength	No	Yes	Yes
Morning stiffness	No	No	Yes
Global disease activity			
Physician evaluation	Yes	Yes	Yes
Patient evaluation	Yes	No	No
Pain			
Physician evaluation	No	No	Yes
Patient evaluation	No	No	Yes

*Kremer J, Lawrence D, Jubiz W.
Reproduced with permission from *The Journal of Musculoskeletal Medicine*, May, 1989.

ulation also increased significantly in all 3 groups. Production of IGA *in vitro* in the absence of mitogen stimulation decreased significantly in both fish-oil groups from baseline, but IgG production was not affected after mitogen stimulation.

This investigation established that salutary clinical benefits after fish oil ingestion in patients with rheumatoid arthritis are more commonly observed after treatment periods of at least 18 weeks. This observation was of significance in that the previous studies had only examined potential clinical benefits over periods of 6-14 weeks. In addition, it appears that higher doses of fish oil are associated with an increased frequency of significant clinical improvements after fish-oil ingestion (Table 20-4). Moreover, fish-oil ingestion is associated with significant decreases in ionophore-stimulated neutrophil leukotriene B_4 and macrophage production of IL-1. Both of these effects could contribute to the amelioration of disease activity through a variety of mechanisms involving the inflammatory reaction [13] and the immune system [7].

Fish Oil in Rheumatoid Arthritis: The Next Step
Most clinicians are loathe to recommend fish oil supplements to their patients with rheumatoid arthritis because of understandable confu-

sion about a) the amount to prescribe; b) the overall effectiveness; and c) the additional expense of an 'unproven' remedy. There is therefore a need to better define the overall therapeutic value of fish oil and place these dietary supplements in their appropriate niche in relation to non-steroidal and anti-inflammatory drugs (NSAIDs) and slow acting antirheumatic drugs (SAARDs). Studies are therefore required to determine whether patients consuming fish oil for a long enough period of time to establish their clinical benefits ($\geq$ 18 weeks) could discontinue NSAIDs without a deterioration in their clinical status. The investigation should monitor inflammatory and immune parameters of disease and correlate these measures with clinical outcome. This type of study would allow investigators to determine whether NSAIDs enhance or inhibit the inflammatory and immune changes induced by fish oil. The proposed hypothetical investigation will allow investigators to determine whether higher dose fish oil supplementation for periods of at least 18 weeks could provide equivalent clinical benefits to NSAIDs and thus allow patients to discontinue these potentially dangerous medications without clinical deterioration. It is likely that fish oil will not be widely employed by physicians treating patients with rheumatoid arthritis until its role in the therapeutic hierarchy can be established as in the hypothetical investigation described.

References

1. Panush, R.S., Carter, R.L., Katz, P., Lowsari, S., and Finnie, S., (1983) Arthritis Rheum. 26, 462-469.
2. Kremer, J.M., Bigauoette, J., Michalek, A.U., et al., (1985) Lancet 1, 184-187.
3. Kremer, J.M., Jubizm, W., Michalekm, A., et al., (1987) Ann. Intern. Med. 106, 497-503.
4. Sperling, R.I., Weinblatt, M., Robin, J.L., et al., (1987) Arthritis Rheum. 30, 988-997.
5. Cleland, L.G., French, J.K., Betts, W.H., et al., (1988) J. Rheumatol. 15, 1471-1475.
6. Endres, S., Ghorbani, R., Kelley, V., (1989) N. Engl. J. Med. 302. 265-271.
7. Areand, W.P., and Dayer, J.M., (1990) Arthritis Rheum. 33, 305-315.
8. Kremer, J., Lawrence, D.L., Jubiz, W., et al., (1990) Arthritis Rheum. 33, 810-820.
9. Traill, K.N., and Wick, G., (1984) Immunol. Today 5, 70-75.
10. Johnston, P.V. (1985) Adv. Lipid Research 21, 103-141.
11. Del Buono, B.J., Williamson, P.L., and Schlegel, R.A., (1986) J. of Cell. Physiology 126, 379-388.

12. Erickson, K.L., (1986) Int. J. Immunopharmac. 8, 529-543.
13. Lee, T.H., Hoover, R.L., Williams, J.D., et al., (1985) N. Engl. Med. 312, 1217-1224.

Chapter Twenty-one

Therapeutic Effects of Gamma-linolenic Acid (GLA) as Evening Primrose Oil in Atopic Eczema and Diabetic Neuropathy

David F. Horrobin

Efamol Research Institute
P.O. Box 818
Kentville, Nova Scotia, Canada, B4N 4H8

Linoleic acid and alpha-linolenic acid are the main dietary essential fatty acids. But in order to exert most of their biological effects they must be converted to other fatty acids and their oxygenated derivatives, by a series of reactions which begins with 6-desaturation. Brenner's group, whose findings have been confirmed by many others, has demonstrated that the first 6-desaturation step is severely rate-limiting (1-4). Moreover, this slow step can be further impaired by a range of other factors, among which is diabetes mellitus (5,6).

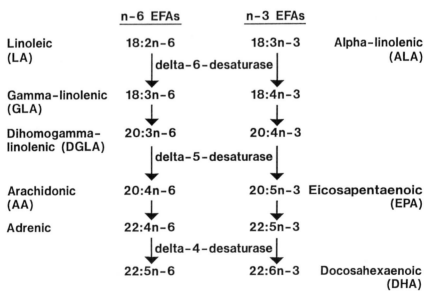

It is not always appreciated that it is the rate-limiting nature of the 6-desaturation step which provides the main rationale for the therapeutic and nutritional uses of eicosapentaenoic acid (EPA) a derivative of alpha-linolenic acid (Fig. 21-1). Without this limitation, many if not most could obtain all the EPA they need by conversion within the body of dietary alpha-linolenic acid. Everyone who advocates the possible use of EPA is by implication admitting the rate-limiting nature of the steps by which it is normally derived from alpha-linolenic acid.

It is therefore surprising that there is not a similar widespread recognition of the possible value of direct administration of a 6-desaturated derivative of linoleic acid, such as gamma-linolenic acid (GLA). If the rate of conversion of alpha-linolenic acid to its derivatives such as EPA may be inadequate for normal health, then equally the rate of conversion of linoleic acid must also be potentially inadequate. The rationale for the use of GLA is identical to the rationale for the use of EPA.

In 1956, Sinclair proposed that many diseases, particularly those associated with a "Western" lifestyle, might result from inadequate intake of EFAs (7,8). This concept was almost entirely ignored because it seemed to most people that intakes of linoleic acid and alpha-linolenic acid were for the most part more than adequate. It was not then appreciated that even in the presence of an adequate intake of the main dietary EFAs, an internal deficit might develop as the result of inadequate metabolism.

Building upon work by Brenner's group and others, in recent years it has been suggested that Sinclair may well have been right in principle. However, the EFA deficiency may not be of inadequate intake but of inadequate metabolism (4,9,10). Like Sinclair's earlier proposal, the idea that some diseases might be caused by inadequate 6-desaturation of linoleic acid has met with rather less than universal approval! However, there is now substantial evidence that at least two conditions, atopic eczema and diabetic neuropathy are associated with reduced GLA formation and can be treated by administering GLA in an appropriate form.

Gamma-Linolenic Acid (GLA)

GLA is derived from linoleic acid by 6-desaturation. It is present in most human and animal tissues in only trace amounts because, having been formed slowly by a rate-limiting step, it is very rapidly elongated to dihomogammalinolenic acid (DGLA) which is in turn converted to further metabolites.

GLA and DGLA are present in trace amounts in many foods, in slightly larger amounts in organ meats such as liver, kidneys and adrenals, and in substantial quantities in human milk (9,11,12,13). GLA is present in quite large amounts in various oils notable those derived from certain fungi, and from the seeds of the evening primrose, blackcurrant and borage plants (9). The fatty acid compositions of the oils derived from the wild plants vary widely presenting great difficulties for those interested in evaluating their nutritional or therapeutic properties (14). Just as research on fish oil was advanced greatly when the standardized oil "Maxepa" became available, so therapeutic research on GLA has depended on the provision of a standardized evening primrose oil of constant composition, "Efamol". Efamol is derived from strains of Oenothera spp selected to yield oil of constant and reliable composition. This oil has been subjected to full toxicity testing as would be required for any drug (15,16). It has been approved for the addition to infant milks in Japan and, under the trade name "Epogam" as a drug in the UK, available for the treatment of atopic eczema in adults and children. The clinical work on atopic eczema and diabetic neuropathy described in this paper has all been conducted on Efamol.

Atopic Eczema

Atopic eczema is a characteristic form of dermatitis which has a strong hereditary component. The skin is healthy at birth but the typical skin rash develops usually within 2-6 months. The dermatitis can be very severe with itch as the outstanding sympton. The illness fluctuates in intensity, often becoming less evident as a child grows older and disappearing around puberty, only to return at times of stress. Genetically the disease is associated with a family history of both eczema and other atopic disorders such as asthma and allergies and a variety of other conditions such as Crohn's disease and premenstrual syndrome. A high risk of developing atopic eczema can be predicted by elevated levels of immunoglobulin IgE in umbilical cord blood.

Biochemistry

Hansen in the 1930s was the first to suggest that atopic eczema might be related to an EFA abnormality. He reported that iodine values in blood from patients were low and also that in those fed linoleic acid, linoleic acid concentration was normal but arachidonic acid concentration was far below normal (17,18). At that time the pathway from linoleic acid to arachidonic acid was unknown but with hindsight it can be seen that this observation indicated a possible block in conversion of linoleic acid to arachidonic.

Over forty years elapsed before this question was re-evaluated by modern gas chromatographic techniques. It was then shown in adults with atopic eczema that Hansen was right. Patients had normal or slightly elevated levels of linoleic acid in plasma phospholipids with reduced levels not only of arachidonic acid but also of gamma-linolenic acid (GLA) and DGLA (19,20). This implied a reduced rate of conversion from linoleic acid to GLA, possibly suggesting a variant 6-desaturase with somewhat reduced activity.

This observation has now been confirmed several times. In children with atopic eczema the abnormal pattern is more marked than in adults, with clearly elevated levels of linoleic acid and reduced concentrations of metabolites (21). In umbilical cord blood, infants with high IgE levels but no atopic eczema as yet, have a similar EFA abnormality with the elevation of linoleic acid being directly proportional to the elevation of IgE (21). The white cells of cord blood from infants with high IgE concentrations also contain low amounts of linoleic acid metabolites (22). Milk from Zimbabwean women with atopic eczema contains elevated linoleic and reduced GLA, DGLA and arachidonic acid as compared with milk from normal Zimbabweans (23). Adipose tissue from people with atopic eczema shows a similar abnormality as compared to normal adipose tissue (24).

Thus it now seems probable that atopic dermatitis is associated with an abnormal EFA profile indicating a possible reduced conversion of linoleic acid to its metabolites (19-26). There is a similar abnormality in the n-3 pathway (20,21) indicating reduced 6-desaturase activity for both linoleic and alpha-linolenic acids. The abnormality is present at birth in infants with high IgE levels, even prior to the emergence of any skin disease.

Clinical trials

If the rate of GLA formation is reduced, and if that reduced rate is important in contributing to the skin problems, then providing GLA should produce some improvement in the skin condition.

This hypothesis has now been tested extensively in placebo-controlled trials of Efamol involving over 300 patients with atopic eczema (27-33). There is a consistent improvement in the skin condition which is over and above the best that can be achieved by conventional therapy (32).

Two features of the response are of particular importance. First many patients find that they can reduce substantially their usage of steroids, drugs which are widely used for atopic eczema but which have important side effects, notably skin atrophy, when used for long periods and/or in high dosage (28). Second, the itch of atopic eczema, which is the symptom of most concern to patients, can be relieved without causing drowsiness (32). Hitherto only the sedating antihistamines have been reported to relieve the itch of eczema. One trial has reported no effect (34) but there is strong evidence that in this trial active and placebo capsules were mixed with some patients in both groups receiving both active and placebo. This was indicated by the fact that plasma DGLA rose both in those assigned to receive EPO and those assigned to receive placebo (32).

Even the apparently normal areas of skin in patients with atopic eczema are considerable rougher than normal. This can easily be felt by hand and quantified by objective profilometric techniques. Two groups of investigators have now been able to show by such objective methods that administration of Efamol makes the "normal" skin areas in atopic eczema patients smoother (35,36).

Thus the abnormal skin in atopic eczema can be at least partially normalised by the administration of GLA, suggesting that the EFA abnormality contributes to the cause of the disease. Since patients exhibit low levels of both n-3 and n-6 6-desaturated EFAs, it is possible that combined treatment with GLA + EPA will be more benefical than treatment with GLA alone. Such trials are under way.

Diabetic Neuropathy

There are two types of diabetes mellitus, insulin-dependent or type I, and non-insulin dependent, or maturity-onset or type II. In both types major problems result from the development of damage to the eyes, kidneys, cardiovascular system and peripheral nerves. The reasons for these problems are as yet unknown.

Nerve damage (neuropathy) produces clinical symptoms in about half of all patients with both types of diabetes (37). If nerve function is assessed neurophysiologically, almost all patients who have been diabetic for more than five years can be shown to have nerve damage. This produces a variety of symptoms including loss of sensation, weakness, abnormal control of cardiovascular and gastrointestinal systems, and loss of bladder and reproductive function. At present there is no treatment.

The cause of the nerve damage is unknown but could be related to inadequate microcirculation and oxygen supply, to abnormal glycosylation of proteins, to loss of normal inositol metabolism, to accumulation of glucose, fructose and sorbitol or to other factors (37,38). It has recently been proposed that inadequate conversion of linoleic acid to GLA and futher metabolites are required for the normal structure of nerve membranes, for the normal control of the microcirculation and for the normal fluidity of red cell membranes (38). All three factors could be important in neuropathy.

Biochemistry

Diabetes mellitus is one of the best documented causes of reduced 6-desaturation. The abnormality was first reported by Brenner's group (5,6,39,40) by whom it was also found that administration of arachidonic acid could reverse the testicular atrophy in diabetic animals. Since then, many others have shown that both 6- and 5-desaturation are impaired in diabetic animals, that this is relected in the fatty acid pattern in blood and other tissues and that it can be normalized by insulin (41-52). In humans, diabetics have been found to exhibit impaired 6- and 5- desaturation and below normal concentrations of linoleic acid metabolites (53-59). On treatment with insulin, the concentrations of linoleic acid metabolites in humans increase, indicating improved 6-desaturation (59).

Patients with diabetes have dry, rough skin similar to that found in patients with eczema and, especially in older individuals, the skin may break out into an eczema-like rash. Patients with atopic eczema do not, as far as is known, develop neuropathy. However, it is possible that the neuropathy develops as a result of the simultaneous presence of both abnormalities of glucose, polyol and EFA metabolism. The possible importance of a deficit of GLA can only be tested by controlled trials.

Therapeutic effects of GLA

GLA as Efamol has now been extensively studied in both animal and human diabetic neuropathy. The results are remarkable consistent with no dissenting observations. In every situation in which it has been tested (and over ten medical schools have now been involved in the investigations) administration of GLA has been found to prevent or improve diabetic neuropathy whereas linoleic acid has not.

I suggested to Julu, an expert in animal diabetic neuropathy, that he should look at the effects of feeding Efamol on the condition. He was able to show that Efamol but not coconut oil could prevent the development of neuropathy in motor and sensory nerves and in both large and small myelinated and unmyelinated fibres (38,60,61). Julu has gone on to show that Efamol could reverse already established neuropathy (62) and could also do so faster than insulin (63).

These observations have been repeatedly confirmed. Tomlinson et al. have found that Efamol prevents the development of diabetic neuropathy in animals without interfering with glucose, sorbitol or inositol metabolism (64,65). The effect of GLA is therefore not produced as a consequence of improvement in other aspects of diabetes. However, GLA does improve nerve Na/K ATPase activity, an abnormality which had hitherto been thought to be secondary to disturbed polyol metabolism (66). In another animal model, GLA was found to reduce the insensitivity to painful stimuli usually found in diabetic animals (67).

Cameron, Cotter et al. like the other investigators have found that GLA could prevent the development of diabetic neuropathy whereas linoleic acid had no effect (68,69). One curiosity of diabetic nerves is that they are resistant to the conduction block produced in normal nerves by restriction of oxygen supply and/or blood flow. In crude terms this is believed to be because the impaired microcirculation makes the nerve accustomed to operating under conditions of reduced oxygen tension. Cameron et al. have found that in diabetic animals GLA makes the nerve normally susceptible to the adverse effects of reduced oxygen supply. Moreover, the capillary density in the sciatic nerves of diabetic animals treated with Efamol was significantly greater than that in those treated with linoleic acid.

These observations have been extended to humans. In a pilot study, 22 patients with established diabetic neuropathy were entered into a double-blind, placebo-controlled trial of Efamol (70,71). Motor nerve conduction velocity (MNCV), sensory nerve action potential (SNAP), and thresholds to heat and cold stimuli were measured in upper and lower limbs. All eight parameters improved during treatment with Efamol while all eight either deteriorated or remained unchanged during treatment with placebo. In six of the eight cases the effect of Efamol was significantly better than the effect of placebo.

These results have now been confirmed in a much larger 12 month multi-centre study involving around 90 patients in seven hospitals in the UK and Finland. The results are almost identical to those observed in the earlier pilot study.

The results of both the animal and the human studies are so consistent that there is now little doubt that a defective flow of linoleic acid through to GLA and beyond is a fundamental factor in diabetic neuropathy. The preventive and therapeutic effects are achieved in the absence of any change in diabetic control. The GLA must therefore be counteracting the neurological consequences of diabetes without any effects on the diabetes itself.

Conclusion

In atopic eczema and in diabetic neuropathy there is good evidence both for deficits of GLA and its metabolites and for the therapeutic effects of administering GLA. Matters of great interest are whether the anti-inflammatory effects in eczema can be extended to other inflammatory conditions such as rheumatoid arthritis, and whether those in diabetic neuropathy can be extended to other diabetic complications and to cardiovascular and other diseases. There is an increasingly substantial body of information which suggests that GLA may turn out to have a number of important uses both as a nutritional product and as a therapy (72).

References

1. Brenner, R.R., (1982) Progr. Lipid Res. 20:41-48.
2. Sprecher, H., (1982) Progr. Lipid Res. 20:13-22.
3. Garcia, P.T., Holman, R.T., (1965) J. Am. Oil Chem. Soc. 42:1137-1141.
4. Horrobin, D.F., (1983) Rev. Pure Appl. Pharmacol Sci. 4:339-342.
5. Mercuri, O., Peluffo, R.O., and Brenner, R.R., (1966) Biochim. Biophys. Acta. 116:407-411.
6. Brenner, R.R., Peluffo, R.O., Mercuri, O., Restelli, M.A., (1968) Am. J. Physiol. 215:63-69.
7. Sinclair, H.M., (1956) Lancet i:381-383.
8. Sinclair, H.M., In: Omega-6 Essential Fatty Acids: Pathophysiology and Roles in Clinical Medicine, edited by D.F. Horrobin, New York, Alan R. Liss, 1990 pp1-20.
9. Horrobin, D.F., and Manku, M.S., Clinical biochemistry of essential fatty acids. In: Omega-6 Essential Fatty Acids: Pathophysiology and Roles in Clinical Medicine, edited by D.F. Horrobin, New York, Alan R. Liss, 1990 pp21-43.
10. Horrobin, D.F., Polyunsaturated oils of marine and plant origin and their uses in clinical medicine. In: Dietary n-3 and n-6 Fatty Acids: Biological Effects and Nutritional Essentiality, edited by C. Galli, New York, Plenum Press, 1988.

11. Carter, J.P., (1988) Food Technology, June:72-82.
12. Gibson, R.A., and Kneebone, G.M., (1981) Am. J. Clin. Nutr. 34:252-260.
13. Harzer, G., Haug, M., Dieterich, I., Gentner, P.R., (1983) Am. J. Clin. Nutr. 37:612-622.
14. Hudson, B.J.F., (1984) J. Am. Oil Chem. Soc. 61:540-543.
15. Everett, D.J., Perry, C.F., and Bayliss, P., (1988) Med. Sci. Res. 16:865-866.
16. Everett, D.J., Greenough, R.J., Perry, C.J., McDonald, P., and Bayliss, P., (1988) Med. Sci. Res. 16:863-864.
17. Hansen, A.E., (1937) Am. J. Dis. Child 53:933-946.
18. Brown, W.R., and Hansen, A.E., (1937) Proc. Soc. Exp. Biol. Med. 30:113-116.
19. Manku, M.S., Horrobin, D.F., and Morse, N. et al., (1982) Prostaglandins Leukotrienes Med. 9:615-628.
20. Manku, M.S., Horrobin, D.F., and Morse, N.L., et al., (1984) Br. J. Dermatol. 110:643-648.
21. Strannegard, I.-L., Svennerholm, L., and Strannegard, O., (1987) Int. Arch. Allergy Appl. Immunol. 82:422-423.
22. Galli, E., Picardo, M., and DeLuca, C. et al., (1989) Pediatric Res. 26:519.
23. Wright, S., and Bolton, C., (1989) Br. J. Nutr. 62:693-697.
24. Wright, S., Sanders, T.A.B., Submitted for publication.
25. Wright, S., (1985) Acta. Derm. Venereol (Stockh) Suppl 114:143-145.
26. Melnik, B.C., and Plewig, G., (1989) J. Am. Acad. Dermatol. 21:557-563.
27. Wright, S., and Burton, J.L., (1982) Lancet 2:1120-1122.
28. Schalin-Karrila, M., Mattila, L., Jansen, C.T., and Uotila, P., (1987) Br. J. Dermatol. 117:11-19.
29. Bordoni, A., Biagi, P., Masi, M. et al., (1987) Drugs Exptl. Clin. Res. XIV:291-297.
30. Biagi, P.L., Bordoni, A., and Masi, M., et al., (1988) Drugs Exptl. Clin. Res. XV:285-290.
31. Meigel, W., (1986) Z. Hauktr 61:473-478.
32. Morse, P.F., Horrobin, D.F., Manku, M.S., and Stewart, J.C.M., (1989) Br. J. Dermatol. 121:75-90.
33. Guenther, L., and Wexler, D., (1987) J. Am. Acad. Derm. 17:860.
34. Bamford, J.T.M., Gibson, R.W., Renier, C.M., (1985) J. Am. Acad. Dermatol. 13:956-959.
35. Nissen, H.P., Wehrmann, W., Kroll, U., and Kreyser, H.W., (1988) Fat. Sci. Tech. 7:247-288.
36. Marshall, R.J., and Evans, R.W., In: Omega-6 Essential Fatty Acids: Pathophysiology and roles in clinical medicine, edited by D.F. Horrobin, New York, Alan Liss, 1990 pp 81-98.
37. Dyck, P.J., Thomas, P.K., Asbury, A.K., et al. Diabetic Neuropathy. Philadelphia, WB Saunders, 1987.
38. Horrobin, D.F., (1988) Prostagl. Leukotr. EFAs 31:181-197.
39. De Alaniz, M.J.T., De Gomez Dumm, I.N.T., and Brenner, R.R., (1976) Mol.

Cell Biochem. 12:3-8.
40. De Alaniz, M.J.T., and Brenner, R.R., (1969) Acta. Physiol. Latinoam 19:1-15.
41. Friedman, N., Gellhorn, A., and Benjamin, W., (1966) Israel J. Med. Sci. 2:677-682.
42. Faas, F.H., and Carter, W.J., (1980) Lipids 15:953-961.
43. Faas, F.H., and Carter, W.J., (1983) Lipids 18:339-342.
44. Holman, R.T., Johnson, S.B., and Gerrard, J.M., et al. (1983) Proc. Nat. Acad. Sci. USA 80:2375-2379.
45. Huang, Y.-S., Fujii, K., and Takahashi, R., et al., (1985) IRCS. J. Med. Sci. 13:1145-1146.
46. Peluffo, R.O., Ayala, S., and Brenner, R.R., (1970) Am. J. Physiol. 218:669-673.
47. Poisson, J.-P., (1985) Enzyme 34:1-14.
48. Poisson, J.-P., Blond, J.-P., (1985) Diabete Metab. 11:289-294.
49. Poisson, J.-P., Blond, J.-P., and Lemarchal, P., (1979) Diabete Metab. 5:43-46.
50. Poisson, J.-P., Lemarchal, P., and Blond, J.-P., et al., (1978) Diabete. Metab. 4:39-45.
51. Wilder, P.J., and Coniglio, J.G., (1984) Proc. Soc. Exp. Biol. Med. 177:399-405.
52. Huang, Y.-S., Horrobin, D.F., Manku, M.S., Mitchell, J., and Ryan, M.A., (1984) Lipids 19:367-370.
53. Mikhailidis, D.P., Kirtland, S., Barradas, M.A., and Dandona, P., (1986) Progr. Lipd Res. 25:303-304.
54. Mikhailidis, D.P., Kirtland, S.J., and Barradas, M.A., et al., (1986) Diabetes. Res. 3:7-12.
55. El Boustani, S., Descomps, B., and Monnier, L., et al., (1986) Progr. Lipid Res. 25:67-71.
56. Jones, D.B., Carter, R.D., Haitas, B., and Mann, J.I., (1983) Br. Med. J. 286:173-175.
57. Tilvis, R.S., and Miettinen, T.A., (1985) J. Clin. Endocr. Metab. 61:741-745.
58. Tuna, N., Frankhausen, S., and Goetz, F.C., (1968) Am. J. Med. Sci. 255:120-130.
59. Tilvis, R.S., and Helve, E., Miettinen, T.A., (1986) Diabetologia 29:690-694.
60. Julu, P.O.O., (1988) Diabetic Complications 2:185-188.
61. Julu, P.O.O., Gamma-linolenic acid: a novel remedy for diabetic neuropathy in experimental animals. In: Omega-6 Essential Fatty Acids: Pathophysiology and Roles in Clinical Medicine, edited by D.F. Horrobin, Alan Liss, 1990 pp 465-476.
62. Hono, R.G., Julu, P.O.O., and Kunzekweguta, W.S., J. Physiol., in press.
63. Julu, P.O.O., and Mutumba, A., J. Physiol., in press.
64. Tomlinson, D.R., Robinson, J.P., Compton, A.M., and Keen, P., (1989) Diabetologia 32:655-659.

65. Tomlinson, D.R., Robinson, J.P., and Compton, A.M. The effects of gamma-linolenic acid treatment on motor nerve conduction velocity and axonal transport of substance P in diabetic rats. In: Omega-6 Essential Fatty Acids: Pathophysiology and Roles in Clinical Medicine, edited by D.F. Horrobin, New York, Alan Liss, 1990 pp 457-463.
66. Calcutt, N.A., Fernandes, K.L.J., and Tomlinson, D.R., Dietary supplementation with essential fatty acids attenuates deficient Na+/K+ - ATPase activity in sciatic nerve homogenates from streptozotocin-diabetic rats. Submitted for publication.
67. Wiesenfeld-Hallin, Z., and Eneroth, P., The effects of evening primrose oil on streptozotocin diabetic rats. In: Omega-6 Essential Fatty Acids: Pathophysiology and roles in clinical medicine, edited by D.F. Horrobin, New York, Alan Liss, 1990 pp 477-486.
68. Cotter, M.A., Robertson, S., Cameron, N.E., Essential fatty acid dietary supplementation prevents the development of resistance to ischaemic conduction block and conduction velocity deficits in streptozotocin-diabetic rats. British Diabetic Association, Annual Meeting, 22nd-24th March 1990.
69. Cameron, N.E., Cotter, M.A., and Robertson, S., Essential fatty acid supplementation can improve nerve function and vascular supply in diabetic rats. European Association for the study of diabetes, Summer 1990.
70. Jamal, G.A., Carmichael, H.A., and Weir, A.I., (1986) Lancet i:1098.
71. Jamal, G.A., Prevention and treatment of diabetic distal polyneuropathy by the supplementation of gamma-linolenic acid. In: Omega-6 Essential Fatty Acids: Pathophysiology and roles in clinical medicine., edited by D.F. Horrobin, New York, Alan Liss, 1990 pp 487-504.
72. Horrobin, D.F., (ed). Omega-6 Essential Fatty Acids: Pathophysiology and Roles in Clinical Medicine. New York, Alan Liss, 1990.

Chapter Twenty-two

Do *Trans* Acids Have Adverse Health Consequences?

E.A. Emken

Northern Regional Research Center
Peoria, IL 61604

The term *"trans* acids" is an all-encompassing term that is used to refer to the large number of isomeric fatty acid structures formed by catalytic hydrogenation of vegetable oils. The gas chromatogram (GC) of a margarine base stock (Figure 22-1) shows the complexity of the fatty acid composition and illustrates the best separation that can be

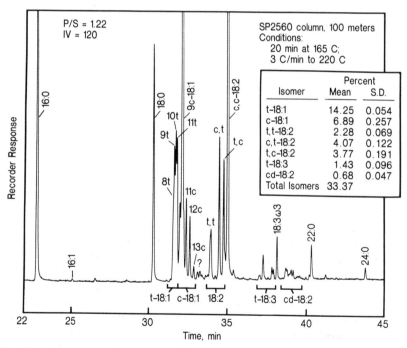

Fig. 22-1. Partial gas chromatogram of a partially hydrogenated soybean oil (margarine base stock).

achieved by normal GC analysis. GC analysis alone cannot separate all of the over 25 *trans* and *cis* isomers that have been identified in partially hydrogenated vegetable oils (PHVO) (1-4). Many of the individual isomers are present at only 0.1-0.5% of the total sample and need to be partially separated and concentrated by other methods before they can be separated by fused silica capillary columns.

The total *trans* isomer content of PHVO varies between 5% and 45%. The actual percent *trans* is dependent on the properties of the nickel catalyst, hydrogenation conditions and the iodine value of the hydrogenated oil. Food company specifications require PHVO feed stocks that have a wide variation in physical properties. As a result the total isomer content and overall fatty acid composition of PHVO is highly variable. One major reason for some of the inconsistency between results from early biological studies is that the PHVO used contained different isomer and fatty acid compositions or the PHVO used was essential fatty acid deficient (EFAD).

When an EFAD-PHVO is the only dietary fat source, the biological effects are much different than when a non-EFAD PHVO is fed. This problem is now recognized and most recent studies use non-EFAD PHVO or only specific fatty acid isomers are added to diets that are not EFAD.

This review covers studies pertinent to the metabolic fate and biochemistry of fatty acid isomers present in PHVO and reports related to coronary heart disease and cancer. These metabolic and health-related studies reflect those areas where much of the concern about *trans* acids has centered. References 5-10 represent other reviews on this topic and contain additional references not cited in this review.

Metabolism and biochemistry

A major reason for the concern about *trans* fatty acid structures was the realization that a *trans* double-bond alters the conformation of the fatty acid structure. This structural change is responsible for the higher melting point of *trans* fatty acids compared to *cis* fatty acids. The effect of a *trans* bond on fatty acid conformation is illustrated by the comparison in Figure 22-2 of minimum energy conformations for stearic, elaidic, oleic, linoleic and linolenic acid isomers. The *trans* fatty acid isomers tend to have a "straighter" structure than *cis* fatty acids. These computer-generated structures, which represent the lowest energy conformation state calculated by the program Alchemy II (Tripos Associates, Inc., St. Louis, MO), suggest that the *trans* isomers are less like saturated

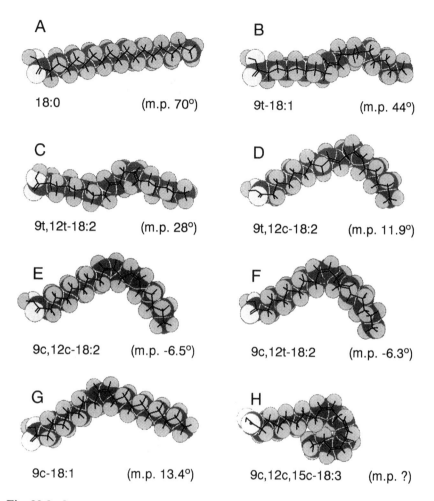

Fig. 22-2. Comparison of melting points and orthogonal projections for minimum energy conformations of isomeric and non-isomeric 18-carbon fatty acids.

fatty acids than predicted by simple ball and stick molecular models. Because these isomers have different configurations, biochemists correctly reasoned, and subsequently demonstrated, that the *trans* bond has a significant effect on the binding constants of many enzymes involved in the metabolism of fatty acid isomers. Experimental data suggest that the biological properties of the *trans* isomers are somewhere

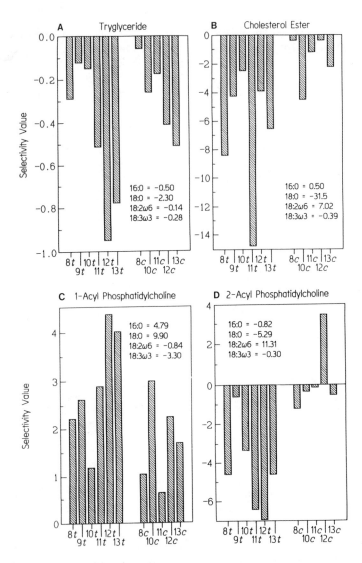

Fig. 22-3. Comparison of human plasma (A) triglyceride, (B) cholesterol ester, (C) 1-acylphosphatidylcholine, (D) 2-acylphosphatidylcholine selectivity values for incorporation of deuterium-labeled *trans* and *cis* positional isomers relative to oleic acid. Values for palmitic (16:0), stearic (18:0), linoleic (18:2), and linolenic (18:3) acid are included for comparison.

between those of saturated fatty acids and their *cis* fatty acid counterparts and are associated with the computer-calculated structures and melting point data. Since the *trans* isomers are not biologically similar to stearic or oleic acid, how should they be classified?

The plots in Figure 22-3 for human plasma lipid data illustrate the relative *in vivo* selectivity of triacylglycerol acyltransferase, phosphatidylcholine acyltransferase and lecithin:cholesterol acyltransferase for most of the *cis* and *trans* 18:1 positional isomers in PHVO (11-17). Relative selectivity values for palmitic, stearic, oleic, linoleic and linolenic acid are also included for comparison. These data were obtained by feeding mixtures of triglycerides containing approximately equal amounts of deuterium-labeled 9c-18:1 and two or more other deuterated fatty acids to normal young adult male subjects. The deuterated oleic acid served as a common internal standard to which data from different studies can be compared.

The triglyceride data shows lower selectivity values for the 18:1 isomers relative to 9c-18:1, which suggest lower incorporation and/or more rapid removal. The cholesterol ester data show that there is a strong discrimination against incorporation of the *trans* 18:1 isomers. The phosphatidylcholine data for the 1- and 2-acyl position show that the *trans* isomers are preferentially incorporated at the 1-acyl position and partially exluded from the 2-acyl position. These data agree well with both *in vivo* and *in vitro* data from animal studies. The distribution pattern for the 18:1 isomers and saturated fatty acids have some similarities, but there are considerable differences depending on which specific 18:1 isomers are compared. Data of this type are often cited as evidence that *trans* isomers are equivalent to saturated fatty acids. This generalization is an over-simplification. The plasma selectivity values (Figure 22-3) suggest that both double-bond position and geometric configuration influence fatty acid metabolism and that the metabolism of the 18:1 isomers is intermediate between saturated fatty acids and 9c-18:1.

Small amounts of *trans* 18:2 and 18:3 are present in partially hydrogenated soybean and canola oil. Earlier studies with c,t- and t,c-18:2 indicated that only c,t-18:2 was converted to a "c,t" 20:4 isomer in rat liver (18-19). However, the rate of conversion was not determined nor compared to the conversion of linoleic acid. Recently reported *in vivo* conversion rates for mice fed t,c- , c,t- and c,c-18:2 to 20:4 are included in Figure 22-4 (20). The overall conversion rate for c,t-18:2 is nearly identical to the conversion rate for c,c-18:2. However, the individual relative

c,c-18:2 Diet $K_{20:4}$ = 0.47 mg/g/day

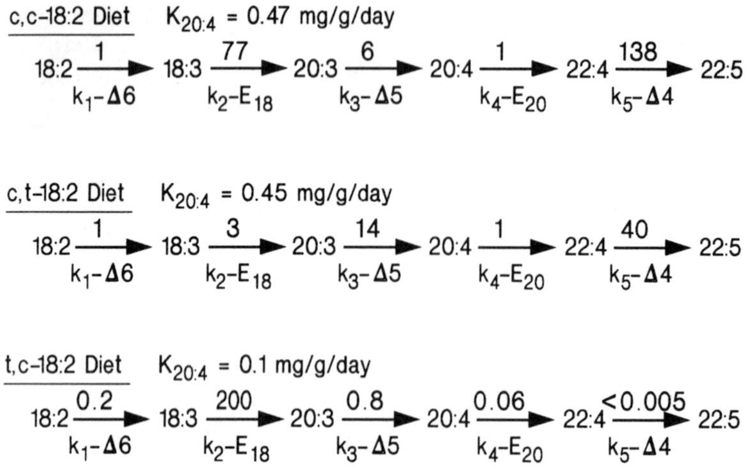

$$18:2 \xrightarrow[k_1-\Delta 6]{1} 18:3 \xrightarrow[k_2-E_{18}]{77} 20:3 \xrightarrow[k_3-\Delta 5]{6} 20:4 \xrightarrow[k_4-E_{20}]{1} 22:4 \xrightarrow[k_5-\Delta 4]{138} 22:5$$

c,t-18:2 Diet $K_{20:4}$ = 0.45 mg/g/day

$$18:2 \xrightarrow[k_1-\Delta 6]{1} 18:3 \xrightarrow[k_2-E_{18}]{3} 20:3 \xrightarrow[k_3-\Delta 5]{14} 20:4 \xrightarrow[k_4-E_{20}]{1} 22:4 \xrightarrow[k_5-\Delta 4]{40} 22:5$$

t,c-18:2 Diet $K_{20:4}$ = 0.1 mg/g/day

$$18:2 \xrightarrow[k_1-\Delta 6]{0.2} 18:3 \xrightarrow[k_2-E_{18}]{200} 20:3 \xrightarrow[k_3-\Delta 5]{0.8} 20:4 \xrightarrow[k_4-E_{20}]{0.06} 22:4 \xrightarrow[k_5-\Delta 4]{<0.005} 22:5$$

Fig. 22-4. Overall conversion rates and relative rate constants for liver metabolites from mice fed c,c-, c,t-c, and t,c-18:2 for 4 days. Calculations assume delta-6 desaturase was the rate-limiting step for both 18:2 isomers. E18 or E20 refer to elongation steps and delta 4, 5, and 6 refer to desaturation steps.

rate constants for elongation and desaturation suggests that the position of the *trans* bonds influence the binding constants of the enzymes responsible for these metabolic conversions. The relative rate constants were calculated by assuming that delta-6 desaturase is the rate limiting step in the conversions of both 18:2 isomers. These data suggest that c,t-18:2 may be a stronger competitive inhibitor than t,c-18:2 for the conversion of c,c-18:2 to 20:4. The data are consistent with reports that *trans* monoene and diene isomers in PHVO inhibit desaturase activity and reduce 20:4 levels in tissue lipids (21-25). Recent radioisotope studies in rats have confirmed that *trans* acids inhibit conversion of 9c,12c-18:2 to 20:4, but 20:4 percentages in liver phosphatidylcholine were only slightly reduced (26). This result suggests that acyltransferase specificity rather than desaturase activity controls the 20:4 level in tissue phospholipids.

The *in vivo* conversion in rats of 9c,12c,15t-18:3 to *trans* 20:5ω3 and *trans* 22:6ω3 has also been reported (27). It is not known if the conversion rate of this *than* 18:3 isomer is similar to linolenic acid. It is not known if the c,t- and t,c-18:2 isomers are a potential source of biologically active *trans* eicosanoids or if they have any influence on health. The health consequences of the metabolites of the mono-*trans* 18:2 and 18:3 isomers in humans are probably minimal, since they have not been detected in tissue lipids.

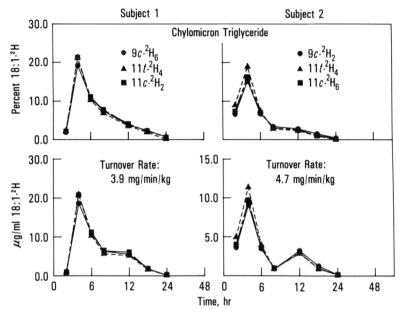

Fig. 22-5. Chylomicron triglyceride data from subjects fed deuterium-labeled 9c-18:1, 11t-18:1, and 11c-18:1. Data are plotted as percent isotopic enrichment and as ug/ml plasma.

Absorption

Deuterated *trans* and *cis* 18:1 isomers are well absorbed (90-100%) in man (11-17). These data were calculated from chylomicron triglyceride data by assuming 98% absorption for the deuterium-labeled oleic acid that was fed at the same time. Figure 22-5 illustrates a set of typical chylomicron triglyceride data used for these calculations. Absorption of the even-numbered *trans* positional isomers was good despite their melting points of about 50 C, which is well above body temperature. These results are consistent with data that has shown pancreatic lipase activity is not sensitive to the *trans* fatty acid structure (28).

Oxidation

Four different sequence of steps are involved in beta-oxidation of *cis* and *trans* positional isomers. The pathway depends on whether the double-bond has a *trans* or *cis* configuration and whether it is located at an even or odd numbered carbon (9). The *in vitro* activity of the hy-

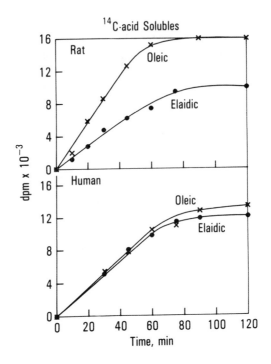

Fig. 22-6. Beta-oxidation rates for positional isomers of *cis* and *trans* octadecenoate CoA esters by rat liver mitochondria and melting points of octadecenoic fatty acid isomers.

dratase, isomerase, and epimerase enzymes involved in beta-oxidation have some sensitivity to double-bond position or geometrical structure (9,27) (Figure 22-6). In contrast to *in vitro* rat heart data homogenized human heart tissue oxidized 9t-18:1 at nearly the same rate as 9c-18:1 (Figure 22-7) (30). This difference suggests that human enzymes may have broader specificities than rat enzymes.

Fatty acid composition data for human tissues show that there is little difference between isomer distribution patterns in tissue lipids and PHVO (31-33). However, recent data for human heart lipids report that the 10t- and 10c-18:1 isomers are present at lower levels than in PHVO or adipose tissue (34). This result is consistent with tissue fatty acid data from rats fed 10c-18:1 (35). The *trans* content of human tissue lipids (liver, aorta, brain, heart, plasma and red cell) range from 0.1 to

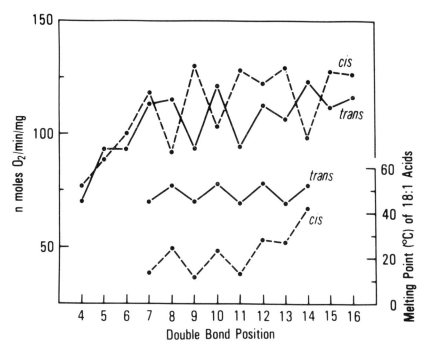

Fig. 22-7. Oxidation of uniformly carbon-14 labelled oleic and elaidic acids by rat and human heart homogenates.

3.9%. These human tissue data from numerous studies have been summarized previously (36). Since PHVO supplies approximately 6% of the total fat in the U.S. diet (7,37-38), the low *trans* content of human tissue lipids is indirect evidence for preferential oxidation. *In vivo* oxidation of *trans*- and *cis*-18:1 and 18:2 isomers by isolated rat liver supports this indirect evidence and the overall premise that isomers in PHVO are readily oxidized (39).

Human studies, which used 18:1 fatty acid isomers labeled with deuterium, show that *trans* fatty acids were removed more rapidly than oleic acid from human plasma triglycerides. In these studies, retroconversion of the 18:1 isomers to 16:1 isomers was higher than for 9c-18:1 (11-17). An example is illustrated in Figure 22-8 for the 10t- and 10c-18:1 isomers. These results are consistent with the evidence that the *trans* acids do not accumulate in tissue lipids and, therefore, they must be readily oxidized.

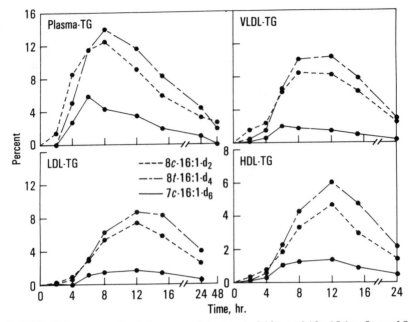

Fig. 22-8. Retroconversion in humans of deuterated 10t- and 10c-18:1 to 8t- and 8c-16:1 compared to retroconversion of 9c-18:1 to 7c-16:1. Data are plotted for total plasma and individual lipoprotein triglyceride fractions.

Long-term Animal Studies

Long-term studies have been reported for rats, mice, rabbits, and swine fed PHVO. Results from studies with rats fed 9-11 wt% PHVO (35%t) diets for about 45 generations detected no problems associated with growth, organ size or development, reproduction, tumors or longevity (40). Serum cholesterol levels were slightly lower for the PHVO fed rats compared to the cottonseed oil fed rats. Histological examination of organs from rats and mice fed 30 wt% PHVO diets (3 levels of trans) for 18 months and rabbits fed for 10 years found no abnormalities (41-43). Female swine fed diets containing PHVO (36%t) diets from 3 weeks to 2 years of age reported no effects on growth, organ weights, or reproduction (44-45). There was no overall effect on fatty acid composition of organ lipids of the sows or their piglets. Brain and nerve functions in the piglets were not altered compared to lard fed control groups.

Coronary Heart Disease and Risk Factors

The influence of PHVO and *trans* fatty acids on serum cholesterol has received much attention because serum cholesterol is considered an important risk factors associated with coronary heart disease (CHD). Results from three human studies are summarized in Table 22-1 (46-48). PHVO, containing three levels of total *trans*, were compared to unhydrogenated oil diets. No measurable effect on plasma cholesterol or triglyceride levels were observed. Other studies in humans, which compared diets containing *trans* acids to saturated fatty acids, found that *trans* acids in PHVO increase cholesterol less than saturated fatty acids (49-50).

The lack of a cholesterol increasing effect in humans is supported by the animal data (provided the diets contain about 4% linoleic acid) summarized in Table 22-2 (51-53). For example, Vervet monkeys fed 14% PHVO diets (23% and 43%t) had lower serum cholesterol levels than monkeys fed a mixture of olive and corn oil. In fact, diets containing only 2 en% linoleic acid prevented arteriosclerosis-related problems in rats (54). Importantly, the animal data provided no evidence that *trans* fatty acids enhance the development of arterial lesions or lipid infiltration into the endothelia cells (51-53). Also, the anti-thrombotic effect of *trans* acid fed rats was not different from *cis* acids (63).

TABLE 22-1

Influence of Hydrogenated Vegetable Oils (PHVO) on Serum Cholesterol and Triglyceride Levels in Humans[1]

Diets	Dietary Fat Composition						
	PHVO	SBO	PHVO	CNTRL	PHVO	SBO	PALM
% *trans*	7.7	0	44	0	16	0	0
% 18:2ω6	31	35	10	16	33	41	9.6
P/S Ratio	1.6	1.6	0.34	0.64	1.5	2.0	0.22
% (wt.) Fat	20	20	18	18	17	17	17
Wks Fed	5	5	3.5	3.5	3	3	3
Serum Lipids:							
Chol, mg/dL[2]	217	215	189	188	161	169	188
TG, mg/dL[2]	110	110	108	108	64	48	59
# Subjects	6	6	17	17	12	12	12

[1]Data adapted from references 46, 47, and 48.
[2]Chol = Cholesterol; TG = Triglyceride

TABLE 22-2
Influence of Partially Hydrogenated Vegetable Oils (PHVO) on Serum Lipids and Atherosclerosis in Animals[1]

Diets	Rabbit[1]		Monkey[2]		Swine[3]	
	PHVO	Control	PHVO	Control	PHVO	Control
% *trans*	23	0	43	0	39	0
% 18:2ω6	10	23	15	23	12	16
P/S Ratio	0.33	1.6	0.33	1.8	0.64	2.58
% (wt.) Fat	14	14	14	14	21	21
Wks Fed	20	20	48	48	24	24
Serum Lipids:						
Chol, mg/dL[2]	87	72	163	166	115	116
TG, mg/dL[2]	39	29	55	62	73	97
Difference in Arterial Score	none		none		none	

[1]Data adapted from references 51, 52 and 53.
[2]Chol = Cholesterol; TG = Triglyceride

Low and high density lipoprotein levels (LDL and HDL) are another widely publicized CHD risk factor. The information available on the influence of PHVO on LDL and HDL levels is mainly limited to data from animal experiments (Table 22-3). Swine and rats studies suggest that *trans* acids in PHVO do not increase LDL cholesterol levels (55-58). These studies indicate that PHVO may lower HDL cholesterol levels. The results from rats fed 10 wt% PHVO (42.5%t) diets indicate the levels of HDL protein (apolipoprotein A-I) increased compared to olive and safflower oil fed rats (59). A PHVO diet was reported to lower serum cholesterol levels compared to a high oleic acid control diet in rats (59). A possible reason for this result was the 35% reduction in cholesterol absorption observed for the rats fed PHVO. Other data related to human lipoproteins are from studies which show that incorporation of deuterium-labelled 18:1 isomers into the various lipoprotein lipid fractions is not particularly different from data for the total plasma lipid fractions (11-17).

Platelet aggregation is a third recognized CHD risk factor. *In vitro* studies show that 9t-18:1 and 9c-18:1 have little effect on human platelet aggregation and that t,t-18:2 and c,c-18:2 enhance aggregation to a similar extent (60-61). In rats fed PHVO diets containing 22% and 40% *trans* acids, a 10% to 2 fold increase in platelet aggregation occurred

TABLE 22-3
Influence of Partially Hydrogenated Vegetable Oil Containing Diets on Lipoprotein Cholesterol Levels in Animals

Model	Fat Source	Diet trans (%)	Fat wt%	Chol.	Total Lipoprotein (mg/dl)			Ref.
					VLDL	LDL	HDL	
Rat	PHVO	48	20	—	11	29	13	55[1]
	Tallow	0.5	20	—	12	23	25	
	Corn	0	20	—	11	37	20	
Rat	PHVO	25	10	—	8	9	83	58
	Corn	0	10	—	8	13	80	
Swine	PHVO	48	15	124	11	66	47	56
	Tallow	0.5	15	119	5	71	43	
	Basal	0	3	99	5	64	36	
Swine	PHVO	48	15	163	18	44	34	57
	PHVO	25	15	178	16	42	38	
	High oleic	0	3	155	16	39	42	

[1]Lipoprotein data from reference 55 is for cholesterol ester only.

(62). In contrast, platelet aggregation was similar for rats fed 24 wt% PHVO (58%t) or olive oil diets (63). Bleeding times reflect platelet aggregation. In rats fed 5-15% 9t,12t-18:2, bleeding times increased slightly (64), but in another similar study, a 6.3% 9t,12t-18:2 diet produced no effect on hemalogical properties (65). In terms of health effects, the importance of the 9t,12t-18:2 isomer is minimal because of the low (<0.3%) amounts generally present in PHVO (66).

Eicosanoids (PGE_2, prostacyclin, thromboxin A_2, etc.) influence platelet aggregation, formation of arterial lesions and vascular constriction. In rats, the production of the eicosanoids were not altered by diets containing PHVO (54,67) but 9t,12t-18:2 reduced the levels of a variety of eicosanoids (68). The prostacyclin levels in swine fed PHVO vs lard diets were similar, but lower than in animals fed safflower oil (53). The influence of PHVO on eicosanoid production is small and appears inconsistent with the desaturase inhibition and conversion data for the *trans* 18:2 and 18:3 isomers. For example, a lower concentration of 20:4 would be expected to reduce the amount of eicosanoid metabolites produced.

The correlations between cardiovascular risk factors and specific fatty acid isomers in human adipose tissue are summarized in Table 22-4 (33). The only 18:1 isomer that had a positive correlation with CHD risk

TABLE 22-4
Correlations between Adipose Tissue Fatty Acid Isomers and Risk Factors Associated with Coronary Heart Disease. (n = 76; p<0.05)

Risk Factor	trans acids	Correlation Coefficient	cis Acids	Correlation Coefficient
Triglyceride	—	—	14:1-7c[1]	-0.255
Cholesterol	14:1-5t?	-0.301	16:1-7c?	0.252
	18:1-11t	-0.230	18:1-11c	0.239
VLDL-C	14:1-5t?	-0.321	—	—
LDL-C	18:1-11t	-0.310	16:1-7c?	0.263
	—	—	18:1-11c	0.243
LDL-C/HDL-C	—	—	16:1-9c	0.277
Diastolic	—	—	14:1-7c?	-0.263
	—	—	18:1-13c	-0.305
Systolic	—	—	16:1-7c?	0.286
Age	18:1-12t+8c	0.259	—	—

[1]Question mark indicates position of double bond was not rigorously established.

factors was 11c-18:1. It is not known if this correlation is related to the presence of this isomer in animal fats or to an enhanced biosynthesis of 11c-18:1.

Cancer

The scientific literature is replete with studies on the effects of dietary fat on tumor growth and development. However, relatively few studies have focused on the effect of PHVO diets and specific fatty acid isomers on cancer and immune function.

Available data is based on rodent models and the results are inconsistent. Results from five rat studies that used carcinogens to induce colon and mammary tumors are summarized in Table 22-5. Elaidic acid (25% of diet) produced a higher incidence of colon cancer in rats than a diet containing 25% oleic acid when linoleic acid was not included in the diet (69). However, the difference was not statistically significant. No differences were found for the number of carcinogen induced colon or mammary tumors in rats fed trans acid containing diets compared to 0% *trans* control diets (70-73). Also, in the absence of added carcinogens, there was no difference in total tumor frequency or distribution in lifespan studies with mice and rats fed soybean oil and PHVO diets (41,42).

TABLE 22-5

Carcinogen Induced Tumor Studies with Rats

Tumor	Dietary Fat	Trans (%)	Fat Wt.%	Incidence Tumors (%)	Ref.
Colon	9t-18:1	100	25	23	69
	9c-18:1	0	25	37	
Colon	PHVO	40	5	75	70
	High Oleic Safflower	0	5	71	
Mammary	PHVO	45	10	63	71
	Olive	0	10	67	
Colon	PHVO	42	10	35	72
	Olive	0	10	31	
Mammary	PHVO	38	5 & 20	16 & 32	73
	Corn	0	5 & 20	44 & 80	
	Olive/Plus Cocoa butter	0	5 & 20	24 & 40	

Results from mice fed *trans*, *cis* or saturated fatty acid diets show no differences in the promotional effects of these fatty acids on liver or mammary tumors (74). Tumor growth and metastasis was investigated by intravenous injection and transplantion of mammary tumor cells into mice receiving 5 wt% and 20 wt% total fat diets containing 0% or 42% *trans* acids. In this study, no significant differences were observed for transplanted tumor growth rate, but the *trans* fat diets were less effective than the *cis* diets for promotion of metastasis. (75). Results of mutagenicity (Ames) tests (Table 22-6) with tissue from rats fed PHVO and *cis* diets did not show a difference in mutagenic response to known carcinogens (76-77).

It has not been established whether total fat or polyunsaturated fat (caloric effect vs. PUFA effect) is primarily responsible for an increased risk for cancer in humans. If total fat intake is primarily responsible for higher cancer risk, then whether a fat contains *trans* isomers or not would make little difference. If high PUFA diets are found to be associated with higher cancer risk, then PHVO, which contains less 18:2, would be less likely to enhance carcinogenesis than the corresponding unhydrogenated oil. This rational is consistent with the experimental data and the concept that *trans* acids in PHVO are unlikely to increase the risk of cancer.

TABLE 22-6
Influence of Partially Hydrogenated Vegetable Oil (PHVO) on Mutagenicity and Tumor Growth

Test	Dietary Fat	Trans %	Wt% Fat	Response to Mutagentic Agent			Ref
				Benzo-Pyrene	Flourine Acyl	Flourine Amino	
Ames	High Oleic	0	16	66	271	900	76
	PHVO	43	15	67	228	1432	
				Afla-toxin	Flourine Amino		
Ames	Lard-Olive	0	20	1400	425		77
	PHVO-Olive	18	20	1100	425		
	PHVO-Olive	37	20	800	200		
				Tumor Volume			
Tumor	Olive-Coconut	0	20	730			75
Growth	PHVO	42	20	570			

Conclusion

In general, studies conducted 20-30 years ago tended to report results that suggested PHVO produced adverse health effects. Most studies published in the last 10 years do not suggest adverse health effects are produced by PHVO. When results from numerous biochemical and metabolic studies with isomeric fatty acids are combined with results from a variety of studies with non-isomeric dietary fatty acids, the main health consequence of hydrogenating vegetable oils appears related to the reduction in linoleic and linolenic acids content rather than to the *trans* and positional isomers.

Addendum

After this review was prepared, Mensink and Katan reported a comparison of the influence of diets containing saturated, *trans*, or oleic acids on lipoprotein cholesterol levels in 59 young adult subjects (78). Compared to the oleic acid diet, the *trans* diet had about 50% of the total serum cholesterol increasing effect as the saturated fat diet. However, the *trans* diet increased LDL cholesterol by nearly as much as the saturated diet and lowered the HDL cholesterol level by 6.6 mg/dl. Thus, based on the change in LDL/HDL ratio, the *trans* diet had at least as much of an unfavorable effect as the saturated fat diet.

References

1. Scholfield, C.E., Davison, V.L., and Dutton, H.J. (1967) J. Am. Oil Chem. Soc. 44: 648-651.
2. Grandgirard, A., Piconneaux, A., Julliard, F., and Sebedio, J.L. (1987) J. Am. Oil Chem. Soc. 64: 1434-1440.
3. Mutter, M., and Homan, H.R. (1987) J. High. Resolut. Chrom. 10: 6672-673.
4. McDonald, R.E., Armstrong, D.J., and Kreishman, G.P. (1989) J. Agric. Food Chem. 37: 637-642.
5. Emken, E.A., and Dutton, H.J., editors. (1979) Geometrical and Positional Fatty Acid Isomers. American Oil Chemist's Society, Champaign, Illinois.
6. Emken, E.A. (1984) Ann. Rev. Nutr. 4: 339-376.
7. Senti, F.R., editor (1985) Health Aspects of Dietary trans Fatty Acids. Life Science Research Office, Federation of American Societies for Experimental Biology, Bethesda, Maryland. FDA223-83-2020
8. Applewhite, T.H. (1981) J. Am. Oil Chem. Soc. 58: 260-269.
9. Emken, E.A. (1983) J. Am. Oil Chem. Soc. 60: 995-1004.
10. Perkins, E.G. and Visek, W.J., editors, (1983) Dietary Fats and Health. American Oil Chemist's Society, Champaign, Illinois.
11. Emken, E.A., Rohwedder, W.K., Adlof, R.O., Dejarlais, W.J., and Gulley, R.M. (1985) Biochim. Biophys. Acta 836: 233-245.
12. Emken, E.A., Adlof, R.O., Rohwedder, W.K., and Gulley, R.M. (1989) Lipids 24: 61-69.
13. Emken, E.A., Adlof, R.O., Rohwedder, W.K., and Gulley, R.M. (1983) J. Lipid Res. 24: 34-46.
14. Emken, E.A., Rohwedder, W.K., Adlof, R.O., Dejarlais, W.J., and Gulley, R.M. (1986) Lipids 21: 589-595.
15. Emken, E.A., Dutton, H.J., Rohwedder, W.K., Rakoff, H., Adlof, R.O., Gulley, R.M., and Canary, J.J. (1980) Lipids 15: 864-871.
16. Emken, E.A., Rohwedder, W.K., Adlof, R.O., and Gulley, R.M. (1987) Lipids 22: 495-504.
17. Emken, E.A., Rohwedder, W.K., Dutton, H.J., DeJarlais, W.J., Adlof, R.O., Mackin, J., Dougherty, R.M., and Iacono, J.M. (1979) Metabolism 28: 575-583.
18. Privett, O.S., Stearns, E.M., and Nickell, E. (1967) J. Nutr. 92: 303-310.
19. Anderson, R.L., Fullmer, C.S., and Hollendbach, E.J. (1975) J. Nutr. 105: 393-400.
20. Beyers, E.C., and Emken, E.A. (1989) J. Am. Oil Chem. Soc.66:439.
21. Cook, H.W., and Emken, E.A. (1990) Biochem. Cell Biology, 68:653-660.
22. Hill, E.G., Johnson, S.B., and Holman, R.T. (1979) J. Nutr. 109: 1759-1765.
23. Mahfouz, M.M., Johnson, S.B., and Holman, R.T. (1981) Biochim. Biophys. Acta 663: 58-68.
24. Lawson, L.D., Hill, E.G., and Holman, R.T. (1985) Lipids 20: 262-276.
25. Astrog, P.O., and Chevalier, J. (1988) Nutr. Reports Internatl. 38: 885-895.

26. Zevenbergen, J.L., and Houtsmuller, U.M.T. (1989) Biochim. Biophys. Acta 1002: 312-323.
27. Grandqirard, A., Piconneaux, A., Sebedio, J.L., O'Keefe, S.F., Semon, E., and LeQuere, J.L. (1989) Lipids 24: 799-804.
28. Jensen, R.G., Sampugra, J., and Pereira, R.L. (1964) Biochim. Biophys. Acta 84: 481-482.
29. Lawson, L.D. and Holman, R.T. (1981) Biochim. Biophys. Acta 665: 60-65.
30. Lanser, A.C., Emken, E.A., and Ohlrogge, J.B. (1986) Biochim. Biophys. Acta 875: 510-515.
31. Ohlrogge, J.B., Emken, E.A., and Gulley, R.M. (1981) J. Lipid Res. 22: 955-960.
32. Adlof, R.O., and Emken, E.A. (1986) Lipids 21: 543-547.
33. Hudgins, L.C., Hirsch, J. and Emken, E.A. (1991) Am. J. Clin. Nutr. 53: in press.
34. Rocqulein, G., Guenot, L., Astorg, P.O., and David M. (1989) Lipids 21: 775-780.
35. Wood, R. (1979) in Geometrical and Positional Fatty Acid Isomers, (Emken, E.A. and Dutton, H.J., editors), Ch. 9, pp 213-218, American Oil Chemist's Society, Champaign, Illinois.
36. Ohlrogge, J.B. (1983) in Dietary Fats and Health. (E.G. Perkins and W.J. Visek, editors), Ch. 20, pp 359-374. American Oil Chemist's Society, Champaign, Illinois.
37. Emken, E.A. (1981) J. Am. Oil Chem. Soc. 58: 278-283.
38. Hunter, J.E., and Applewhite, T.H. (1986) Am. J. Clin. Nutr. 44: 707-717.
39. Ide, T., and Sugano, M. (1984) Biochim. Biophys. Acta 794: 281-291.
40. Alfin-Slater, R.B., Wells, P., Aftergood, L., and Deuel, H.J. (1957) J. Nutr. 63: 241-261.
41. Vles, R.O., and Gottenbos, J.J. (1972) Voeding 33: 428-433.
42. Vles, R.O., and Gottenbos, J.J. (1972) Voeding 33: 455-465.
43. Vles, R.O., and Gottenbos, J.J., Van Pijpen, P.L. (1977) Bibl. Nutr. Dieta 25: 186-196.
44. Opstvedt, J., and Pettersen, J. (1988) Lipids 23: 713-719.
45. Pettersen, J., and Opstvedt, J. (1988) Lipids 23: 720-726.
46. Erickson, B.A., Coots, R.H., Mattson, F.H., and Kligman, A.M. (1964) J. Clin. Invest. 43: 2017-2025.
47. Mattson, F.H., Hollenbach, F.J., and Kligman, A.M. (1975) Am. J. Clin. Nutr. 28: 726-731.
48. Laine, D.C., Snodgrass, C.M., Dawson, E.A., Ener, M.A., Kuba, K., and Frantz, I.D. (1982) Am. J. Clin. Nutr. 35: 683-690.
49. Anderson, J.T., Grande, F., and Keys, A. (1961) J. Nutr. 75: 388-394.
50. Vergroesen, A.J., and Gottenbos, J.J. (1975) The role of fats in human nutrition. Vergroesen, A., editor. Ch.1, pp 1-32. Academic Press, London.
51. Ruttenberg, H., Davidson, L.M., Little, N., Klurfeld, D.M., and Kritchevsky, D. (1983) J. Nutr. 113: 835-844.

52. Kritchevsky, D., Davidson, L.M., Weight, M., Kriek, N.P., and Du Plessis, J.P. (1984) Atherosclerosis 51: 123-133.
53. Royce, S.M., Holmes, R.P., Takagi, T., and Kummerow, F.A. (1984) Am. J. Clin. Nutr. 39: 215-222.
54. Zevenbergen, J.L. and Haddeman, E. (1989) Lipids 24: 555-563.
55. Eqwim, P.O., and Kummerow, F.A. (1972) J. Nutr. 102: 783-792.
56. Jackson, R.L., Morrisett, J.D., Pownall, H.J., Gotto, A.M., Kamio, A., Imai, H., Tracy, R., and Kummerow, F.A. (1977) J. Lipid Res. 18: 182-190.
57. Elson, C.E., Benevenga, N.J., Centy, D.J., Grummer, R.H., Lalich, J.J., Porter, J.W., and Johnson, A.E. (1981) Atherosclerosis 40: 115-137.
58. Sugano, M., Ryu, K., and Ide, T. (1984) J. Lipid Res. 25: 474-485.
59. Sugano, M., Watanabe, M., Kohno, M., Cho, Y., and Ide, T. (1983) Lipids 18: 375-381.
60. Seifert, R., Schachtele, C., and Schultz, G. (1987) Biochim. Biophys. Res. Comm. 149: 762-768.
61. Pozdniakov, A.L., Lovich, N.A., Kulakova, S.N., Korf, I.I., and Levacvhev, M.M. (1984) Voprosy Pitaniia 6: 56-61.
62. Goranov, I.M. (1983) Zywienie Czlowieka Metab. 15: 10-18.
63. Hornstra, G., and Lussenburg, R.N. (1975) Athersclerosis 22: 499-516.
64. Raccuglia, G. and Privett, O.A. (1970) Lipids 5: 85-89.
65. Bruckner, G., Trimbo, S., Goswami, S., and Kinsella, J.E. (1983) J. Nutr. 113: 704-713.
66. Mossoba, M.M., McDonald, R.E., Chen, J.Y.T., Armstrong, D.J., and Page, S.W. (1990) J. Agric. Food Chem. 38: 86-92.
67. Hwang, D.H., Mathias, M.M., Dupont, J., and Meyer, D. (1975) J. Nutr. 105: 995-1002.
68. Hwang, D.H., and Kinsella, J.E. (1978) Prostaglandins and Medicine 1: 121-130.
69. Hogan, M.L. and Shamsuddin, A.M. (1984) J. Natl. Cancer Inst. 73: 1293-1296.
70. Sugano, M., Watanabe, M., Yoshida, K., Tomioka, M., Miyamoto, M., and Kritchevesky, D. (1989) Nutr. Cancer 12: 177-187.
71. Watanabe, M., and Sugano, M. (1986) Nutr. Reports Intrnl. 33: 163-169.
72. Watanabe, M., Koga, T., and Sugano, M. (1985) Am. J. Clin. Nutr. 42: 475-484.
73. Selenska, S.L., Ip, M.M., and Ip, C. (1984) Cancer Res. 44: 1321-1326.
74. Brown, R.R. (1981) Cancer Res. 41: 3741-3742.
75. Erickson, K.L., Schlanger, D.S., Adams, D.A., Fregeau, D.R., and Stern, J.S. (1984) J. Nutr. 114: 1834-1842.
76. Ponder, D.L., and Green, N.R. (1985) Cancer Research 45: 558-560.
77. Ostlund-Lindqvist, A., Albanus, L., and Croon, L. (1985) Lipids 20: 620-624.
78. Mensink, R.P., and Katan, M.B. (1990) N. Engl. J. Med. 323: 439-445.

List of Contributors

Dr. Susan Carlson
The Newborn Center
Department of Pediatrics and
 Obstetrics and Gynecology
853 Jefferson Avenue
The University of Tennessee
Memphis, TN 38103

M.T. Clandinin
Nutrition and Metabolism, Research
 Group
Departments of Foods & Nutrition
 and Medicine
University of Alberta
Edmonton, Alberta, Canada T6G 2C2

Dr. Robert Colvin
Department of Pathology
Massachusetts General Hospital and
 Harvard Medical School
Boston, MA 02114

E.A. Emken
Northern Regional Research Center
1815 North University Street
Peoria, IL 61604

Nancy Ernst
National Heart, Lung, and Blood
 Institute
National Institutes of Health
7550 Wisconsin Avenue, Room 204
Bethesda, MD 20892

C.J. Field
Nutrition and Metabolism, Research
 Group
Departments of Foods & Nutrition
 and Medicine
University of Alberta
Edmonton, Alberta, Canada T6G 2C2

M.L. Garg
Nutrition and Metabolism, Research
 Group
Departments of Foods & Nutrition
 and Medicine
University of Alberta
Edmonton, Alberta, Canada T6G 2C2

Dr. Scott Grundy
Center for Human Nutrition
University of Texas Southwestern
 Medical Center at Dallas
5325 Harry Hines Boulevard
Dallas, TX 75235-9052

Dr. William S. Harris
Lipid Laboratory
University of Kansas Medical Center
3800 Cambridge
Kansas City, KS 66103

D.M. Hegsted
New England Regional Primate
 Research Center
Harvard Medical School
Southboro, MA 01772

Dr. Maureen Henderson
Head, Cancer Prevention Research
 Program
Fred Hutchinson Cancer Research
 Center
1124 Columbia Street, MP-702
Seattle, WA 98104

Bruce Holub
Department of Nutritional Sciences
University of Guelph
Guelph, Ontario, Canada N1G 2W1

List of Contributors

David Horrobin
Efamol Research Institute
P.O. Box 818
Kentville, Nova Scotia, Canada B4N 4H8

James Iacono
Western Human Nutrition Research
  Center
USDA-ARS
P.O. Box 29997
Presidio of San Francisco, CA 94129

Rashida Karmali
Memorial Sloan-Kettering Cancer
  Center
1275 York Avenue
New York, NY 10021

Darshan Kelley
Western Human Nutrition Research
  Center
Agricultural Research Service, USDA
P.O. Box 29997
Presidio of San Francisco, CA 94129

Dr. Howard Knapp
Department of Internal Medicine
University of Iowa
Iowa City, IA 52242

Christopher Knoell
Arthritis Unit of the Department of
  Medicine
Massachusetts General Hospital and
  Harvard Medical School
Boston, MA 02114

Dr. Joel Kremer
Department of Medicine
Division of Rheumatology
Albany Medical College
Albany, NY 12208

William E.M. Lands
Department of Biological Chemistry
University of Illinois at Chicago
1853 West Polk Street, A312-CMW
Chicago, IL 60612

Bozena Libelt
Department of Biological Chemistry
University of Illinois at Chicago
1853 West Polk Street, A312-CMW
Chicago, IL 60612

Joseph Loscalzo
Department of Medicine
Brigham and Women's Hospital and
  Harvard Medical School
Boston, MA 02114

Dr. Simin Nikbin Meydani
Nutritional Immunology Laboratory
USDA Human Nutrition Research
  Center on Aging at Tufts
  University
711 Washington Street
Boston, MA 02111

Anna Morris
Department of Biological Chemistry
University of Illinois at Chicago
1853 West Polk Street, A312-CMW
Chicago, IL 60612

Robert Nicolosi
Department of Clinical Sciences
University of Lowell
Lowell, MA 01854

Walter Olesiak
c/o Sono Aibe, 904 Koizumi Building
3-29-11 Nishiwaseda
Shinjuku-Ku, Tokyo 169, Japan

List of Contributors

Bandaru Reddy
Division of Nutritional
   Carcinogenesis
American Health Foundation
Valhalla, NY 10595

Dr. Dwight Robinson
Arthritis Unit of the Department of
   Medicine
Massachusetts General Hospital and
   Harvard Medical School
Boston, MA 02114

Norberta Schoene
Lipid Nutrition Laboratory
Beltsville Human Nutrition Research
   Center
U.S. Department of Agriculture
Beltsville, MD 20705

Howard Sprecher
Department of Physiological
   Chemistry
The Ohio State University
Columbus, OH 43210

Arthur F. Stucchi
Department of Clinical Sciences
University of Lowell
Lowell, MA 01854

Dr. Sumio Tateno
Sakura National Hospital
National Kidney Transplantation
   Center of Japan
2-36-2 Ebaradai Sakura
Chiba, Japan Code No. 285

A.B.R. Thomson
Nutrition and Metabolism, Research
   Group
Departments of Foods & Nutrition
   and Medicine
University of Alberta
Edmonton, Alberta, Canada T6G 2C2

M. Toyomizu
Nutrition and Metabolism, Research
   Group
Departments of Foods & Nutrition
   and Medicine
University of Alberta
Edmonton, Alberta, Canada T6G 2C2

Dr. Li-Lian Xu
Arthritis Unit of the Department of
   Medicine
Massachusetts General Hospital and
   Harvard Medical School
Boston, MA 02114

Index

1-acyl-2-*sn*-glycero-3-phosphocholine 18
1,2-dimethylhydrazine 159-160
2,4-dienoyl-CoA reductase 16
3,2'-demethyl-4-amino-biphenyl (DMAB) 159
delta 3-*cis*-delta 2-*trans* enoyl-Co A isomerase 16
delta 4 desaturase 36-37
5-hydroperoxyeicosatetraenoic acid 174
7,12-dimethylbenz(a)anthracene (DMBA) 150, 162

A

Acetylcoenzyme A 23
Acyl-Co A 15, 34-35
Acyltransferase 220, 249
Adipocytes
   relationship of diet fat, plasma membrane and insulin stimulated functions 209-222
American Heart Association 53, 81
Amyloidosis 179
Angiotensin II 102
Antihistamines 238
Apolipoproteins 79, 84, 256
Arachidonic acid 19, 44-49, 123, 125, 129, 132
   importance of in infant growth 44-49
   metabolites in control of immune system 168-169
Arteriosclerosis 255
Aspirin 99, 130
Atherosclerosis 50-67, 96, 122, 130, 170
Atopic eczema
   therapeutic effects of gamma-linolenic acid 234-244
Australia 143
Autoimmune disease (see Immune system)
Autoimmune glomerulonephritis 203-204
Azoxymethane 159-160, 162

B

beta-keto acyl-Co A 14
Beef 3, 85

Beef fat (Lard) 3, 85, 88, 160-161, 204-205, 210
Black currant oil 153-155, 236
Blood 24, 26, 35, 44-49, 50
   coronary heart disease, dietary fatty acids and serum cholesterol 50-66
   dietary fatty acids and platelet function 129-135
   effect of dietary fats and eicosanoids on immune system 168-183
   effect of dietary fatty acids on blood pressure 94-106
   pregnancy-induced hypertension 100
   effect of omega-6 FA on blood pressure 107-121
   effect of omega-3 FA on blood platelet reactivity 122-128
   effect of trans fatty acids on coronary heart disease 255-258
Blood pressure (see Blood)
Brain lipids 14, 18
Butter (see Dairy products)

C

cDNA 13
Calcium 119, 124, 132
Canadian 158
Cancer 167
   correlations between FA intake and incidence 136-148
   FA metabolism and biochemical mechanisms 150-156
   omega-3 FA as anticancer agents 157-166
   effect of trans fatty acids on 258-260
Canola oil 127, 249
"Carbohydrate-induced hypertriglyceridemia" 57
Cardiovascular disease 107, 122
Caproic acid
   effect on cholesterol 90
Caprylic acid
   effect on cholesterol 90
Cell-mediated immune response 167-183
   effect of dietary fatty acids 185-200
Cereals 6, 9
Chain elongation of fatty acids 14-15, 23,

37, 46, 129, 250
Chain elongating enzymes 12
Chemotaxis 184, 199
Cholesterol 122, 145, 255
   dietary fatty acids and coronary heart disease 50-66
   dietary fatty acids, triglyceride and lipoprotein distribution 69-76
   dietary cholesterol and LDL metabolism 77-82
   effect of saturated fatty acids 83-93
   role of overnutrition 91-92
Cocoa butter 88
Coconut oil 7, 59, 62, 78, 86, 87, 133, 150, 160-161, 196, 240
Collagen 123, 124, 133
Concanavalin 175-183, 184-200
Corn oil 40, 60, 64, 78, 133, 150-156, 160-165, 170
Coronary heart disease (CHD) 73, 77, 144, 255
   dietary fatty acids and serum cholesterol 50-66
   effect of *trans* fatty acids 255-258
Crohn's disease 236
Cyclooxygenase 100, 125, 130, 150-156, 164, 167, 170, 174
Cytochrome b5 13
Cytochrome b5 reductase 13
Cytochrome P-450 101
Cytokine production
   effect of N-3 fatty acids 174-178

D

Dairy products 4-9
   butter 9, 85, 90, 112
   cheese 4-9, 112
   milk 4-9, 112
Denmark 97
Dermatiitis 236-238
Desaturases (4-, 5-, 6-, and 9-desaturase) 12, 13-14, 36-37, 209, 237
Desaturation 13-14, 18, 23, 46, 129, 209, 220, 234, 239, 250
Diabetes 130, 210
   diabetic neuropathy; therapeutic effects of gamma-linolenic acid 234-244
Diet
   annual U.S. consumption 137-138
   deficiency of essential fatty acids 31-32
   factors associated with fat intake 8-9
   trends in consumption of fats 1-3
   trends in fats avaliable in food supply 3-4
   trends in available foods; fat intake 4-7
   trends in contribution of fats; individual foods 7-8
   trends in consumption of foods; fat intake 8-9
Dietary fatty acids (see also: Fatty acids or Essential)
   cholesterol, triglyceride and lipoprotein distribution 69-76
   quantity vs. quality ; affect lipids and lipoprotein 69-70
   correlation between FA intake and cancer incidence 136-148
   effect; and eicosanoids on immune system 167-183
   effect on cell mediated immune system 184-200
   effect on LDL metabolism 77-82
   effect of omega-6 FA on blood pressure 107-121
   effect of omega-3 FA on blood platelet reactivity 122-128
   effect on blood pressure 94-106
   endogenous n-7 and n-9 FA 32-33
   function of essential FA 21-40
   mechanism of platelet function 129-135
   metabolism and biochemical mechanisms in cancer 150-156
   metabolism of 12-19
   omega-3 fatty acids as anticancer agents 157-166
   plasma membrane composition and insulin stimulated functions in adipocytes 209-222
   saturated fatty acids and cholesterol 83-93
   serum cholesterol and coronary heart disease 50-66
Dietary fiber 157, 159
Dihomogamma-linolenic acid 235
Discriminant learning 43
Docosahexaenoic acid (DHA) 42, 44, 123-124, 133, 152, 161, 174-179, 185, 205, 207, 224
   exogenous DHA and preterm infant 44-45
   importance of 45-49

E

"Efamol" 236, 238-239
Eggs 4-9, 62
Electroretinogram 43
Eicosapentaenoic acid (EPA) 74, 98, 122-124, 127, 133, 152, 161, 185, 205, 207, 224, 235
Eicosanoids 23, 30, 38, 98, 126, 250, 257
  and effect of dietary fats on immune system 167-183
Epidemiology 77, 129, 136, 157-159
  of dietary FA on blood pressure 94-106
  of omega-6 on blood pressure 107-121
"Epogam" 236
Erythrocytes 26
Eskimos 40, 72, 39, 71, 161, 169
Essential fatty acids
  deficient 246
  function of 21-40
    marginal supplies 31-32
  serum cholesterol and coronary heart disease 50-66
Estradiol 145-147
Evening primrose oil
  therapeutic effects of gamma-linolenic acid in atopic eczema and diabetic neuropathy 234-244

F

Fatty acids
  composition of present day diets 1-10
  correlation between FA intake and cancer incidence 136-148
  effect of saturation on LDL metabolism 77-82
  function of essential fatty acids 21-40
    composition of triglycerides 24-26
    composition of phospholipids 26-29
  general categories of 30-31
  metabolism and biochemical reactions in cancer 150-156
  metabolism of dietary fatty acids 12-19
  serum cholesterol and coronary heart disease 50-66
  cholesterol, triglyceride and lipoprotein distribution 69-76
  saturated FA and cholesterol 83-93
  trans fatty acids: adverse health consequences? 245-263
Flax seed oil 199
Fluorescence polarization 79

Fiber (see Dietary fiber)
Fibrinogen 124
"Field trials": dietary FA, serum cholesterol and coronary heart disease 55-57
Finland 65, 110, 114, 240
Fish 3, 102
Fish oil (see Marine oils)
"Food group" consumption 7
Food supply (see Diet)
Fruits 6

G

Gamma-linolenic acid 153
  therapeutic effects in atopic eczema, diabetic neuropathy 234-244
Gemfibrozil 74
Glucose 239-240
  transport and metabolism: diet, insulin binding 215-218
  incorporation into lipids 218-219
Greece 159
GTP-binding proteins 129, 132, 134

H

Heart disease (see Coronary heart disease)
Hepatocytes 18
High density lipoproteins (HDL) 52, 84, 256, 260
  serum cholesterol and coronary heart disease 65-66
  effect of dietary FA on lipoprotein distribution 69-76
Highly unsaturated fatty acids
  (see also: Docosahexaenoic acid, Eicosapentaenoic acid) 21-40, 161
  maintance in phospholipids 35-37
Human milk 44, 236
Humoral immunity 167-183
Hydrogenation 54, 245-246
Hydroxyeicosatetraenoic acid 168-169
Hypertension 94, 107, 132
  pregnancy-induced 100

I

Immune system 223
  effect of dietary fats and eicosanoids 167-183

effect of dietary fatty acids on cell mediated 184-202
suppression of autoimmune disease by purified N-3 FA 203-207
Indomethacin 164, 170
Infants
  omega-3 fatty acids for growth and development 42-47
"Ingredient group" consumption 7
Inositol 239-240
Insulin 13
  insulin stimulated functions in adipocytes: diet fat, plasma membrane composition 209-222
Interleukin 169, 227
Italy 65, 69, 110, 144, 159

J

Japanese 39, 57, 97, 122, 137, 144, 151, 158

L

Lard (see Beef fat)
Lauric acid
  effect on cholesterol 87-88, 91
Lecithin 35
Leukotrienes 99, 168, 225
Linoleic acid 12, 14, 16, 42, 127, 150, 160, 234, 246
  conversion to 20-carbon acids 18-19
Linolenic acid 3, 12, 14, 16, 42, 127, 246
  conversion to 20-carbon acids 18-19
Linseed oil 210
Lipoproteins (see Low density; High density)
  distribution: effects of dietary FA 69-76
  postprandial 74-75
Lipoprotein lipase 33
Lipoxins 169-170
Lipoxygenase 133, 152, 164, 167, 170, 174
Low density lipoproteins (LDL) 52, 84, 123, 256, 260
  effect of dietary FA on lipoprotein distribution 69-76
  effect of dietary fat saturation on LDL metabolism 77-82
Lupus erythematosus 203
Lymphocyte proliferation
  effect of N-3 fatty acids 174-178

M

mRNA 13, 78
Malonyl-Co A 14, 15
Marine oil (fish oil) 44-47, 122, 130, 133, 204-205
  dietary supplementation with rheumatoid arthritis 225-233
  effect on lipoprotein levels 71-76
  effect on blood pressure 94-106
  vascular reactivity 101-103
  effect on natural killer cells 170-174
  effect on cytokine production, lymphocyte proliferation 174-183
  FA metabolism and biochemical mechanisms in cancer 150-156
  omega-3 FA as tumor inhibitors 159-165
  suppression of thromboxane A_2 synthesis 125-127
"Maxepa" 236
Membrane lipids 12, 15-16, 16-19
  fluidity 79, 126
  plasma composition: diet fat, and insulin stimulated functions in adipocytes 209-222
Menhaden oil 81, 99, 161-165, 204
"Metabolic studies": dietary FA, serum cholesterol and coronary heart disease 55-57
Methylazoymethanol acetate 159
Methylnitrosourea 159, 161
Monounsaturated fatty acids 2-3, 7, 117, 137, 161, 214
  serum cholesterol and coronary heart disease 53-63
  effect on LDL metabolism 81
Myristic acid
  effect on cholesterol 86-87, 92

N

NADH 15
NADPH 15
National Food Consumption survey 1
National Health and Nutrition Examination survey 1
National Heart, Lung, and Blood Institute survey 2
Natural killer cell 169-174, 184-200
Neutrophil leukotriene (see leukotriene)
Norway 98

O

Oils (see individual)
Olive oil 59, 62, 64, 151, 159-161, 194, 225, 256
Omega-3 fatty acids 3
   as anticancer agents 157-166
   for growth and development 43-50
   fish oils and lipoprotein levels 71-75
   effect on LDL metabolism 80-81
   effect on blood platelet reactivity 122-128
   dietary supplementation with rheumatoid arthritis 223-233
Omega-6 fatty acids 157, 161
   (see also: Linoleic acid)
   effect on blood pressure 107-121
Osteoporosis 179
Oxidation 16, 251-254

P

Palm oil 7, 45, 86, 150
Palm kernel oil 7, 86, 87
Palmitic acid
   effect on cholesterol 84-86, 92
Partially hydrogenated vegetable oils 246-260
Peripheral blood lymphocytes 185-200
Phagocytosis 184, 199
Phenformin 194
Phenylephrine 102
Phosphatides 212-214
Phosphoglycerides 13, 16, 125, 153
   liver ethanolamine 18
Phospholipids 32, 42-47, 125, 206-207, 237
   fatty acid composition of 26-29
   maintenance of highly unsaturated FA 35-37
Phytohemagglutinin 175-183, 184-202
Piroxicam 164
Platelet factor-4 131
Polyunsaturated fatty acids 2-3, 7, 46, 53, 131, 136, 142, 150, 163, 223
   biosynthesis & metabolism 12-19
   desaturation 13-14
   chain elongation 14-15
   retroconversion 15-16
   regulation of 22-carbon unsaturated fatty acid biosynthesis 16-18
   conversion of linoleate and linolenate to 20-carbon acids 18-19
   "cholesterol-lowering" effect 57

effect of on immune response 167-183
effect of omega FA on blood platelet reactivity 122-129
effect of omega-6 FA on blood pressure 107-121
effect of on LDL metabolism 77-82
lowering of HDL 70-71
purified N-3 FA; suppression of autoimmune disease 203-207
serum cholesterol and coronary heart disease 65-66
Potassium
   role in regulating blood pressure 119
Poultry 4-10
Prostacyclin 103, 126, 152, 257
Prostaglandins 99-106, 150-156, 164-165, 168-179, 203, 257
Protein kinase 126

R

Regulation
   of 22-carbon unsaturated fatty acid biosynthesis 16-18
Restenosis 73
Retina lipids 14, 18, 42
Retinal physiology 44
Retroconversion 15-16
Rheumatoid arthritis 179, 203
   dietary supplementation with omega-3 FA 223-233

S

Safflower oil 59-64, 89, 99, 102, 151, 160-161, 196, 205, 210, 256-257
Saturated fatty acids (SFA) 2, 7-8, 21-22, 69, 117, 137, 205, 224, 246, 249, 255
   serum cholesterol and coronary heart disease 53-66
   effect of on LDL metabolism 77-82
   plasma cholesterol levels 83-93
Shellfish 4-9
Smoking 50-52, 132
Sodium
   role in blood pressure 107
Soybean oil 89, 125-127, 249, 258
Spain 159
Sphingomyelin 125, 212
Stearic acid 3, 13, 63, 160, 248
   effect on cholesterol 88-91
Streptozotocin 210

Sunflower oil 127, 133, 194

T

Taiwanese 97
Thrombin 126, 132-133
Thrombosis 65, 255
Thromboxins (thromboxanes) 99, 123, 129, 152, 257
Thromboxane synthase 99
Thromboglobulin 131
"*Trans* acids" *trans* unsaturated fatty acids
  adverse health consequences? 245-263
  effect on cholesterol 90-92
Triglycerides 205, 248-249
  fatty acid composition of 24-26
  synthesis, transport, and storage 34-36
  effect of dietary fatty acids on 69-76
  effect on LDL metabolism 77-82
Tripalmitin 64
Tristearin 64
Tropical oils (see Coconut, Palm, Palm kernel)

Tumor (see Cancer)
Type IIb hyperlipidemia 72

U

Unsaturated fatty acids 21-40, 129

V

Vitamin A 75
Vegetables 6-7
Very low density lipoproteins 74, 77, 84

W

World Health Organization 122

Z

Zimbabwean 237